Cases in
Health Services
Management

Cases in Health Services Management

SIXTH EDITION

Edited by

Kurt Darr, J.D., Sc.D., LFACHE
The George Washington University

Tracy J. Farnsworth, Ed.D., MHSA, M.B.A., FACHE
Idaho State University

Robert C. Myrtle, D.P.A.
University of Southern California

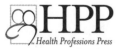
Health Professions Press

Baltimore • London • Sydney

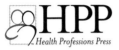

Health Professions Press, Inc.
Post Office Box 10624
Baltimore, Maryland 21285-0624

www.healthpropress.com

Manufactured in the United States of America by Versa Press, East Peoria, Illinois.
Cover and interior designs by Erin Geoghegan.
Typeset by Absolute Service, Inc., Towson, MD.

This casebook can be used alone or in conjunction with other texts. To help instructors use the cases most effectively in the classroom, the editors have prepared an instructor's guide, *Instructor's Manual for Cases in Health Services Management*, available to faculty as a downloadable PDF file from Health Professions Press (see website and address above or call 1-888-337-8808 or 1-410-337-9585). *Cases in Health Services Management* can also be used in conjunction with the textbook, *Managing Health Services Organizations and Systems*, also published by Health Professions Press.

The cases presented in this volume are based on the case authors' field research in a specific organization or are composite cases based on experiences with several organizations. In most instances, the names of organizations and individuals and identifying details have been changed. Cases are intended to stimulate discussion and analysis and are not meant to reflect positively or negatively on actual persons or organizations.

Library of Congress Cataloging-in-Publication Data
Names: Darr, Kurt, editor. | Farnsworth, Tracy J., editor. | Myrtle, Robert
    C., editor.
Title: Cases in health services management / edited by Kurt Darr, Tracy J.
    Farnsworth, Robert C. Myrtle.
Description: Sixth edition. | Baltimore : Health Professions Press, Inc.,
    [2017] | Preceded by: Cases in health services management / edited by
    Jonathon S. Rakich, Beaufort B. Longest, Kurt Darr. 5th ed. c2010. |
    Includes bibliographical references. | Description based on print version
    record and CIP data provided by publisher; resource not viewed.
Identifiers: LCCN 2017008811 (print) | LCCN 2017010156 (ebook) | ISBN
    9781938870736 (epub) | ISBN 9781938870620 (pbk.)
Subjects: | MESH: Hospital Administration | Health Services Administration |
    Total Quality Management | Organizational Case Studies | United States
Classification: LCC RA971 (ebook) | LCC RA971 (print) | NLM WX 150 | DDC
    362.10973—dc23
LC record available at https://lccn.loc.gov/2017008811

British Library Cataloguing-in-Publication data are available from the British Library.

To the Alumni of the GWU MHA Program
(Dedication of Dr. Darr)

To my wife, Michelle;
parents Karl and Jackie;
and children, Lindsey (Dan), Taylor (Jill), Rachel (Steven), and Dallin
(Dedication of Dr. Farnsworth)

To my students, who made this work possible
(Dedication of Dr. Myrtle)

Contents

PART I   POLICY ENVIRONMENT OF HEALTH SERVICES DELIVERY

Alexandra Piriz Mookerjee and Kurt Darr

Led by a new CEO, the efforts of a mid-Atlantic acute care hospital to develop a vertically integrated, clinic-driven health services system result in allegations of antitrust, excessive healthcare costs, disruption of physician referral patterns, and use of harsh collection practices, all of which cause a negative reaction in its service area.

Mary K. Feeney and Abigail Peterman

Flu vaccine shortages in 2004–2005 caused by a major manufacturer's problems with quality control result in federal and state efforts to secure supplies of the vaccine and raise public policy and resource-allocation issues that users can role-play in three scenarios.

Kimberly A. Rucker, Nora G. Albert, and Kurt Darr

A pharmaceutical manufacturer encounters significant negative stakeholder reaction to its introduction of a new medication for the human immunodeficiency virus despite having

met expectations for clinical rigor and carefully assessing
stakeholders and the external environment.

A new CEO urges his board to move toward becoming an
accountable care organization and promoting regional population health, which demands choosing among three common
approaches to navigating the challenges and opportunities of
developing a clinically integrated network.

A healthcare executive facing continual public policy
restructuring of Hawaii's Health Systems Corporation must
develop strategic options for his board to consider in response
to this environmental uncertainty.

The CEO of a 350-bed hospital explores strategic alternatives
to enhance its financial situation and reputation by asking the
hospital board to approve a worksite wellness program to be
marketed to area companies to improve workers' health and
decrease employers' healthcare costs.

The new CEO of a 30-bed, not-for-profit rural hospital faces a
turnaround situation to make the hospital profitable after 3 years

of losses. Problems include challenging payer mix, employee overstaffing, and difficulty recruiting physicians.

8   **Klamath Care: Targeting and Managing Growth and Company-Wide Development** 121

Tracy J. Farnsworth, Leigh W. Cellucci, and Carla Wiggins

The CEO of a growing system of urgent care centers recounts the organization's development over a decade while considering strategies and options for future growth in an increasingly crowded marketplace with an analysis that uses financial, market share, and demographic data.

9   **Hospital Consolidation** 133

Tracy J. Farnsworth

This case focuses on the relationship healthcare providers have with their local and regional markets and the need to balance organization and community interests when making decisions that affect the healthcare marketplace.

10   **Service Area Management** 141

Tracy J. Farnsworth

Users are challenged to analyze, prioritize, and use disparate information common to a dynamic and competitive healthcare marketplace as part of an organization's strategic planning and marketing processes.

11   **Western Healthcare Systems: A Healthcare Delivery Continuum.** 157

Robert C. Myrtle

Western Healthcare Systems was creating an integrated delivery system when an opportunity to acquire a large multispecialty group arose, but it may be imprudent to proceed because of hospital and multispecialty group physician resistance.

PART III   ORGANIZATIONAL MANAGEMENT

Kent V. Rondeau, John E. Paul, and Jonathon S. Rakich

The VP for nursing services of a 285-bed for-profit hospital must decide what actions to take regarding her in-box, which includes e-mail, correspondence, and phone messages that communicate various challenges, such as two angry nurses, a wandering patient, staff shortages, and increasing numbers of OR infections. Emphasizes priority setting, decision making, and delegation.

Kurt Darr

Management of a community hospital is unwilling to recognize and address major problems in its radiology department, which is directed by a radiologist whose disruptive behavior and preoccupation with income and stock market speculation have diminished the quality of radiograph readings with tragic results.

Kent V. Rondeau

The future of a total quality management initiative is threatened when the CEO has to overcome more than the expected barriers and pitfalls in a chain of seven nursing homes and the initiative becomes entangled in negotiations with the union representing nurses.

Cynthia Mahood Levin and Kurt Darr

A tax district community hospital has major problems with its governance structure because of historical animosities among internal stakeholders, medical staff politics, weak and ambivalent senior management, and a disruptive member of the medical staff who has ambitions to attain major power in the hospital.

A change initiative introduced to democratize decision making and improve clinical care in a healthcare organization is met with staff suspicion, derision, and resistance.

PART IV   ORGANIZATIONAL EFFECTIVENESS

After the merger of two hospitals, planning must include how to consolidate duplicated services and realign units, including a burn center, while considering the center's financing and community and organizational impact.

A not-for-profit pediatric dental care center that has struggled financially for years as it serves a Medicaid population is offered the opportunity to become part of a federally qualified health center, but to do so requires expanding services and significantly changing its governance structure.

Efforts to provide pharmacy services in a rural community are successful because of creative thinking, perseverance, political deal making, and using telepharmacy in a unique and effective way.

An academic medical center must decide how to structure and fund hospitalist services in the context of its relationship with an affiliated school of medicine; the history and content of hospitalist functions; and other revenue that might be derived from hospitalist services, even while considering several alternate strategies.

A negotiation simulation allows participants to assume union and hospital roles to work toward an acceptable collective bargaining agreement.

Several years after initiating healthcare services for diverse, underserved communities, hospital leadership is planning how to take its activities to a level with greater impact and sustainability.

PART V   LEADERSHIP CHALLENGES

A software company supplying information technology services to Ontario (CN) hospitals has an ill-defined structure and controls that frustrate a new employee with conflicting demands from the firm's managers, including expectations inconsistent with her job description.

Declining physical health forces an accomplished retired professor to enter a life care community in which his diminished independence leads to conflicts with management and staff even as further health problems result in an apparently willed death.

About the Editors

Kurt Darr, JD, ScD, LFACHE, is Professor Emeritus of Hospital Administration, and of Health Services Management and Leadership, Department of Health Services Policy and Management, School of Public Health, The George Washington University. Dr. Darr holds the Doctor of Science from The Johns Hopkins University and the Master of Hospital Administration and Juris Doctor from the University of Minnesota. His baccalaureate degree was awarded by Concordia College, Moorhead, MN.

Dr. Darr completed an administrative residency at the Rochester (MN) Methodist Hospital and subsequently worked as an administrative associate at the Mayo Clinic. After being commissioned in the U.S. Navy during the Vietnam War, he served in administrative and educational assignments at St. Albans Naval Hospital (NY) and Bethesda Naval Hospital (MD). He completed postdoctoral fellowships with the U.S. Department of Health and Human Services, the World Health Organization, and the Accrediting Commission on Education for Health Services Administration.

Dr. Darr is admitted to practice before the Supreme Court of the state of Minnesota and the Court of Appeals of the District of Columbia. He was a mediator for the Civil Division of the Superior Court of the District of Columbia and has served as a hearing officer for the American Arbitration Association. Dr. Darr is a member of hospital committees on quality improvement and on ethics in the District of Columbia metropolitan area. He is a Life Fellow of the American College of Healthcare Executives.

Dr. Darr's teaching and research interests include health services management, administrative and clinical ethics, hospital organization and management, quality improvement, and applying the Deming method in health services. Dr. Darr is the editor and author of numerous books, articles, and cases used for graduate education and professional development in health services.

Tracy J. Farnsworth, EdD, MHSA, MBA, FACHE, is President and Chief Executive Officer of the Proposed Idaho College of Osteopathic Medicine. Dr. Farnsworth has served as Director and Associate Dean of the School of Health Professions, Division of Health

Sciences, Idaho State University (ISU [Pocatello]) since 2010. He is Associate Professor in the Health Care Administration Program at ISU and has served as Program Director.

Dr. Farnsworth is a graduate of Brigham Young University. He received master's degrees in Business and Health Services Administration from Arizona State University and the Doctor of Education in Educational Leadership from ISU. In 2014, Dr. Farnsworth was awarded the Kole-McGuffey Prize for excellence in education research, and in 2016 he received the J. Warren Perry Distinguished Author Award from the Association of Schools of Allied Health Professions.

Prior to becoming an educator, Dr. Farnsworth had executive-level appointments with Intermountain Healthcare, Catholic Healthcare West, the City of Hope National Medical Center, and other public and private healthcare systems.

A Fellow of the American College of Healthcare Executives, Dr. Farnsworth has written and spoken widely on subjects related to hospital and health systems performance improvement, healthcare reform, medical education, healthcare leadership and governance, and inter-professional education/collaboration.

Robert C. Myrtle, DPA, is Professor Emeritus of Health Services Administration, Sol Price School of Public Policy, University of Southern California. Dr. Myrtle received a bachelor's degree in business administration from the California State University, Long Beach, and a master's and doctoral degree in public administration from the University of Southern California. During 41 years at the University of Southern California (USC), Dr. Myrtle co-authored two books on management; 18 book chapters; 51 articles in journals, including *Health Care Management Review, Health Policy and Planning, Public Administration Review, Social Science and Medicine*, and *The Gerontologist*; and 70 conference papers and professional reports. He has academic appointments in the Leonard Davis School of Gerontology and the Marshall School of Business and is a Visiting Professor in the Institute of Health Policy and Management at the National Taiwan University.

Dr. Myrtle's key research interests are leadership, executive development, and organizational and management effectiveness. Current research includes the influence of managers' behavior on perceptions of overall leadership effectiveness; examining factors influencing the performance of surgical teams; and assessing factors influencing organizational legitimacy during and following major natural disasters.

Dr. Myrtle is the recipient of the Academy of Management's Health Care Division's Teaching Excellence Award and the American Society for Public Administration's Los Angeles Chapter Harry Scoville Award for

Academic Excellence. He was named Professor of the Year at USC and has three times been named Most Inspirational Business Professor. He is the recipient of the American College of Healthcare Executives Regents Award, and the Hubert H. Humphrey Award for best article of the year appearing in the *Journal of Health and Human Services Administration*.

Dr. Myrtle was chair of the Los Angeles County Hospitals and Health Services Commission. He was board chair for SCAN Health Plan and was a member of the board of directors for the Huntington Medical Foundation. He has served as board chair of Health and Human Services for the City of Long Beach (CA).

Professor Emeritus Darr coauthored the textbook, *Managing Health Services Organizations and Systems, Sixth Edition* (2014), with Beaufort B. Longest, Jr., published by Health Professions Press. This health services management textbook should be used as a complement to *Cases in Health Services Management*.

Contributors

Nora G. Albert, MHA
Project Manager
Children's National Health System
111 Michigan Ave, NW
Washington, DC 20010

Douglas Archer, MHA
Hospital Administrator
Sutter Health-Memorial
  Hospital–Los Banos
520 West I St.
Los Banos, CA 93635

**Alexander R. Bolinger, PhD,
  MBA**
Associate Professor of
  Management
Idaho State University
921 S. 8th Ave.
Pocatello, ID 83209-8020

Leigh W. Cellucci, PhD, MBA
Professor and Program Director
Department of Health Services
  and Information Management
East Carolina University
Greenville, NC 27858-668

Stephen Cheung, MHA, DDS
School of Dentistry
State Capital Center
School of Policy, Planning,
  and Development
University of Southern California
Sacramento, CA 95811

George S. Cooley
Long Green Associates, Inc.
Long Green, MD 21092

Kathryn H. Dansky, PhD
Associate Professor Emerita
Department of Health Policy and
  Administration
College of Health and Human
  Development
Pennsylvania State University
201 Main
University Park, PA 16802

Kurt Darr, JD, ScD, LFACHE
Professor Emeritus, Hospital
  Administration
Dept. of Health Services
  Management & Leadership
The George Washington
  University
2175 K Street, NW
Suite 320
Washington, DC 20037

**Cara Thomason Embry, MSG,
  MHA, RN**
Sol Price School of Public
  Health
University of Southern California
Los Angeles, CA 90089-0626

Bonnie Eng-Suess, MHA
Director of Hospital Risk
  Contracting and Operations
Dignity Health
251 S. Lake Ave., Ste 700
Pasadena, CA 91101

Bruce D. Evans, MBA
Professor of Management
University of Dallas
Satish & Yasmin Gupta College
  of Business
1845 E. Northgate Dr.
Irving, TX 75062

**Tracy J. Farnsworth, EdD,
  MHSA, MBA, FACHE**
Associate Dean and Director
Kasiska School of Health
  Professions
Division of Health Sciences
Idaho State University
921 South 8th Ave.
Pocatello, ID 83209-8090

Mary K. Feeney, PhD
Associate Professor and Lincoln
  Professor of Ethics in Public
  Affairs
School of Public Affairs
Arizona State University
411 N. Central Ave., Suite 450
Phoenix, AZ 85004

Julie Frischmann
Instructor/Academic Coach
Student Success Center
Idaho State University
921 S. 8th Ave.
Pocatello, ID 83209-8010

Elizabeth M. A. Grasby, PhD
c/o Richard Ivey School of
  Business
The University of Western
  Ontario
1151 Richmond Street North
London, Ontario N6A 3K7
CANADA

Earl G. Greenia, PhD, FACHE
Professor, Healthcare
  Administration & Management
Colorado State University–Global
  Campus
7800 E. Orchard Road
Greenwood Village, CO 80111

Michael J. King, MHA
Chief Financial Officer, Shared
  Services Division
Tenet Healthcare Corporation
1445 Ross Ave., Suite 1400
Dallas, TX 75202

Eleanor Lin, MHA, DDS
Children's Dental Health Clinic
455 E. Columbia St.
Long Beach, CA 90806

Cynthia Mahood Levin, MHSA
Healthcare Consultant
Palo Alto, CA

Nova Ashanti Monteiro, MD
Children's National Medical Center
111 Michigan Avenue NW
Washington, DC 20010

Robert C. Myrtle, DPA
Professor Emeritus, Health
  Services Administration
Sol Price School of Public Policy
University of Southern California
105 Siena Drive
Long Beach, CA 90803

John E. Paul, PhD, MSPH
Clinical Professor and Associate
  Chair for Academics
Department of Health Policy and
  Management
Gillings School of Global Public
  Health
University of North Carolina at
  Chapel Hill
135 Dauer Drive.
Chapel Hill, NC 27599

Abigail Peterman
Center for Science, Technology
  and Environmental Policy
  Studies
Arizona State University
University Center
411 N. Central Ave.
Phoenix, AZ 85004

**Alexandra Piriz Mookerjee,
  MHSA**
Administrator
Westminster Communities of
  Florida
Magnolia Towers
100 E. Anderson St.
Orlando, FL 32801

Brent C. Pottenger, MD, MHA
Dept. of Physical Medicine &
  Rehabilitation
Johns Hopkins Medicine
707 North Broadway
Baltimore, MD 21205

Jonathon S. Rakich
Professor Emeritus
Indiana University Southeast
4201 Grant Line Road
New Albany, IN 47150

Kent Rondeau, PhD
Associate Professor
School of Public Health
University of Alberta
Faculty of Extension, Enterprise
  Square
10230 Jasper Ave., Room 2-216
Edmonton, Alberta T5J 4P6
CANADA

Barry Ross, MPH, MBA
Vice President, Healthy
  Communities
St. Jude Medical Center
101 E. Valencia Mesa Dr.
Fullerton, CA 92835

Kimberly A. Rucker
Healthcare Consultant
Washington, DC

**Carla Jackie Sampson, MBA,
  FACHE**
Graduate Research Associate
Florida Center for Nursing
12424 Research Pkwy, #220
Orlando, FL 32826

Jessica Silcox, RN, MSN
Staff Development Educator &
  Stroke Coordinator
Sentara Northern Virginia
  Medical Center
2300 Opitz Blvd.
Woodbridge, VA 22191

Jason Stornelli
c/o Richard Ivey School of
  Business
The University of Western
  Ontario
1151 Richmond Street North
London, Ontario N6A 3K7
CANADA

Neil Tocher, PhD
Professor of Management
Idaho State University
921 S. 8th Ave.
Pocatello, ID 83209-8020

Gillian Gilson Watson, MHA
Department of Hospital Medicine
University of North Carolina
  Hospitals
101 Manning Dr.
Chapel Hill, NC 27599-7085

**Cherie A. Hudson Whittlesey,
  ML**
Director, Organizational
  Learning and Effectiveness
St. Jude Medical Center
101 E. Valencia Mesa Dr.
Fullerton, CA 92835

Carla Wiggins, PhD
Professor and MHA Program
  Director
Weber State University
3875 Stadium Way, Dept. 3911
Ogden, UT 84408

Preface

Like its predecessors, the sixth edition of *Cases in Health Services Management* describes management problems and issues in various healthcare settings. The primary criterion to select a case was that it had to be rich in applied lessons. Case selection was tempered by the editors' 90 years of combined experience in teaching and using the case method. The result is a comprehensive set of health services management cases in one volume.

Cases vary in length and complexity and are grouped into six parts. Of the 28 cases in this edition, 14 are new. There are two new ethics incidents. Cases and ethics incidents that have stood the test of time and use were retained in this edition. All have been updated and edited to make them as streamlined as possible. Consistent with the evolving healthcare delivery system, half the cases are set outside of acute care hospitals. Those include a long-term care facility, a health network, a continuing care retirement community, an emergency department, a hospital burn unit, a dental clinic, a pharmaceutical company, a city health department, a home health agency, and a software company.

Acute care hospital cases include a range of sizes, types, ownerships, and geographic locations, including rural and inner-city settings. One hospital case is set in a multi-institutional system; another applies the principles of continuous quality improvement. An in-box exercise set in a hospital simulates the time pressures that confront managers and the importance of prioritizing the issues, and a labor relations role-play case creates a powerful learning experience that emphasizes the challenges and dynamics of any negotiated relationship.

Depending on depth of analysis and time available for out-of-class preparation, most cases can be analyzed in two hours, or less. A few cases are short and have one issue. Most, however, are integrative and complex and involve multiple problems and issues. As a result, analyses will often require applying concepts from different disciplinary fields and knowledge areas. This may require users to synthesize and apply knowledge, skills, and experience from the social and health sciences in their analyses and discussions.

The primary use of this book of cases is the education of health services managers. Case analysis bridges theory and practice. In this regard, students studying health services management, as well as experienced managers, will find the cases informative as they hone analytical and problem-solving skills. These cases can also be used in continuing professional development for practicing managers.

By their nature, cases present events, situations, problems, and issues. The dynamics of the analysis, including the group discussion, make the case method a powerful and rich tool for learning. Users are urged to review the Introduction, which describes the case method and case analysis.

The cases included in this volume are intended to stimulate discussion and analysis. In most instances, the names of organizations and individuals are disguised. In all instances, authors of the cases have prepared well-written, factual situations that are based on field research in a specific organization, or a composite case based on experience with several organizations. No case is meant to reflect positively or negatively on actual persons or organizations, or to depict either effective or ineffective handling of administrative situations.

The 28 cases and 12 ethics incidents are organized into six parts:

Part I: Policy Environment of Health Services Delivery (five cases)

Part II: Strategic Management (six cases)

Part III: Organizational Management (five cases)

Part IV: Organizational Effectiveness (six cases)

Part V: Leadership Challenges (six cases)

Part VI: Ethics Incidents (12 statements of fact that show ethics issues)

The case synopses in the table of contents identify organizational setting, dominant themes, and managerial problems. The core task of teaching effective health services management is to hone the ability to identify and define problems as well as sharpen the judgment and ability to apply the skills and methods to solve them. As experiential learning in health services management education has given way to more discipline-based didactic preparation, and as younger, less-experienced students have entered graduate programs, cases that apply didactic work have become more important. Using these cases following a comprehensive academic grounding in the health services and management disciplines will prepare users for the types of problems they will encounter as health services managers. With instructor or seminar-leader guidance, cases such as those in this volume can make an important contribution to that goal.

TEXTBOOK SUPPLEMENT
AND INSTRUCTOR'S MANUAL

A useful supplement for instructors using the case method is *Managing Health Services Organizations and Systems, Sixth Edition*, published by Health Professions Press. This textbook grounds students in the health services system and gives them the knowledge needed for case analysis. Chapter 6, "Managerial Problem Solving and Decision Making," is especially helpful in preparing to use the case method.

An Instructor's Manual, available as a downloadable PDF file from Health Professions Press, can be used by faculty in teaching from *Cases in Health Services Management, Sixth Edition*. It contains the teaching notes prepared by the case authors and is available without charge to instructors who adopt the casebook. Use the following web address to request the Instructor's Manual: http://www.healthpropress.com/instructor-materials/

The Instructor's Manual also contains follow-up case supplements to the following cases in the casebook:

1. Hartland Memorial Hospital (Part 2: Organizational Diagnosis and Social-Networking Exercise)—follow up to case #12

2. Hospital Software Solutions (B)—follow up to case #23.

Instructors who use the follow-up cases are invited to reproduce them for classroom use.

Acknowledgments

The editors gratefully acknowledge the contribution of authors whose cases are included. The authors are listed alphabetically beginning at page xix. We thank them for allowing us to use their cases. In addition, thanks are owed to the publishers who granted permission to reprint the cases to which they hold copyright.

We are indebted to the staff of Health Professions Press for their help in producing this casebook, specifically Mary Magnus, Director of Publications; Cecilia González, Editorial and Production Manager; Kaitlin Konecke, Marketing Manager; and Lisa Minick, Sales and Brand Manager.

The editors gratefully acknowledge the contributions made by two of the editors who collaborated in preparing previous editions of this casebook, Jonathon S. Rakich, Ph.D., and Beaufort B. Longest, Jr., Ph.D. Professor Emeritus Rakich, Professor Longest, and Professor Emeritus Darr edited the first five editions of *Cases in Health Services Management*, which were published over three decades. The participation and historic roles of Drs. Rakich and Longest in setting direction, selecting cases, and working as part of a team to produce a high-quality casebook can be seen even in this edition. The editors of the Sixth Edition thank them.

Introduction

For decades, the case method has played an essential role in the study of law, medicine, and business. It has become an established part of education in healthcare management programs and similar types of educational activities. The cases in this volume were selected for use in healthcare management education because they describe problems and situations managers have faced in the past and provide meaningful learning opportunities for the managers of tomorrow. This discussion uses "student(s)" in its broadest definition to include all who are learning to become managers of health services, or learning to improve their ability to manage.

The cases facilitate the following:

- Assist students to develop the assessment, analytical, and conceptual skills necessary for effective problem solving and decision making

- Support students as they synthesize and integrate theory and its application

- Encourage dynamic and interactive discussion among students that challenges their experience and values

- Allow students to quickly acquire knowledge and insights.

Traditional didactic education provides background and foundation in disciplines and methodologies relevant to health services management. Fellowships, residencies, internships, and similar types of field experience supplement didactic learning for many students. Case studies blend didactic and experience-based learning; both are enhanced in the process.

This introduction (1) describes the types of cases in this volume, (2) lists benefits of the case method, (3) discusses the roles of students and instructors in using cases, and (4) outlines a methodology for case analysis.

TYPES OF CASES

Cases are situation-specific descriptions of management issues and problems that students identify and evaluate. By definition, cases describe past events. They do, however, reflect contemporary situations, issues, and problems that confront managers. Thus, cases impart valuable lessons and insights that are relatively unfettered by temporal change. The lessons learned analyzing and evaluating cases have enduring value and are applicable throughout a manager's career.

Some cases in this volume are comprehensive and integrative and reflect functional areas as well as issues and problems that affect the whole organization. Others are narrowly focused. The cases enable students to do the following:

- Operationally define the issue(s) or problem(s) present

- Identify facts and distinguish them from assertions, opinions, and hearsay

- Separate facts important to solving the problem from facts that are unimportant

- Distinguish relevant facts from irrelevant facts

- When necessary, make assumptions that are supported by facts

- Apply relevant management disciplines and methodologies

- Take the role of managers or external consultants when considering alternatives, offering recommendations, and planning implementation

In sum, case studies and the case method offer a disciplined approach to, and methodology for, problem solving and thereby enrich the learning experience.

BENEFITS OF THE CASE METHOD

The case method has numerous benefits. None is more important than giving students the opportunity to develop and sharpen their analytical skills and thought processes. The essence of case analysis is assessment and problem solving. Thus, cases enable students to hone skills in situation assessment, problem diagnosis and definition, alternative solution evaluation and selection, and development of plans to implement solutions and evaluate the solution(s) after implementation. Students must articulate and justify their recommendations; this enhances logic, argumentation, and communication skills, as well.

The case method requires students to synthesize and integrate knowledge. Compartmentalized subject areas and underlying disciplines, such as organizational behavior, accounting, economics, marketing, finance, and law must be linked, blended, and applied holistically during case analysis. Cases require that students apply management principles to actual settings. A case study is an opportunity to practice being a manager—it puts students at the scene of the events depicted and requires application of management theory. A case study exposes students to various organizational settings and managerial problems and provides a vehicle to introduce and discuss complementary subject matter relevant to the case, but not included in it.

Finally, cases allow students to learn and practice group interactive skills. The case method is used in group forums. Whether structured or unstructured, all participants discuss the case, present their analyses, and critique the analyses of others. The flow of facts, perceptions, and values results in productive student learning, including learning to work effectively in a group.

ROLES OF INSTRUCTORS AND STUDENTS

In using the case method, instructors leave the usual role of lecturer and become discussion leaders and facilitators. The instructor's task in the case method is to encourage students to think independently and to formulate and defend their analyses. The task of learning is the students'. Learning takes place most effectively in the case method if students use the opportunity provided by analysis and discussion to sharpen their skills.

Instructors are essential to the case method and contribute in several ways: selecting cases and the order in which they are assigned; structuring a teaching approach that permits students (in a classroom setting or online) to gain maximum benefit from the case analysis and interactive discussions; and giving direction to class discussion by expanding or contracting it, or changing the direction and focus, as appropriate. To effectively facilitate use of the case method, instructors must be thoroughly knowledgeable about the case—to the point of memorizing important facts and key elements. Only then can instructors correct misunderstandings and misperceptions, as well as provide information and facts that students may have missed or misunderstood. Instructors may also define and address collateral issues. Instructors can provide direction in the analyses by using the Socratic method to pose questions and focus analysis. Following discussion, the instructor should critique the group's work by commenting on class discussion, the analytical process, elements ignored or those over- or underemphasized, and the quality of findings and recommendations. Critiques improve learning and the ability of students to use the case method effectively.

Instructors may use several criteria to evaluate student performance:

- Mastery of the facts in the case—as well as of facts acquired by the student from other sources—and their use(s)

- Application of discipline-specific knowledge and analytical methodologies

- Soundness of assumptions, as supported by facts, and the logic of a student's inductive or deductive reasoning

- Accuracy of identifying problems and the clarity and precision with which they are articulated

- Consistency and compatibility of analysis, recommendations, and whether the solution will solve the problem

- Quality of alternative solutions to the problem(s) identified and the comprehensiveness of decision criteria by which alternative solutions are judged

- Means to implement and evaluate the solution

- Degree to which the solution and implementation are feasible and relevant to the issue(s) involved and whether they consider internal and external forces, including stakeholders

Pedagogically, instructors may choose an unstructured or structured approach when using the case method. In the unstructured approach, the instructor assigns a case. Students read and prepare an analysis of the case for class discussion. The instructor initiates discussion by asking open-ended questions of the class in general, or of specific students: What is the problem in the case? What contextual aspects should be considered? What facts are there? Which facts are important, unimportant? If you were the decision maker, what would you do? Why? How would you implement your recommendation(s)?

The structured approach is more formal and requires that each student prepare a written report using a specific format or outline. The instructor initiates discussion by asking one or two members of the class to present their analysis. Alternatively, the instructor assigns the case to groups of students. Each group prepares a written analysis of the case. One group presents its analysis to the class, and this analysis is the basis for discussion.

The pedagogical technique an instructor uses will be influenced by factors such as personal preference; class size and length of class period; and academic mix and previous experience of students, including their familiarity with the case method and their grounding in the underlying disciplines. Over time, the instructor's approach may change from structured to unstructured depending on learning objectives, the degree to which the instructor introduces corollary subject matter through lectures or through controlled and directed discussion, and the progress students make in adapting to the case method.

Whatever the approach, two attributes of case study sometimes surprise students. First, it is impossible for case writers to include all relevant facts and circumstances of a situation. This means cases are incomplete.

These gaps can be partially filled by making assumptions supported by facts available in the case. This situation is typical for managers, who rarely have all the facts they would like to have before making a decision.

Second, it is not uncommon that problems identified in cases have no right or wrong answers. This attribute makes case study dynamic, interesting, integrating, and powerful. Initially, students may be frustrated because answers to the problems in a case are elusive. Greater experience with case study will show them, however, that small differences in situation assessment, assumptions, or problem definition can lead to very different conclusions and recommendations.

The students' role in case study is demanding. Because of the joint responsibility present in learning, this is as it should be. An often anxiety-laden aspect of the case method is that students must present their analyses and recommendations to the class and have their peers and the instructor challenge their work. If class discussion is to be productive, students must be well prepared and actively participate. Effective participation means contributing substance, not merely talking or restating points made by others.

METHODOLOGY FOR CASE ANALYSIS

There are several effective case analysis models. Instructors may have developed their own. Commonly, instructors require students to assume they are part of the organization or setting of the case, take a manager's perspective, and apply a systematic, analytical approach from that perspective.

Typically, students begin their analysis by assessing the facts of a case and organizing them by category. Categories may include organizational objectives; expectations about performance held by internal and external stakeholders; past and present results of operations; internal organizational strengths and weaknesses; external influences, such as regulations or the actions of competitors; and similar, relevant aspects of the case. In some cases, each category may be important. For others, only some categories are important. Regardless, the initial task is to gather and organize facts, which allows the problem statement to be formulated.

The problem statement is the starting point for analysis. The case may have one problem or several, and problems may be explicit or implicit. Correctly stating the problem is a crucial aspect of the case method; it is a skill essential to effective management. It is not easy to state the problem, but that skill can be learned and is facilitated by prior use of the case method and work experience. Success depends on thoroughly and effectively assessing the facts in the case. Figure I.1 is a model of the problem-solving process.

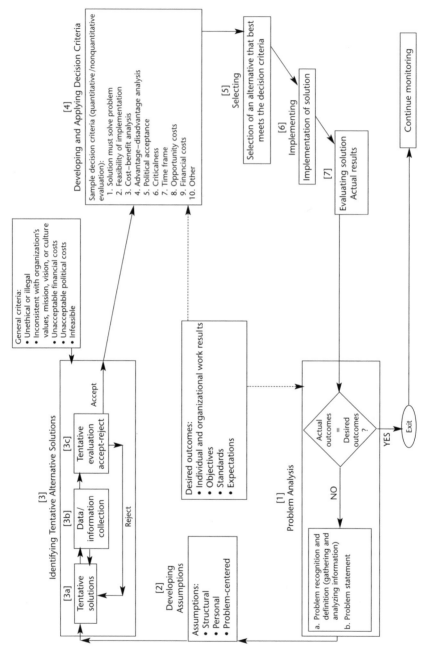

Figure I.1. Problem-solving process model under the condition of deviation.

Care must be taken to distinguish the symptoms of a problem from its root causes. Exhibits and figures in a case must be thoroughly assessed. Data should be analyzed—to the point of performing calculations—so the case and the problems present can be understood.

Making assumptions relevant to the problem statement follows. There are three types of assumptions: structural, personal (about the problem solver), and problem centered. Facts must be available to support assumptions, which are inferences drawn from facts using deductive or inductive reasoning. Assumptions allow the problem solver to extend and enhance what is known from the facts in a case. Table I.1 provides further explication of the three types of assumptions.

The next step in case analysis is formulating alternative solutions that can solve the problem(s). Facts that delimit or distinguish infeasible alternatives from those that can be considered further are especially useful here. Facility expansion, for example, may be infeasible if assessment of the current financial situation shows capital funds are unavailable, or the organization's

Table I.1.   Attributes of the three types of assumptions

Assumptions	Attributes
Structural	Relate to context of problem—boundary assumptions
	Within (outside) manager's authority
	Additional resources are (are not) available
	Other departments cause problem
	Problem caused by uncontrollable external factor(s)
Personal	Conclusions and biases decision makers bring to problem
	Risk taker; risk averse
	Likely reactions of superiors, subordinates, stakeholders
	Anchoring—adjustments from past starting point
	Escalating commitment—unwilling to admit past mistakes
	Confirmation bias—notice more, give greater weight, or seek evidence that confirms a claim/position
Problem Centered	Perceived relative importance of problem
	Degree of risk from problem
	How urgently solution is needed
	Economic cost and benefit
	Political cost and benefit
	Degree to which subordinates or superiors will accept solution
	Likelihood of success if solution implemented

market area will not sustain growth in capacity. Quantitative and financial analytical methods should be used to compare alternatives, as appropriate.

After tentative alternative solutions have been developed, the analyst must evaluate them. Evaluating alternative solutions requires the application of decision criteria that judge relative merit and effectiveness in solving the problem. Figure I.1 shows two levels of applying decision criteria. In Part [3], general criteria are applied. For example, is the alternative unethical or illegal? Is it consistent with the organization's values (philosophy), culture, and mission? Are there unacceptable financial or political costs? Is the alternative infeasible?

Part [4] of Figure I.1 shows application of relevant, specific criteria to the tentative alternative solutions that have met the general criteria of Part [3]. Arraying the decision criteria and alternative solutions in a matrix facilitates comparison. Categories of criteria include the following:

- Which alternative provides the greatest benefits of all types?

- What are the relative quantitative and nonquantitative costs of each alternative?

- Are internal capabilities to implement alternatives equal?

- Will external influences constrain or support implementation of alternatives differently?

Answers to these and similar questions will determine which solution is selected. Table I.2 is a sample decision matrix.

Once chosen, the solution must be implemented. The plan of implementation should identify the means, methods, and staff to evaluate the solution when implemented. Evaluation must answer the question, How will we know the problem has been solved? The primary focus of some cases is implementation. Others emphasize evaluating alternative solutions and choosing one. Implementation of solutions is addressed more generally in this volume. Regardless of emphasis, however, the analysis must give attention to implementation and evaluation of the solution. This makes case analysis more realistic, which is, after all, the central reason for using the case method.

OTHER RESOURCES IN USING THE CASE METHOD

A generic model for case analysis includes the following:

1. Students must identify their role in the analysis because their perspective of the problem will be a function of whom they are.

2. State the problem to be solved: "In what ways can I (we) . . . ?"

Table I.2.   Decision matrix from evaluating alternative solution[a]

Decision criteria	Alternative solution 1	Alternative solution 2	Alternative solution 3
Must meet these requirements			
1. Solution effectively solves the problem	3	5	5
2. Feasibility of implementation	5	3	5
3. Cost–benefit analysis	5	5	3
4. Advantage–disadvantage analysis	3	3	5
Want to meet these requirements			
5. Political acceptability	1	3	3
6. Criticalness	1	3	5
7. Time frame	1	3	5
8. Opportunity costs	5	1	3
9. Monetary costs	3	5	5
Total score	27	31	39

Conclusion: Alternative solution 3 accepted.

Adapted from Arnold, John D. *The Complete Problem Solver: A Total System for Competitive Decision Making*, 62. New York: John Wiley & Sons, 1992.

[a]Key:

5 = Solution *fully* meets decision criterion.

3 = Solution *partially* meets decision criterion.

1 = Solution *fails* to meet decision criterion.

3. Summarize, organize, and number the facts relevant to the problem statement.

4. Draw inferences (make assumptions [as shown in Table I.1]) relevant to the problem statement:

    a. Structural assumptions (context, resources, constraints, laws, regulations)

    b. Personal assumptions about the problem solver (biases, risk taker, risk averse, escalating commitment, anchoring, confirmation bias)

    c. Problem-centered assumptions (urgency, time frame, importance, degree of risk)

5. Link the facts to the inferences (assumptions) by citing the numbers of the facts that support the inferences.

6. Identify tentative alternative solutions.

7. Use general, broad-based criteria to perform initial screening of tentative alternative solutions (Part [3] in Figure I.1).

8. Develop a decision matrix—see Table I.2—to compare and apply specific decision criteria to select the solution to be implemented (Part [4] in Figure I.1).

9. State in general terms how *and* by whom the solution will be implemented.

10. Identify how *and* by whom the solution will be evaluated after it is implemented.

Additional information about problem solving and using the case method can be found in Chapter 6, "Managerial Problem Solving and Decision Making," of *Managing Health Services Organizations and Systems, Sixth Edition* (2014, Longest & Darr), published by Health Professions Press, Baltimore, MD.

PART I

Policy Environment of Health Services Delivery

1

Carilion Clinic

Alexandra Piriz Mookerjee
Westminster Communities of Florida, Orlando, FL

Kurt Darr
The George Washington University, Washington, D.C.

CASE HISTORY/BACKGROUND

Nestled in the Commonwealth of Virginia between Salem and Vinton is the city of Roanoke, whose population was approximately 98,000 in 2010.[1] The metropolitan area population was about 309,000.[1] Bisected by the Roanoke River and circled by the Blue Ridge Mountain Parkway, Roanoke is the commercial and cultural hub of western Virginia and southern West Virginia.[1,2]

The community that became Roanoke was established in 1852.[1] Early economic development of Roanoke resulted from its importance as the junction point for the Shenandoah Valley Railroad and the Norfolk and Western Railway.[2] These railroads were essential for transporting coal from western Virginia and West Virginia.[2] Roanoke's service area includes a regional airport, shopping malls, a regional hub for United Parcel Service, and manufacturing plants for General Electric, Yokohama tires, and Dynax, a maker of friction-based automobile parts.[2,3]

CARILION CLINIC

Carilion Clinic employs almost 12% of Roanoke's population. The Clinic includes 9 freestanding hospitals, 7 urgent care centers, and 220 (and increasing) practice centers, and it employs over 650 physicians in more than 70 specialties.[4] The Clinic has 1,026 licensed beds, not including 60 neonatal intensive care unit beds.[4] The Clinic had 48,659 admissions in fiscal year 2014–15.[4]

The Clinic's joint ventures and related companies include the following:

Carilion Clinic Physicians, LLC (real estate holding company)

Carilion Emergency Services, Inc.

Carilion Behavioral Health, Inc.

In March 2010, the same month and year the Affordable Care Act became law, the Clinic was ordered by the Federal Trade Commission to divest itself of an outpatient surgical center and an imaging center.[5] Both had been acquired as it sought to re-create "The Mayo Clinic" medical delivery model.

Led by Edward G. Murphy, M.D., from 1998 to 2011, Carilion Health System became Carilion Clinic, a vertically integrated health-care system. During Murphy's tenure the system expanded to include graduate and undergraduate medical education programs, a school of medicine (through a partnership with Virginia Polytechnic Institute and State University Virginia Tech), and, perhaps most impressively, Carilion established an accountable care organization in partnership with Aetna insurance company.[4,5]

Dr. Murphy's total compensation was almost $2.3 million in 2007. Nancy Agee, the Clinic's chief operating officer at the time, earned the next highest salary of about $800,000.[6] When Murphy resigned in 2011, Ms. Agee was promoted to president and CEO. In fiscal 2014, Carilion Clinic net revenue was $1.5 billion.[5] Agee's salary was $1.9 million.[7]

CONTROVERSY IN ROANOKE

Despite its philanthropic mission and positive effect on Roanoke, Carilion Clinic has not always enjoyed a good relationship with its community. (Carilion Clinic's mission, vision, and values are shown in Appendix 1.)

In May 1988, the U.S. Justice Department's Antitrust Division sought to prevent the merger of Roanoke's two hospitals: Memorial Roanoke Hospital and Community Hospital of Roanoke Valley. The lawsuit sought to block the merger because of the monopoly it alleged would result. Less than one year after the suit was filed, the Fourth Circuit U.S. Court of Appeals found for defendants Memorial Roanoke Hospital and Community Hospital of Roanoke Valley.

> [T]he merger between defendant hospitals would not constitute an unreasonable restraint of trade under the Sherman Act §1. The merger would strengthen the competition between the hospitals in the area

because defendant hospitals could offer more competitive prices and services.[8]

In the two appeals that followed, courts found for defendant hospitals, which then merged and were named Carilion Health System. The decision provided a legal basis for what is now the Carilion Clinic.

IN A MARKET: WHAT CONSTITUTES A MONOPOLY?

A monopoly occurs when one or more persons or a company dominate an economic market. This market domination results in the potential to exploit or suppresses those in the market or those trying to enter it (supplier, provider, or consumer).[9]

During the 19th century, the U.S. government began prosecuting monopolies under the common law as "market interference offenses" to block suppliers from raising prices. At the time, companies sometimes sought to buy all supplies of a certain material or product in an area, a practice known as "cornering the market."

In 1887, Congress passed the Interstate Commerce Act in response to railway companies' monopolistic practices in small, local markets.[10] This legislation protected small farmers who were being charged excessive rates to transport their products. Congress addressed monopolistic practices further by passing the Sherman Antitrust Act of 1890, which limited anticompetitive practices of businesses. The act blocked transfer of stock shares to trustees in exchange for a certificate entitling them to some of the earnings.[10] The Sherman Act was the basis for the Clayton Antitrust Act of 1914, the Federal Trade Commission Act of 1914, and the Robinson–Patman Act of 1936, which replaced the Clayton Act.[9]

Antitrust or competition laws address three main issues:

1. Prohibit agreements or practices that restrict free trade and competition among business entities

2. Ban abusive behavior by a firm dominating a market, or anticompetitive practices that tend to lead to such a dominant position

3. Supervise the mergers and acquisitions of large corporations, including some joint ventures[10]

The Herfindahl–Hirschman Index (HHI) helps implement these laws by providing a mathematical method to determine market "density," or the concentration of the market. Antitrust laws and methods of calculating market density, such as the HHI, are imperfect and can leave gaps that may be exploited. The HHI is discussed in Appendix 2.[11]

Since its establishment, the mission of the Federal Trade Commission has remained largely unchanged. Laws affecting private enterprise and government agencies have not. It is possible this mal juxtaposition underlies many of the difficulties in the healthcare industry.

VERTICAL INTEGRATION: THE MAYO CLINIC MODEL

The Mayo Clinic is the leading example of vertical integration in the delivery of healthcare in the United States. Founded in Rochester, Minnesota, in 1863, the Mayo Clinic began as the medical practice of William Worrall Mayo and his two sons, who were also physicians. It grew to include a comprehensive array of specialties.[12] Mayo developed different levels of care across the health services continuum. The result was a vertically integrated health system.[12] Mayo physicians are salaried at market levels, and they control the management structure.[12]

Mayo Clinic is headquartered in Rochester, Minnesota; it has satellite clinics elsewhere in the United States. In addition, Mayo and various medical centers worldwide have consulting and referral relationships. Mayo provides excellence and dedication in delivery of services with a constant, and self-admittedly stubborn, commitment to core values, which include that the needs of the patient come first, the integration of teamwork, efficiency, and mission over profit.[13]

Mayo has been long recognized for high performance, research, and innovation. It has ranked at or near the top of "Honor Roll" hospitals through the history of *U.S. News and World Report's* best-hospital rankings. In 2015–2016, Mayo Clinic had more number one rankings than any U.S. hospital or system. Eight specialties were ranked number one: diabetes and endocrinology, gastroenterology and gastrointestinal surgery, geriatrics, gynecology, nephrology, neurology and neurosurgery, pulmonology, and urology.

FORESHADOWING A MAYO CLINIC CLONE

Even before Murphy took the helm in 2001, Carilion Health System actions had stirred significant, but manageable, controversy in the community. Much of the controversy resulted from the antitrust case in 1988. After the court ruled that the merger did not violate federal law because it posed no threat of monopoly, the hospital continued its previous work in the community.

After becoming CEO, Murphy began to vertically integrate the Carilion Health System. His formal plan was presented in fall 2006. Part of evolving to a Mayo-style organization included acquiring physician practices in the community; some were closed after acquisition.

WHO IS EDWARD G. MURPHY, M.D.?

Edward G. Murphy earned his BS from the University of Albany, New York, and his medical degree (with honors) from Harvard University Medical School.[7] Although he never practiced medicine, Murphy was a clinical professor at the University of Albany School of Public Health and an adjunct assistant professor at Rensselaer Polytechnic Institute School of Management.[14] Before leaving New York state he was also a member of the New York State Hospital Review and Planning Council, and he served on its executive committee as the vice chair of the fiscal policy council.[14]

From 1989 to 1991, Murphy served as the vice president of clinical services at Leonard Hospital, a 143-bed facility north of Albany, New York.[15] In 1991, he was promoted to president and CEO of Leonard Hospital until it merged with St. Mary Hospital to form Seton Health System in 1994. Murphy became president and CEO of that new health system and stayed with Seton until 1998, when he relocated to Roanoke to head Carilion Health System.[14,16]

During his tenure at Carilion Clinic, Murphy managed the growth of that two-hospital health system into a vertically integrated model of healthcare delivery anchored by a 500-physician specialty group practice that included nine not-for-profit hospitals, undergraduate medical programs, an array of tertiary referral services, and a multistate laboratory service.[14] In 2007, Murphy announced plans for The Virginia Tech Carilion School of Medicine, which opened in 2010.[17] In 2010, Murphy was paid $2.27 million ($1.37 million in salary and $900,000 in benefits).[18]

Murphy's other roles in the Roanoke community included memberships on the boards of Healthcare Professionals Insurance Company and Trust; Luna Innovations, Inc.; and Home Town Bank. He is past chair of the Art Museum of Western Virginia. He also served in an influential position with the Council on Virginia's Future, which works to frame the growth and progress of the state, including businesses, people, and the health of the population.[14]

Murphy left Carilion to become chairman of Sound Physicians, a national provider of intensivist and hospitalist services. In 2012, he became the operating partner of Radius Ventures, a venture capital firm that invests in health-related companies.[19,20]

VERTICAL INTEGRATION: BECOMING A "CLINIC"

Murphy was always clear about his plans for Carilion Health System. In an August 2006 interview, he stated, "Right now . . . our core business is hospital services. In the new model, the core business will be physician services; the hospital will become ancillary."[21] In a 2007 interview for *Health Leaders Magazine*, Murphy explained, "I've been enamored of this model of healthcare delivery for a long time."[21]

In Fall 2006, Murphy, his staff, and the leadership board of Carilion Health System announced their plan to create a new model for Carilion's management characterized by teamwork and salaried physicians and other caregivers focused on patients across the spectrum of care.[22] Murphy explained:

> The essence of the clinic model is that hospitals stop becoming independent businesses and start becoming ancillary services to the physician practice. . . . If hospitals eventually want to provide better and more cost-effective healthcare, it's a necessary shift.[22]

The transformation was planned for seven years with an 18-month phase-in of its new name, *Carilion Clinic*. Plans for Carilion Clinic included a 50–50 partnership with Virginia Tech University in Blacksburg, Virginia, to establish a private, not-for-profit clinical research institute and a new medical school. Further, from 2007 to 2012 Carilion Clinic would add four or five fellowships for physicians to support its mission.[22]

Ground was broken for the much-anticipated university in early 2008.[23] On July 20, 2009, the Virginia State Council for Higher Education approved the Virginia Tech Carilion School of Medicine as a postsecondary institution.[24] It's first class matriculated in fall 2010.[24]

THE *WALL STREET JOURNAL* EXPOSÉ

Usually, an organization is pleased if the *Wall Street Journal* publishes an article about it. That is, of course, unless the story ignites a firestorm that leads to separate citizen and physician coalitions working against the organization and raises the specter of a word from Carilion Clinic's prehistory: *monopoly*.

"Nonprofit Hospitals Flex Pricing Power. In Roanoke, Va., Carilion's Fees Exceed Those of Competitors: The $4,727 Colonoscopy" was published on the front page of the *Wall Street Journal* August 28, 2008 (see Appendix 3). The author, John Carreyrou, explored Carilion's history, including the 1989 antitrust case, its expanding "market clout," and the strides toward its goal of vertical integration. The article suggested that some of the means used were questionable.[25]

Carreyrou asserted that skyrocketing healthcare costs in Roanoke were partially caused by, or possibly even led by, Carilion Clinic.[25]

In a press release, Carilion Clinic denied monopolistic practices or exploitative pricing and claimed it faced robust competition from Lewis-Gale Medical Center located in nearby Salem, Virginia.[26] (See Appendix 4, and the link to general information about Lewis-Gale Medical Center in Appendix 5.) Carilion Clinic defended its pricing practices by noting it must cross-subsidize emergency departments and care for the uninsured.[26]

Unsettling to some, however, was Carilion's practice of suing patients for unpaid medical bills. After Carilion obtains a court judgment, a lien is placed against the patient's home. A lien on real property puts a "cloud" on the title, which prevents the owner from conveying the property with a clear title until the lien has been satisfied. Responding in the *Wall Street Journal*, Murphy stated,

> Carilion only sues patients and places liens on their homes if it believes they have the ability to pay. . . . If you're asking me if it's right in a right-and-wrong sense, it's not. . . . But Carilion cannot be blamed for the country's "broken" healthcare system.[24]

Murphy asserted that Carilion's efforts to protect its financial interests meet legal requirements, but may be morally flawed. This position appears inconsistent with Carilion's mission that "Patient Care Comes First."

WHERE WERE THE LOCAL MEDIA?

As reported by Carreyrou, Carilion Clinic complained several times to editors of the *Roanoke Times* regarding reporter Jeff Sturgeon's coverage of the system. Shortly after the complaints, and mainly in response to a May 2008 article by Sturgeon, Carilion greatly reduced advertising in the *Roanoke Times*. About the same time, Sturgeon, the paper's longtime health issues writer, was reassigned. (See the article referenced in Appendix 6.)

Even after Sturgeon's reassignment, Carilion continued to be front-page news in the *Roanoke Times*. Reporter Sarah Bruyn Jones covered community reaction to the *Wall Street Journal* article and the impetus it gave to local coalitions. Her articles included the following: "Carilion Critics Draw Hundreds to Meeting" (September 2008); "Fed Agency Looks into Carilion Purchase" (September 2008); "Carilion Footprint Expands in Deal" (August 2008); and "Carilion to Buy Cardiology Practice" (August 2008). Jones's reporting put Carilion's practices at the forefront for Roanoke's citizens, but, as noted by Carreyrou, Carilion's growth seemed unstoppable.

THE BACKLASH

The August 2008 *Wall Street Journal* article resulted in a community uproar and fueled physicians' efforts to air their concerns about Carilion, including its anticompetitive actions and unfair pricing, and their desire to have open referrals for patients from outside Carilion's health network.[27] Citizen and physician coalitions met in hotel conference rooms and community centers to discuss the "unfair practices and behaviors" of Carilion Clinic. One, the Citizens Coalition for Responsible Healthcare, sponsored a petition that read as follows:

> To Dr. Murphy and the Carilion Health System Board of Directors:
>
> Please reconsider your Carilion Clinic plans. I want to keep my right to choose my doctor, even if he or she is an independent physician. Please rethink spending $100 million of my community's money on a Clinic model that could ruin our hospitals! Monopolies are never good for healthcare.[27]

The coalition's website offered copies of the *Wall Street Journal* article, video recordings of their meetings, information about a new forum program, and a membership form for those who wished to join their efforts.

The citizen coalitions stated they intended to focus on the negative impact of Carilion's transformation to a physician-led clinic that they asserted will increase costs and drive out many local physicians.[27] Murphy's plan was to bring into Carilion as many physicians as possible; all of whom will be salaried. The concerns of citizen coalitions stemmed from the scope of the effort, which resulted in closure or sale of many physician practices. Unaffiliated physicians asserted they could not compete. Further, Carilion's system of internal referrals, added to the purchase of existing practices, gave many specialists no choice but to leave, or stay and fight.[27]

Despite the controversy, Carilion has shown no signs of slowing; it has stayed the course outlined in Fall 2006.

CARILION'S RESPONSE

On August 28, 2008, less than 24 hours after publication of Carreyrou's *Wall Street Journal* article, Carilion responded. Statements published in newspapers and posted on Carilion's website, as well as press releases, stated the allegations and conclusions drawn from them were misleading and misinformed.

In response, Carilion directed readers' attention to the Virginia Hospital and Healthcare Association PricePoint website. It showed that Carilion's prices are comparable to surrounding hospitals and are generally lower than its closest competitor, Lewis-Gale Medical Center in neighboring Salem, Virginia.[26] To support their position on pricing,

Carilion stated, "Medical care in hospitals is more expensive . . . having staff and technology at the ready has its costs."[25] Also mentioned was Carilion's Life-Guard helicopter, which is a subsidized service.[26] Carilion provided $42 million in charity care in 2007 and an additional $25 million in free care (bad debt written off), thus illustrating its dedication and support of its service area.[26] Carilion supports research and education—substantial resource commitments that add major costs to the organization and provide subsidized services to the community.[26]

In explaining the policy to sue patients, Carilion stated that efforts are made to qualify patients for public programs, as needed. Further, Carilion said only "a small fraction of the nearly 2 million" patient billings each year go to court.[26]

> Court filings are a final resort, and we try to be flexible. If the judgment includes a lien on an individual's property, we do not foreclose on the lien. The lien is satisfied if and when the property is sold.[26]

In response to concerns about its internal referral practice, Carilion stated that referrals are sent from physician to physician in the system with the intention of sending patients to better, more-qualified physicians who have "earned" the referral. This "earn, not force" mentality contributes to the goal of well-coordinated care and service, which is the first choice of patients.[26]

Carilion's press release closed by describing a wasteful and poorly organized U.S. healthcare system that it hoped to improve with the vertically integrated clinic model of providing care.[26] The hope is that comprehensive, high-quality, and cost-effective care will put the patient first. The reader of the press release is reminded that what happened at Mayo could be replicated at Carilion.

CURRENT SITUATION IN ROANOKE

As noted, Carilion Clinic has a medical school partnership, an expanding physician practice with a robust specialty list, and its own accountable care organization, which continues to show progress and increased membership.

Three decades after the hospital merger controversy began in Roanoke, Virginia, the economic and healthcare environments have changed, the population is increasing, and healthcare costs are rising.[25] When the antitrust case was brought in 1988, Roanoke had among the lowest health insurance premiums in Virginia; now, they are among the highest.[28,29]

DISCUSSION QUESTIONS

1. Identify the problems Carilion Clinic faces as it seeks to become a comprehensive, vertically integrated healthcare provider. Rank these problems in terms of their difficulty of solution.

2. Develop arguments to *support* Carilion Clinic's efforts to become a comprehensive, vertically integrated healthcare system.

3. Identify reasons why competition is useful *and* why it is not useful in terms of healthcare cost, quality, and access.

4. Why could Mayo Clinic develop a comprehensive, vertically integrated healthcare system, whereas Carilion Clinic has had so much difficulty?

5. Identify the advantages and disadvantages of developing specialty services internally to achieve vertical integration compared with obtaining the same services by acquiring existing providers.

APPENDIX 1

Carilion Clinic

Mission
Improve the health of the communities we serve.

Vision
We are committed to a common purpose of better patient care, better community health, and lower cost.

Values

- **CommUNITY**—Working in unison to serve our community, our Carilion family, and our loved ones

- **Courage**—Doing what's right for our patients without question

- **Commitment**—Unwavering in our quest for exceptional quality and service

- **Compassion**—Putting heart into everything we do

- **Curiosity**—Fostering creativity and innovation in our pursuit of excellence

Retrieved May 9, 2016 from https://www.carilionclinic.org/about-carilion-clinic#sthash.pvG4Jrd2.dpuf

APPENDIX 2

Herfindahl–Hirschman Index

The Herfindahl–Hirschman Index (HHI) is a commonly accepted measure of market concentration. The HHI is calculated by squaring the market share of each firm competing in the market and then summing the products. For example, for a market consisting of four firms with shares of 30, 30, 20, and 20 percent, the HHI is 2,600 ($30^2 + 30^2 + 20^2 + 20^2 = 2,600$).

The HHI considers the relative size distribution of the firms in a market. It approaches zero when a market is occupied by numerous firms of relatively equal size and reaches its maximum of 10,000 points when a market is controlled by a single firm. The HHI increases both as the number of firms in the market decreases and as the disparity in size among the firms increases.

The agencies generally consider markets in which the HHI is between 1,500 and 2,500 points to be moderately concentrated and consider markets in which the HHI exceeds 2,500 points to be highly concentrated (see U.S. Department of Justice and the Federal Trade Commission, *Horizontal Merger Guidelines* § 5.2, 2010). Transactions that increase the HHI by more than 200 points in highly concentrated markets are presumed likely to enhance market power under the *Horizontal Merger Guidelines*.

Retrieved May 5, 2016, from https://www.justice.gov/atr/herfindahl-hirschman-index. (Updated July 29, 2015.)

APPENDIX 3

On August 28, 2008, the front page of the *Wall Street Journal* carried an article entitled "Nonprofit Hospitals Flex Pricing Power. In Roanoke, VA., Carilion's Fees Exceed those of Competitors: The $4,727 Colonoscopy." Written by John Carreyrou, the article reported the large price discrepancies for a diagnostic procedure in Roanoke, Virginia, and highlighted the role of the Carilion Clinic. It detailed how delivery of healthcare in Roanoke evolved into a market dominated by the Carilion Clinic and discussed the financial burden that healthcare costs, such as the headline-making colonoscopy, can place on the community.

Published August 28, 2008. *The Wall Street Journal*. Retrieved from http://online .wsj.com/article/SB121986172394776997.html?mod=googlenews_wsj

APPENDIX 4

Carilion Clinic's Press Release
in Response to the *Wall Street Journal* Article

Friday, August 29, 2008

On Thursday, Aug. 28, the *Wall Street Journal* targeted Carilion Clinic in an article about not-for-profit healthcare providers. We would like to address some of the key issues raised by the *Journal*, and hopefully answer some of the questions you may have in relation to the article.

Insurance Rates and Costs   The article implies that Carilion is the reason that insurance premiums are rising in our part of the state. It is misleading to infer that Carilion is the cause when premiums—set by insurance companies—contain many factors outside our control. The hospital component of the premium is just 40 percent; other factors include drug costs, utilization by the population, insurance overhead, and insurance profits. About 60 percent of hospital utilization in this region occurs at Carilion facilities.

If you compare Carilion's hospital charges to Lewis-Gale Medical Center and to HCA Richmond hospitals, we are generally lower, as evidenced on the Virginia Hospital & Healthcare Association (VHHA) PricePoint consumer website at www.vapricepoint.org.

Yes, medical care in hospitals is more expensive than in outpatient settings. Having staff and technology at the ready has its cost. Also, it is no secret that care for the uninsured and for unprofitable services—such as the Carilion Life-Guard helicopter ambulance service and Emergency Room care—has to be subsidized. Carilion is the safety net for many people in our community who have no means to pay for services, and this burden is borne in part by paying patients.

Community Benefits   As stated in the article, we provided $42 million in charity care (at cost) in 2007 to qualifying patients. An additional $25 million in free care was written off as bad debt. The total amount far exceeds U.S. Senator Chuck Grassley's proposed 5 percent requirement for not-for-profit hospitals.

In addition, we support medical residency teaching programs, provide financial assistance to nursing education and allied health programs in the region, and give significant resources to area not-for-profit organizations such as the Roanoke Rescue Mission, Child Health Investment Partnership (CHIP), and Free Clinics. These are important investments in the community's health.

Collections We have a generous charity care policy, and we actively work to qualify the poor, uninsured, and underinsured for free and discounted care. Part of our collection process does include filing court judgments against individuals who do not qualify for charity care and do not pay their bills. This represents a small fraction of the nearly 2 million patient visits that occur per year. It is only fair to patients who do pay their bills that we collect from those who are able to pay but choose not to. Court filings are a last resort, and we try to be flexible. If the judgment includes a lien on an individual's property, we do not foreclose on the lien. The lien is satisfied if and when the property is sold.

Referrals Our position all along has been to *earn*, not force, referrals to our physicians. It is our intent through well-coordinated, high-quality care and service to be the first choice of patients for their medical care.

Board Activities We have a conflict-of-interest policy to which our board members are held accountable. Jay Turner, President of J.M. Turner Construction, is not involved in contracting decisions and abstains from any vote that might involve work by his company, in keeping with the Board's policy. We have always voluntarily disclosed on our Form 990 filings the value of the work Mr. Turner's company contracts with Carilion.

Closing We share national concerns about the rising cost of healthcare. One reason we are reorganizing into a physician-led Clinic is to more effectively and efficiently provide medical care. It is estimated that 30 percent of all medical tests and procedures are unnecessary. Carilion Clinic is on a path to improve healthcare outcomes, to reduce medical waste, and to make a positive difference in the lives of our patients. We have a lot of important work to do to reach our vision of creating a healthier and more vibrant region.

APPENDIX 5

Lewis-Gale Medical Center

The Lewis-Gale Medical Center resulted from the 1996 merger of Lewis-Gale Hospital and Lewis-Gale Psychiatric Center. It is a 506-bed medical center and serves as the hub of the Hospital Corporation of America Virginia Health System's southwestern region. The Hospital Corporation of America is composed of locally managed facilities that include 165 hospitals and 115 outpatient centers in 20 states and England.

Updated May 9, 2016, retrieved from http://www.hcavirginia.com/ and http://www.lewis- gale.com/

APPENDIX 6

This article was published after it was discovered that more than $19 million in construction contracts was awarded to J.M. Turner & Co., whose chairman and CEO and co-owner was a member of the Carilion Clinic board. The article explored the possibly unethical management and decision making involved in those contracts, as well as the pattern of behavior that led to them.

Carilion, Board Members Collaborate

By Jeff Sturgeon

Carilion Clinic awarded $19.3 million worth of construction work over a three-year period to the company of a builder who sits on its board of directors.

Roanoke-based J.M. Turner & Co., Inc., received $582,724, $9 million, and $9.7 million in 2006, 2005, and 2004, respectively. The company's chairman, chief executive officer, and co-owner is Jay Turner, a Carilion board member during each of those years. Turner said Carilion lets board members work for or sell products and services to the system, with oversight, and confirmed that his company provides needed health care construction services.

Carilion's hiring of the firm has not been his decision or a decision he influenced, he said, though he is pleased the company named after his father is a Carilion contractor.

Carilion said it values having business-minded individuals drawn from the community on its board.

"I'm not sure you could have a business-oriented board and not have somebody's company doing business at some level with Carilion in some way. You'd have to bring board members in from outside the state," Carilion spokesman Eric Earnhart said.

For protection, a conflict-of-interest policy exists whose aim, Earnhart said, is to ensure no board member benefits inappropriately from his or her position of power. Carilion spends roughly $1 billion annually in Southwest and Western Virginia.

"We have certainly abided by those rules, and I feel like our company provides a very valuable service," said Turner, 63.

Earnhart said all the work the Turner contracting firm received from Carilion was either competitively bid—meaning the company beat out other contractors for a project with a designated value—or awarded in a "design-build" environment in which only the project manager is chosen upfront after negotiations.

The money represents perhaps 10 percent of Carilion's construction spending during the three years under analysis and would have gone to J.M. Turner & Co. even if the company leader wasn't a board member, Earnhart said.

"We've had excellent experience with J.M. Turner & Co.," he said.

Although its board meetings are closed to the public, Carilion annually identifies board members and key personnel and their family members who have Carilion jobs or business relationships with the health system. Its bylaw also tells how much money the people or their companies received and why.

The law requires not-for-profit, tax-exempt organizations to put the information on a Form 990 that is a public record available from the Internal Revenue Service, the organization itself, and other sources.

Turner topped Carilion's payout lists that detail which system officials benefited financially for 2004 through 2006.

In other examples, Carilion said it bought $1,698 worth of furniture from Grand Home Furnishings, where former Carilion board Chairman George Cartledge is an executive, and paid salary and benefits of $33,297 in 2005 to the spouse of board member and physician James Nuckolls. Nuckolls' wife works at a Carilion-owned medical practice.

It is not publicly known how much business the Turner company received from Carilion last year. A report covering the final three months of 2006 and most of 2007 is due out in late summer or early fall.

Turner has played a role on many Carilion projects

The millions of dollars listed as going to J.M. Turner are not a surprise because the company, while not Carilion's exclusive builder by any means, has played key roles in many projects.

It is currently involved in erecting the large Carilion Clinic physician services building on South Jefferson Street at Reserve Avenue. It will have a role in a new Pearisburg hospital.

Jay Turner also received a fee of $23,000 for his board service from 2004–06, according to reports. Only Cartledge received more—$24,300—during that time.

Carilion uses other construction companies, too.

"Thor Inc. has performed a number of construction projects for Carilion over the last several years, and we have only positive things to say about our relationship with them as our client," company President Allen Whittle said by e-mail.

Despite the scrutiny given Jay Turner's board service, Earnhart said contracting decisions by and large fall to an internal construction team below board level.

As for compliance with the conflict-of-interest policy, Earnhart noted that the board chairman who presides over meetings is James Hartley, a former county prosecutor.

"The board does and always has run a tight ship," Earnhart said.

Turner said if contracting matters reach the board, he will abstain if his company is involved. He said he did abstain when the board hired J.M. Turner contracting to build a planned athletic club at Smith Mountain Lake. For unrelated reasons, the club was not built.

Several steps removed from the Carilion board, J.M. Turner is also picking up business as a subcontractor for a Swedish construction management firm that Carilion has used for various large construction jobs.

The company, Skanska USA Building in Parsippany, N.J., has chosen J.M. Turner to be part of its local construction team on a number of occasions. These payments, the amount of which is not publicly known, are not included in the $19 million Carilion said it paid Turner, according to Earnhart.

So in addition to the disclosed payments, J.M. Turner & Co. indirectly benefits from Carilion's building projects.

Flynn Auchey, an associate professor for Virginia Tech's Department of Building Construction, said companies needing construction services commonly rely on construction services providers with whom they have prior experience, and general contractors do the same with subcontractors.

"Once you find someone you can trust, when you are used to working with someone and communication is good, staying with the same contractors and subcontractors often makes sense," said Auchey, who is also an architect, engineer, and general contractor. "It's not unusual at all."

Concerns about potential conflicts of interest can be quieted, he said, if the client solicits bids from more than one contractor.

Scott Rivenbark, Skanska's on-site project executive in Roanoke, said J.M. Turner has earned all its work received from Skanska through pricing proposals, similar to bids. Skanska has sometimes invited other Southwest Virginia contractors to bid, though not all of the time, and has in some cases chosen other contractors, he said.

Skanska is not under any pressure from Carilion to use J.M. Turner, but "we do so in the best interests of the project when it does make sense," he said.

Published May 31, 2008, *Roanoke Times*. Retrieved from http://www.roanoke.com/business/wb/163971

ENDNOTES

1. U.S. Census Bureau. Retrieved from http://quickfacts.census.gov/qfd/index .html. Updated July 1, 2014. Accessed March 8, 2016.
2. Roanoke. Retrieved from xroads.virginia.edu. Updated September 1, 2009. Accessed April 1, 2016.
3. Roanoke region of Virginia; Roanoke Regional Partnership. Retrieved from http://www.roanoke.org Updated 2009. Accessed July 1, 2009.
4. Carilion Clinic. About us. Retrieved from http://www.carilionclinic.org/ Carilion/About+Us. Updated 2016. Accessed March 8, 2016.
5. Aetna. Aetna and Carilion Clinic announce plans to collaborate on account-able care organization. Retrieved from https://news.aetna.com/news-releases/ aetna-and-carilion-clinic-announce-plans-to-collaborate-on-accountable-care-organization/. Updated 2016. Accessed March 9, 2016.
6. 2006 Carilion Clinic Income Tax Form. Tax Year 10/1/2006–09/30/2007.
7. Hammack, L. (2014). IRS records show salaries of Carilion's high-est-paid executives. Retrieved from http://www.roanoke.com/business/ columns_and_blogs/blogs/med_beat/irs-records-show-salaries-of-carilion-s-highest-paid-executives/article_d3238175-dbd5-54dd-b427-c08a842388cc .html?mode=print. Updated 2016. Accessed March 11, 2016.
8. *United States of America v. Carilion Health System and Community Hospital of Roanoke Valley.* 707 F. Supp. 840.
9. Definition retrieved from http://legal-dictionary.thefreedictionary.com/ Monopoly. Accessed June 20, 2009.
10. Retrieved from http://www.oecd.org Organization for Economic Co-Operation and Development. Updated 2009. Accessed July 1, 2009.
11. Wildermuth, J. (2001, July 1). Will political donations keep Microsoft intact? *San Francisco Chronicle*, p. A-1. Retrieved from http://www.sfgate.com/ cgi-bin/article.cgi?file=/c/a/2001/07/01/MN221539.DTL&type=printable
12. Retrieved from http://www.diavlos.gr/orto96/ortowww/historym.htm. Updated April 12, 1997. Accessed June 21, 2009.
13. Retrieved from http://electronic-engagement.elliance.com/index.php/2009/ 01/11/brand- building-mayo-clinic-style/. Updated 2009. Accessed June 24, 2009.
14. Retrieved from http://www.vtc.vt.edu/about/leadership/ed_murphy.html Updated 2009. Accessed June 23, 2009.
15. Retrieved from http://www.hospital-data.com/hospitals/LEONARD-HOSPITAL-TROY. html Accessed July 6, 2009.
16. Lugar, N. (2008, January/February). Up close with Dr. Edward Murphy. *Roanoker Magazine* Retrieved from http://www.theroanoker.com/features/ EdMurphy_jf08/index.cfm
17. Virginia Department of Game and Inland Fisheries. Retrieved from http:// www.dgif.virginia.gov. Accessed August 14, 2009.
18. Bruyn Jones, S. (2008, September 10). Carilion CEO earned $2.27 million last fiscal year. *Roanoke Times*. Retrieved from http://www.roanoke.com/ business/wb/174762
19. Retrieved from www.radiusventures.com. Accessed March 11 2016.
20. Retrieved from http://www.soundphysicians.com/. Updated 2016. Accessed March 10, 2016.
21. Nason, D. (2006, August). Charting a new course: Dr. Edward Murphy plans a transformation at Carilion Health System. *Virginia Business Magazine*.

Retrieved from http://www.gatewayva.com/biz/virginiabusiness/lifestyle/0806_options/op_pro.shtml

22. Betbeze, P. (2007, June). Keep 'em close. *Health Leaders*. Retrieved from http://www.healthleadersmedia.com/content/90253/topic/WS_HLM2_MAG/Keep-Em-Close.html

23. Retrieved from http://www.vtnews.vt.edu/story.php?relyear=2007&item no=5. Updated 2009. Accessed July 6, 2009.

24. Retrieved from http://www.vtc.vt.edu/about/newsroom/releases/2009-07-20schev certification.html. Updated 2009. Accessed July 22, 2009.

25. Carreyrou, J. (2008, August 28). Nonprofit hospitals flex pricing power. In Roanoke, Va., Carilion's fees exceed those of competitors: The $4,727 colonoscopy. *Wall Street Journal*. Retrieved from http://online.wsj.com/ article/ SB121986172394776997.html?mod=2_1566_topbox

26. Carilion Clinic. (2008, August 29). Statement from Carilion Clinic in response to *Wall Street Journal* article. Retrieved from http://www.carilion-clinic.org/ Carilion/Statement+from+Carilion+Clinic+in+response+to+Wall +Street+ Journal

27. Bruyn Jones, S. (2008, September 10). Carilion critics draw hundreds to meeting: The citizen group says Carilion Clinic is driving up costs. *Roanoke Times*.

28. Retrieved from http://online.wsj.com/public/resources/documents/cigna_email080827.pdf. Updated 2009. Accessed June 28, 2009.

29. Federal Trade Commission. (2009, October 7). Commission order restores competition eliminated by Carilion Clinics acquisition of two outpatient clinics: Hospital must sell all clinic assets acquired in 2008. Retrieved from https://www.ftc.gov/news-events/press-releases/2009/10/commission-order-restores-competition-eliminated-carilion-clinics. Accessed March 10, 2016.

30. Center for American Progress Action Fund. Retrieved from https://www.americanprogressaction.org/issues/regulation/report/2011/09/09/280/health-care-industry-consolidation-focus-needed-on-consumer-protection-and-balanced-antitrust-enforcement/. Updated 2016. Accessed January 1, 2016.

2

Flu Vaccine

Mary K. Feeney
Arizona State University, Phoenix, AZ

Abigail Peterman
Arizona State University, Phoenix, AZ

CASE HISTORY/BACKGROUND

The 2004–2005 U.S. Influenza Vaccine Shortage

Influenza, or the flu, causes roughly 36,000 deaths and 200,000 hospitalizations annually in the United States and costs the American economy more than $83.3 billion each year.[1] The primary method for preventing influenza is the flu vaccine, which is generally available in a variety of settings, including clinics, hospitals, schools, workplaces, and other convenient locations. The vaccine is typically distributed in October and November in anticipation of the winter flu season, which usually begins in late November and peaks in February. For the 2004–2005 flu season, the Centers for Disease Control and Prevention recommended that as many as 185 million Americans receive a flu shot. Among those 185 million, almost half (90 million) are considered high-risk.[2,3] The high-risk population included adults 65 and older, infants 6 to 23 months old, pregnant women, healthcare workers, those who care for children under 6 months old, and people with compromised immune systems or chronic illnesses, such as asthma, lung cancer, and cystic fibrosis.[2,3]

Americans have faced flu vaccine shortages on multiple occasions. For example, at the beginning of the 2000–2001 flu season, demand for the vaccine outstripped supply when problems developing a vaccine for a new viral strain and safety and quality control issues temporarily delayed vaccine delivery by 6–8 weeks.[4,5] The reduced supply resulted in an uneven distribution of available vaccines and sharp price increases as the cost of flu shots more than doubled from the previous season.[5] In 2001–2002, three manufacturers produced 87 million doses, of which almost one-third were not available when demand for the vaccine peaked. The following year supply exceeded demand when only 87% of the 95 million doses produced were purchased. In 2003–2004, demand exceeded supply when 4 million doses were discarded and 87 million doses were inappropriate for that year's flu strain.[3,5,6] As recently as 2013, Americans faced flu vaccine shortages.[7]

The Institute of Medicine noted these recent shortages have "highlighted the fragility of vaccine supply," which is further complicated by declining financial incentives to develop and produce vaccines.[8] The high-risk market (e.g., uncertainty of predicting future demand), long-term, high production costs, and low-profit margins reduced the number of vaccine manufacturers in the United States from more than 25 companies in the 1970s to 5 in 2003.[8] The number increased to 11 in 2015.[1]

Production of the flu vaccine is a risky and long-term venture for numerous reasons.

1.   Opening new manufacturing facilities can take 5 years or longer due to demanding U.S. Food and Drug Administration (FDA) quality standards.

2.   Producing the flu vaccine takes 5 to 6 months, and the formula cannot be altered once production begins.

3.   Manufacturers must reformulate the vaccine annually to address new influenza strains, preventing manufacturers from using supplies from the previous season.

4.   There is extensive risk associated with predicting supply and demand for the flu vaccine because there is no mechanism for predicting the market.

5.   Demand for flu vaccine tends to be fickle, shifting from year to year or month to month based on severity of the flu season, efforts of public health to promote vaccination, and timing of vaccine availability.

6.   Profit margins for the flu vaccine are low because vaccines are sold at a low price relative to the time, risk, and cost of producing safe and efficient vaccines.

7.   Producing vaccines is much less profitable compared to developing pharmaceuticals that patients purchase more frequently.

Precipitating Factors in the 2004–2005 Flu Vaccine Crisis

Chiron and Aventis were the only two U.S.-based producers of vaccine for the 2004–2005 flu season. Their goal was 100 million doses. In

August 2004, Chiron, a California-based company, informed the FDA and the UK Medicines and Healthcare products Regulatory Agency that 48 million doses produced at Chiron's plant in Liverpool were contaminated. Concerns about quality and safety at that plant emerged in 2003 following an FDA inspection. At that time, however, the FDA allowed Chiron to voluntarily fix the problems and, based on assurances from Chiron, the FDA believed the bacterial contamination issue would be resolved. The FDA proceeded to communicate with Chiron via letters, e-mail, and phone. The Medicines and Healthcare products Regulatory Agency took a more proactive approach, including inspections of the plant.[9]

In October 2004, to the surprise of the FDA, the Medicines and Healthcare products Regulatory Agency suspended Chiron's license and closed the Liverpool plant. Dr. Schaffner of the National Vaccine Advisory Committee stated that, "we have been reassured on a regular basis" that the contamination at Chiron was not going to be a major problem.[10] Tommy Thompson, secretary of the U.S. Department of Health and Human Services, reported that "we had no idea" this suspension would occur.[11] In mid-October, the FDA confirmed that none of the Chiron vaccine could be salvaged.

Media frenzy and public outrage followed the announcement that Americans would receive only half the expected 100 million doses of the flu vaccine. Nationwide, long lines formed outside health clinics, others went to Canada for the flu shot. As with the 2000–2001 vaccine shortage, when demand surpassed supply, reports of price gouging immediately appeared. For example, a pharmacist was reportedly offered 10 doses that usually cost $67 for $700.[12] Meanwhile, Shore Memorial Hospital in New Jersey was offered 8,000 doses, which had been illegally smuggled into the United States, at the price of $60 each.[13] In a more extreme case, 620 vaccine doses were stolen from a Colorado pediatrician's office.[14]

In addition to the rising cost of flu shots, distributing available vaccines quickly became a problem. The distribution issues came as no surprise to federal officials or healthcare workers who had long known about the fragility of the U.S. vaccine market. Following the 2000–2001 vaccine shortage the General Accounting Office published a report outlining the issues related to vaccine shortages and recommended policies to prevent future problems. The report's primary concern was that there is "no system to ensure that high-risk people have priority when the supply of vaccine is short."[5] Because the production, sale, and distribution of the flu vaccine are private enterprises, the 2004 vaccine supply was distributed unevenly. Organizations that ordered the vaccine from Chiron had none; those supplied by Aventis had their entire order filled. Distribution is based on the type of healthcare provider, not on level of risk among its patients. Public officials know very little about how flu vaccine supplies are shipped and to whom. This makes it difficult to impossible for the government to affect the distribution of vaccine produced by Aventis, or any supplier.

The CDC responded to distribution concerns by recommending that healthcare providers give priority to high-risk patients. However, because the Centers for Disease Control and Prevention lacked the authority to intervene in the distribution process or enforce guidelines, the recommendation left states, healthcare centers, county health departments, and doctors to determine how to distribute the vaccine. Many flu vaccination providers asked healthy adults to voluntarily forgo vaccination, thus leaving supplies for high-risk individuals. In Maryland, the state immunization center operated as a vaccine broker to ensure that public health agencies received 100% of their orders. Meanwhile, in Virginia, the state divided vaccines proportionate to census data.[15] In rare cases, such as the District of Columbia, flu shots were reserved for high-risk patients.[16] Generally, however, city and state officials did not deny the vaccine to healthy people who wanted it.

In response to price gouging and distribution issues, the Centers for Disease Control and Prevention created a panel to investigate the ethics of distributing the flu vaccine. In addition, a federal task force, the Flu Action Task Force, was convened to manage the federal vaccine supply, coordinate efforts, and prevent price gouging.[17] By mid-October, federal agencies began distributing their store of flu vaccine to high-risk areas. Within one week, 3.2 million doses had been sent to high-priority groups. That same week many hospitals began sharing flu vaccine supplies. The federal government diverted 300,000 doses from federal employees and the military to high-risk civilians.

Once it was confirmed that the entire Chiron supply was unsalvageable, the federal government looked overseas for additional doses. Secretary Thompson announced that Aventis would have 2.6 million more doses of the flu vaccine by January 2005. The United States also began negotiating with ID Biomedical in Canada and GlaxoSmithKline in Germany to purchase additional doses. Unfortunately, those purchases were delayed waiting for FDA approval. By early December, President George W. Bush confirmed that the United States would purchase 1.2 million doses from Germany.[18] The FDA required patients to sign a consent form for the more expensive doses from Germany because they were not licensed in the United States.

State officials began looking for alternatives to obtain the vaccine for high-risk populations. Illinois governor Rod Blagojevich (D) located 750,000 doses overseas and requested permission from the FDA to purchase them. In New York City, Mayor Michael Bloomberg (R) requested 500,000 doses of the flu vaccine from federal health agencies for high-risk residents. When that request was denied, Bloomberg spent $2 million to buy vaccines from manufacturers in Germany and Canada; however, that purchase also required FDA approval.[19]

Unfortunately, previous experience indicates people will not rush to purchase delayed supplies of the flu vaccine. For example, during the 2000–2001 flu season, late shipments went unused or sold at very low prices. Rod Watson, president of Prevention MD, an immunization and medical screening company in Redmond, Washington, canceled numerous flu shot clinics in October, and by December 2004 had excess shots he could barely give away, let alone sell.[20] The same lack of demand occurred in states such as California, Colorado, and Texas, despite the fact that December vaccinations would still protect many people during the peak flu month of February.

CONCLUSION

Appendixes A and B summarize influenza facts and figures and provide a flu timeline for 2004–2005. It is evident that influenza raises a number of healthcare public policy issues, including the following:

- High-risk populations need vaccines.

- The market for flu vaccines is unstable and unpredictable.

- The FDA relies on private companies to provide vaccines but may not monitor them well.

- The federal government is aware of the problems associated with the flu vaccine market, but it has no long-term plan to address them.

- When a vaccine shortage occurs, federal actions are uncoordinated.

- The United States does not have competitive suppliers of flu vaccine.

The following role-play options facilitate the analysis and discussion of these and other issues:

Option 1: The Flu Vaccine Administration Task Force

Option 2: How Will Your State Protect Itself Next Year?

Option 3: Writing a policy brief

The instructor will assign participants to any or all of the options and assign roles within each.

Option 1: The Flu Vaccine Administration Task Force

In the wake of the 2004–2005 flu vaccine shortage, we are convening a federal task force to develop a strategic plan to address the issues in this case. It is your task to discuss and propose policies to ensure the 2004–2005 flu vaccine shortage does not happen again. This may seem an easy task, but you will learn that divergent values and political beliefs make negotiating this plan challenging.

Each group will identify and outline problems the task force will address, as well as the potential solutions they support. Goals to be kept in mind include the following:

1. Protect the health of people in the United States.

2. Ensure fairness in availability and distribution of vaccine.

3. Ensure high-risk populations are protected.

4. Protect market values you support.

5. Protect social values you support.

6. Promote competitiveness in markets.

7. Identify alternatives for flu vaccine production.

Characters

Greg Stanton: You are the mayor of the largest city in your state. You want to purchase vaccines from Germany to ensure high-risk individuals are vaccinated.

Dr. Alex Smith: You are a public health expert working with the Centers for Disease Control and Prevention. Your primary interest is developing rules and procedures for managing flu vaccine production and distribution.

Sam Jones: You are a representative of the Association of Retirement Homes. You are concerned about providing inexpensive (or free) vaccines to older adults. You are also concerned about the distribution issues of getting vaccines to those needing them.

Kelly North: You are a libertarian who believes that government must allow the market to determine vaccine production and distribution.

Tony Brown: You are the leader of the American Coalition for Universal Healthcare. You want the government to ensure vaccines will be available to all citizens, not just to those at high risk.

Option 2: How Will Your State Protect Itself Next Year?

After the 2004–2005 flu vaccine shortage, the federal government decided it would not preempt the flu vaccine market, manage flu vaccine distribution, guarantee purchase of flu vaccines, or pursue alternatives to protect flu vaccine producers.

The governor of your state decided it must develop an emergency plan for future flu vaccine shortages. Your task is to meet with officials and representatives from around the state to develop a plan for purchasing, managing, and distributing flu vaccines in the future. You *cannot* make recommendations for what the federal government should or could do. You are working under the assumption that the state alone must address this issue without assistance from the federal government.

Your task includes the following:

1. Outline the challenges facing the state.

2. Outline the interests of each character.

3. Present the committee's analysis to the class:

   a. Introduce the characters and their interests.

   b. Discuss the plan.

4. Develop an emergency management plan that

   a. Prevents a flu vaccine shortage

   b. Anticipates what the state will do if there is a flu vaccine shortage

5. Participate in a Q&A session with state citizens.

Characters

- Local public health representative
- President of the Public Housing Outreach Organization
- Representative from the State Senior Citizens Association
- State senator (R)
- State senator (D)
- President of the state university
- Owner and operator of Pharma Corporation, the largest producer of vaccines in the United States
- Other (identify your own)

Class Assignment

Other class members are citizens of your state who will participate in a Q&A session following the presentation. As citizens, you will have the opportunity to ask the committee questions and make suggestions. After the Q&A session, citizens and committee members will vote on a plan.

Option 3: Writing a Policy Brief

Following the 2004–2005 flu vaccine shortage and subsequent debate about the need for a long-term plan to address vaccine research, production, and distribution, the U.S. Congress directed the National Academy of Sciences (NAS) to assign the Committee for Innovative Vaccine Research, Production, and Distribution to research the issue and make recommendations for a flu vaccine plan. The committee is developing a report to address the following four areas:

1. Understand market and nonmarket forces that contributed to the previous shortage

2. Develop a plan for the future of vaccine research

3. Ensure the health of all Americans

4. Develop a long-term plan for fair distribution of flu vaccine

You have been invited by the Committee for Innovative Vaccine Research, Production, and Distribution to a panel presentation on the issue of flu vaccines in America. Your preparation includes the following tasks:

1. Visit the website of the NAS and become familiar with its history, mission, units, and committees. Browse a few of their reports to understand the NAS.

2. Choose a character from the list that follows, or develop your own relevant persona.

3. Research the topic and develop your position on the issue. You may choose to speak to one or more of the committee goals.

4. Write a three-page policy brief or position paper presenting your research (the group should send the briefs to their classmates at least 4 days before class).

5. Make a brief presentation to the NAS committee during the class exercise.

6. Answer questions from the NAS committee (i.e., your classmates).

Characters

Association of Public Health Officials (APHO)

Association of Retired Folks (ARF)

Libertarian Organization (LO)

Organization for Free Vaccinations (OFV)

People for a Free Market (PFM)

Scientists for Advanced Technology (SAT)

A university professor

Class Assignment

Other class members are the NAS committee. They should visit the NAS website and become familiar with its history, mission, units, committees, and reports. They will act as members of the committee, listen to the presentations from the panel guests, and ask follow-up questions of the panelists.

APPENDIX A

Influenza Facts and Figures

- Influenza causes roughly 36,000 deaths and 200,000 hospitalizations annually in the United States.

- Nearly 90 million Americans are at high risk of contracting the flu.

- The estimated annual costs of the flu to the U.S. economy are $11–$18 billion.

- As of 2004–2005, two companies, Aventis and Chiron, produced all flu vaccines for the United States and delivered the vaccine in October and November.

- In 2003–2004, the United States had 80 million doses of flu vaccine. (Unfortunately, they were not effective for that year's flu strain.)

- In 2000–2001, delivery of the flu vaccine was delayed until December because of a production problem.

- Health officials have warned about the fragile vaccine situation in the United States for decades.[21]

- "The flu vaccine marketplace has been withering for years."[22]

APPENDIX B

Flu Vaccine Time Line (2004)

Aug. 26, 2004	Bush administration announces first national plan for how the United States can prepare for, and respond to, an influenza pandemic. Tommy Thompson, Secretary of Health and Human Services, states, "A pandemic virus will likely be unaffected by currently available flu vaccines."
Aug. 27, 2004	Chiron announces contamination of 48 million doses of flu vaccine (nearly half the U.S. supply). Chiron is based in California, but manufactures the vaccine in Liverpool, England. About 90% of the vaccines produced by Chiron go to the United States. The U.S. government and Chiron both contend that the flu vaccine problem would be resolved by October or November, when Americans receive flu vaccinations.
Oct. 5, 2004	United Kingdom suspends Chiron's license, which is a surprise to the federal government. "We had no idea," said Secretary Thompson. Dr. Schaffner of the National Vaccine Advisory Committee states, "we have been reassured on a regular basis" that the contamination at Chiron was not going to be a major problem.
Oct. 7, 2004	Centers for Disease Control and Prevention (CDC) recommends rationing flu vaccine to high-risk patients only.
Oct. 8, 2004	CDC says someone will investigate reports of flu vaccine price gouging, but does not specify who. Associated Press reports charges were brought against a Kansas distributor who tried to sell flu vaccine with 1,000% markup.
Oct. 12, 2004	The House Government Reform Committee opens investigation of Food and Drug Administration (FDA) response to August reports of contamination problems at Chiron. CDC and FDA may have known about Chiron's license suspension and shortage as early as Sept. 13th.
Oct. 13, 2004	620 flu vaccine doses are stolen in Colorado.
	Federal government begins to distribute flu vaccine and divert doses to high-risk areas.
Oct. 15, 2004	District of Columbia denies flu shots to non-high-risk people.
Oct. 17, 2004	FDA confirms no flu vaccines from Chiron can be salvaged.
Oct. 18, 2004	Secretary Thompson announces Aventis will have 2.6 million more doses of flu vaccine in January 2005.
	United States begins negotiating with Canada to get 1.5 million doses.

Oct. 19, 2004	Hospitals start sharing flu vaccine supplies. Federal task force, Flu Action Task Force, will manage vaccine supply, coordinate effort, and prevent price gouging.
Oct. 20, 2004	Canadian doctors begin asking for Canadian ID before giving flu vaccine. Canadians argue Bush administration is hypocritical for asking for flu doses, but not allowing Canadian pharmaceuticals into the United States.
Oct. 22, 2004	Secretary Thompson says, "we are prepared," and claims Bush administration increased spending on flu vaccine from $39 million in 2001 to a proposed $283 million for 2002. Thompson argues the United States has a "healthy" supply of flu vaccine, and 61 million doses will be available to the 90 million high-risk Americans.
Oct. 22, 2004	3.2 million flu vaccine doses are sent to high-risk groups.
	Many Americans go to Canada for flu vaccination.
	United States looks to Europe for flu vaccines.
Oct. 28, 2004	CDC creates panel on ethics of flu vaccine distribution.
	Feds divert 300,000 flu vaccine doses from federal employees and military to high-risk civilian populations.
	United States identifies 5 million flu vaccine doses at Canadian and German plants, but awaits FDA approval, which should come in December.
Oct. 30, 2004	Vancouver, British Columbia, Canada, offers special flu vaccination clinic for Americans at $40 per dose.
Nov. 1, 2004	World Health Organization plans a November 11 summit of flu vaccine producers and nations.

Flu Vaccine Time Line (2005)

Aug. 12, 2005	ID Biomedical Corporation's influenza vaccine (Fluviral) receives Food and Drug Administration (FDA) approval for fast track designation. Fast track designation, a result of the FDA Modernization Act of 1997, facilitates and expedites review of new drugs to treat serious or life-threatening diseases and addresses unmet medical needs.
Oct. 6, 2005	Senators Clinton (D-NY) and Roberts (R-KS) introduce legislation to ensure an adequate flu vaccine supply. "Despite three shortages of seasonal flu vaccine since 2000, we still do not have the flu vaccine production and distribution infrastructure we need to ensure a stable supply and demand for seasonal flu vaccine, raising serious concerns about our ability to respond to a flu pandemic or an outbreak of avian flu," states Senator Clinton.
Oct. 11, 2005	Indiana State Medical Association administers its private stock of flu vaccine to high-risk children. The Indiana State Department of Health uses funds from the federal program Vaccines for Children to stockpile doses for uninsured and underinsured children.

REFERENCES

1. Centers for Disease Control and Prevention. (2013, October 23). Adult Immunization. Retrieved from http://www.cdc.gov/workplacehealthpromotion/implementation/topics/immunization.html.
2. Department of Health and Human Services. (2004). Interim influenza vaccination recommendation—2004–05 influenza season. Atlanta, GA: Centers for Disease Control and Prevention.
3. Government Accountability Office. (2004). Infectious disease preparedness: Federal challenges in responding to influenza outbreaks. Washington, DC: United States Government Accountability Office.
4. Cohen, J. (2002, March 15). U.S. vaccine supply falls seriously short. *Science*, 1998–2001.
5. Government Accountability Office. (2001). Flu vaccine: Supply problems heighten need to ensure access for high-risk people. Washington, DC: United States Government Accountability Office.
6. Brown, D. (2004, October 17). How U.S. got down to two makers of flu vaccine. *The Washington Post*, A01.
7. Bindley, K. (2013, January 16). Why there are flu vaccine shortages. *Huffington Post*. Retrieved from http://www.huffingtonpost.com/2013/01/16/flu-vaccine-shortage_n_2482257.html.
8. Institute of Medicine. 2003. Financing vaccines in the 21st century: Assuring access and availability. Washington, DC: The National Academies Press.
9. Brown, D. (2004, November 18). U.S. knew last year of flu vaccine plant's woes. *The Washington Post*, A01.
10. Pollack, A. (2004c, October 29). Vaccines are good business for drug makers. *The New York Times*, C1.
11. Pollack, A. (2004b, October 6). U.S. will miss half its supply of flu vaccine. *The New York Times*, A1.
12. Altman, L. K. (2004b, October 8). U.S. inquiry in price rises for flu shots. *The New York Times*, A23.
13. Associated Press. (2004a, December 13). Flu shot supply grows, but demand withers. Retrieved from http://www.foxnews.com/story/2004/12/13/flu-shot-supply-grows-but-demand-withers.html.
14. Belluck, P. (2004, October 14). A headache and a fever: Long lines for flu shots. *The New York Times*, A1.
15. Levine, S. (2004b, October 15). D.C. plans flu shot crackdown: Only high-risk people get doses under emergency order. *The Washington Post*, 02.
16. Levine, S. (2004a, November 21). A painstaking parceling: Communities agonize over flu vaccine distribution. *The Washington Post*, 01.
17. Harris, G. (2004b, October 28). U.S. Creates Ethics Panel on Priority for Flu Shots. *New York Times*, A18. Retrieved from http://www.nytimes.com/2004/10/28/health/us-creates-ethics-panel-on-priority-for-flu-shots.html.
18. Connolly, C. (2004b, December 8). U.S. to buy German flu vaccine. *The Washington Post*, A02.
19. Connolly, C. (2004a, November 10). N.Y. mayor has plans to import flu shots. *The Washington Post*, A03.
20. Associated Press. (2004b, November 24). Flu vaccine smugglers thwarted. Retrieved from http://www.washingtonpost.com/wp-dyn/articles/A8584-2004Nov23.html.
21. Cowley, G. (2004, November 18). The flu shot fiasco. *Newsweek*. Retrieved from http://www.newsweek.com/flu-shot-fiasco-129367.
22. Simon, H. A., Thompson, V. A., & Smithburg, D. W. (1950). *Public Administration.* New Brunswick, NJ: Transaction Publishers.

3

Merck's Crixivan

Kimberly A. Rucker
Healthcare Consultant, Washington, D.C.

Kurt Darr
The George Washington University, Washington, D.C.

Nora G. Albert
Children's National Health System, Washington, D.C.

INTRODUCTION

Resource allocation, scarcity, pricing, and stakeholder involvement are recurring issues in healthcare. The treatment for HIV discussed in this case is no longer groundbreaking; the lessons remain salient. A current example is Gilead's hepatitis C drug, Sovaldi, that costs $1,000 per pill, or more than $84,000 per patient in a course of treatment. Demand for Sovaldi is high, but its cost causes access problems for many patients. How should a costly, scarce resource be allocated? Does Gilead have a responsibility to increase access to Sovaldi? Merck's Crixivan offers insight into such issues.

ORGANIZATIONAL BACKGROUND

Merck & Co., Inc., is a research-driven pharmaceutical products and services company headquartered in Kenilworth, New Jersey. In 2001, Merck was organized into four major product groups whose goals are to improve human and animal health:

Research: Discovery and development of human and animal health products conducted at eight major research centers in the United States, Europe, and Japan.

Manufacturing: Chemical processing, drug formulation, and packaging operations occurred at 31 plants in the United States, Europe, Central and South America, the Far East, and the Pacific Rim.

Product marketing: Products were sold in the United States, Europe, Central and South America, the Middle East, the Far East, and the Pacific Rim.

Services marketing: The Merck-Medco Managed Care Division managed pharmacy benefits for more than 65 million Americans, encouraged appropriate use of medicines, and provided disease-management programs.

In 2001, Merck's mission statement was:[1]

> The mission of Merck is to provide society with superior products and services—innovations and solutions that improve the quality of life and satisfy customer needs—to provide employees with meaningful work and advancement opportunities and investors with a superior rate of return.

Merck embraced the following values:

- Preservation and improvement of human life

- Commitment to the highest standards of ethics and integrity

- Dedication to the highest level of scientific excellence and commitment of their research to improving human and animal health and the quality of life

- Expectation of profits, but only from work that satisfies customer needs and benefits humanity

- Recognition that the ability to excel—to most competitively meet society's and customers' needs—depends on the integrity, knowledge, imagination, skill, diversity, and teamwork of employees, and we value these qualities most highly

George W. Merck, the company's founder, stated in 1950: "We try never to forget that medicine is for the people. It is not for the profits. The profits follow, and if we have remembered that, they have never failed to appear."[2] In 2015, Merck booked $4.442 billion in net income on sales of $39,498 billion.[3]

THE SITUATION

The History

Merck & Co., had spent years and several hundred million dollars to develop an acquired-immunodeficiency syndrome (AIDS) drug called Crixivan, a promising treatment for HIV infection in adults when anti-retroviral therapy is needed. "It's the largest research and manufacturing project we've ever undertaken," said Raymond Gilmartin, Merck's chairman and chief executive.[4] AIDS was first diagnosed in 1981 in the United States among homosexual men. HIV, the virus that causes AIDS, was identified in 1984.[5] AIDS is a late-stage result of HIV. Individuals with AIDS have severely compromised immune systems that can no longer defend against opportunistic infections and cancers.[6] Deterioration of the immune system causes most deaths associated with AIDS.[7]

Merck began searching for an antiretroviral therapy in 1986. Several years elapsed before it discovered indinavir sulfate, the active ingredient in Crixivan. During those years, Merck experienced several setbacks, none as devastating as the death of Irving Segal, Merck's leading scientific investigator on the project, who died in the bombing of Pan Am flight 103 over Lockerbie, Scotland, in 1988. Despite Segal's death, the project continued, and indinavir sulfate was discovered in 1992. By 1995, Crixivan's clinical trials had progressed to Phase III. Completing Phase III clinical trials is the last step required by the Food and Drug Administration (FDA) before requesting approval for a drug's release for public distribution. In January 1996, Merck's Emilio Emini presented initial data from Phase III studies on protocol 035 at the Third Conference on Retroviruses and Opportunistic Infections. Protocol 035 showed Crixivan alone caused HIV levels to drop to undetectable levels in four of nine (44%) patients after six months of treatment. When Crixivan was combined with AZT and 3TC (two previously developed, but less effective, anti-HIV drugs), the percentage of patients with undetectable blood HIV levels was even more dramatic. Patients receiving the triple-combination therapy resulted in undetectable virus levels in 86% of the cases (six of seven patients), nearly doubling the effectiveness of the drug. These results marked the first instance in which an AIDS drug was shown to decrease the presence of HIV so it became undetectable. Never before had such promising AIDS treatment data been presented; the drug was a breakthrough. Proof of Crixivan's efficacy was an enormous relief to Merck's management.

Two months before obtaining approval to begin Phase III trials, and before knowing if the drug would be successful, Merck's management team took a significant financial risk by beginning expansion of two facilities that would be dedicated to producing Crixivan. Management was elated with the drug's success in Phase III clinical trials. The company could now distribute Crixivan under the FDA's accelerated approval process. The approval came only 42 days after Merck submitted the FDA application—the fastest approval in FDA history. After approval, Merck was eager to begin selling Crixivan, and the company was sure the public would respond positively to a drug that could extend many lives.

The Competition

AZT and 3TC were the antiviral predecessors to Crixivan and the group of anti-HIV drugs that emerged in the mid-1990s. AZT in combination with 3TC was effective, however, the class of drugs known as protease inhibitors—which includes Crixivan—is much more potent. When Merck obtained FDA approval for Crixivan, it was one of three protease inhibitors approved by the FDA available to the public. Merck's competitors, Abbott Laboratories and Roche Holding, LTD, produced the other two drugs, Invirase and Norvir, respectively. All three drugs interrupt the life cycle of the HIV virus. Crixivan had an advantage over the other two drugs because Crixivan was more potent than Invirase and had fewer severe side effects than Norvir.

Because FDA's approval to distribute Crixivan came six months earlier than expected, Merck was months from being able to manufacture the drug at levels to satisfy anticipated demand. Yet, the competitive pressure was mounting. Invirase and Norvir were already on the market. Crixivan's clear advantages in potency and decreased side effects would be insufficient to gain a substantial share of the market if the competing drugs had a significant lead time in availability and use. Merck determined it was essential to market Crixivan as soon as possible and committed itself to doing so. The limited production capability for Crixivan would be difficult to overcome, however.

AIDS Epidemic: The Number of Patients Benefiting from Crixivan

According to the United Nations and World Health Organization, there were more than 3 million new HIV infections in 1996, bringing the total number of people living with HIV/AIDS worldwide to 23 million.[8] It was estimated that from the start of the epidemic until 1996, 1.0 to 1.5 million cumulative HIV infections had occurred in North America. At the time, HIV infection was a major cause of death in persons 25 to 44. It was the leading cause of death in the U.S. among men in this age group. In 1994, HIV infection was the third leading cause of death among 25- to 44-year-old women in the U.S.; an additional estimated 12,000 children were living with the virus. The characteristics of those infected with HIV were changing. In North America, AIDS from heterosexual contact was an increasing proportion of newly diagnosed cases. In 1996, the Centers for Disease Control and Prevention estimated more than 1 million Americans were HIV-positive.[9] Most could benefit from Crixivan.

The large number of persons requiring treatment for AIDS would create high demand for Crixivan when it was learned the drug could substantially extend life without the high dosage and adverse side effects of the other two drugs on the market. High demand for Crixivan would pose numerous problems for Merck. The difficulties resulted from limited production capacity and the medically disastrous consequences if Crixivan patients could not continue treatment because of limited supply.

Production Capacity

A complex molecular structure made Crixivan difficult to mass-produce. Most Merck pharmaceuticals were manufactured in four steps over 2 weeks. Crixivan required a 6-week, 15-step process. Seventy-seven pounds of 30 raw materials produced just 2.2 pounds of the drug, enough for one patient for 1 year.[10] The huge quantities of Crixivan needed to meet patient demand made matters worse. Patients are required to take six 400-milligram pills a day, in combination with other AIDS drugs, to achieve the desired reduction of HIV in the blood. These factors meant the supply of Crixivan would be very limited temporarily. Initially, Merck could only produce enough Crixivan to treat 25,000 to 30,000 patients. Yet, its efficaciousness meant thousands more would likely demand access to Crixivan.

Due to the lack of capacity, Merck could have outsourced manufacture of Crixivan. Earlier, however, Merck had decided to use its own plants in order to control quality. Previously, Merck had outsourced production for less complicated drugs and was displeased with the quality. The company feared the same outcome if it used an external supplier for its most complex production activity to date.

FDA's Conditions

Due to the drug's limited availability, the FDA made approval of Crixivan contingent on Merck's ability to monitor how Crixivan was made available to AIDS patients. This requirement was necessary because of the serious consequences of patients discontinuing the drug or taking fewer than the standard daily dose of 2.4 grams. "If therapy is discontinued, the virus will likely re-emerge, perhaps in a form resistant to the drug. . . . Then the drug will be useless to the patient. . . . Worse, that raises the risk that a drug-resistant strain could cross over into the general population," said a researcher at the Aaron Diamond AIDS Research Center in New York.[11]

Selection of the Distributor: Stadtlanders Pharmacy

Merck executives agonized over the decision of how to distribute Crixivan. One option was to delay distribution until the plants reached full production. However, pressure from AIDS activists to provide the drug as soon as possible, and the competitive pressures from Abbott and Roche Holding, precluded that option.

Nor could Merck consider a broader distribution system because that might lead to disruption of patients' drug regimens. Instead, Merck decided to use a single distributor to control the number of patients who started the drug and guarantee refills for them. Merck representative Michael Watts explained the reasoning behind the distribution strategy: "We selected to go through a single distributor on a temporary basis because the drug is so difficult to make. With a limited supply to work with, Merck needed to make sure that people who began the therapy had a sufficient supply." Watts added, "Going through one distributor is not just a matter of tracking who's on it . . . but [in addition], we can track the amount of drug we have."[12] Merck made the decision to use a single distributor to monitor the number of patients on the drug in the most efficient, effective, and controlled manner.

To quell concerns about the serious consequences of interrupted drug treatment, Merck assured the FDA it would monitor supply and ensure an adequate amount of the drug was available to treat patients who started a Crixivan regimen. To guarantee adequate supply for those starting Crixivan, most prescriptions were to be channeled through a mail-order seller named Stadtlanders. Stadtlanders Pharmacy (acquired by CVS in 2000[13]) provided mail-order pharmaceuticals for customers with special needs. This included patients with HIV and AIDS, organ transplants, or those undergoing fertility treatments who needed assistance to comply with drug regimens. Stadtlanders's services included customer monitoring and counseling and working with insurance plans and assistance programs to help customers with paperwork and billing.[14]

Based on Stadtlanders's specialized services in providing drugs to high-risk patients and the tailored services the pharmacy could provide to patients with AIDS, it was decided that Merck's limited production volume would be monitored primarily through Stadtlanders. In effect, Stadtlanders would have a temporary monopoly.

In spring 1996, Merck spokesperson Jan Weiner explained that limited distribution was a temporary measure: "We intend to use Stadtlanders as a primary distribution outlet until we have adequate supplies. . . . We believe we will have adequate supplies in the fall."[15] Also, some Crixivan would be sold to the Department of Veterans Affairs hospitals and managed care organizations that Merck determined would track and control the patients taking the drug. Those wanting Crixivan had to register with

Stadtlanders, or belong to one of the few VA hospitals or managed care organizations with distribution rights. At full production, Crixivan would be available through retail pharmacies, wholesalers, and other sources.

Pricing Crixivan

When Crixivan was released, pharmaceutical prices were being hotly debated. The Working Group on Pharmaceuticals and National Health Care Reform, an independent committee of academics, advocates, and policy makers, had advocated government controls on pharmaceutical pricing. The group acknowledged research and development costs could not be ignored, but that the entire pharmaceutical industry was too profit-oriented when lives were at stake. The *Fortune 500* listed the pharmaceutical industry as the country's most profitable sector from 1988 to 1994.[16] Merck had a net income of more than $3 billion in 1995, up 11% from the previous year.[17]

Analysts predicted annual sales of Crixivan could be a half billion dollars or more in a few years, but Merck's initial pricing was far lower than expected. Crixivan cost 24% less than Invirase and was 33% below Norvir. A Merck spokesperson said the price was set to be "competitive, to facilitate access, and to assure usage of the product."[18] Jules Levin, who directed the National AIDS Treatment Advocacy Project in New York, praised Merck for its pricing, saying, "Merck has done a very humane thing with the price it's charging."[19]

Stadtlanders added a 37% mark-up to the retail price of the drug. Stadtlanders paid Merck $365 for a patient's 1-month supply of Crixivan that had a list price of $501.88. Stadtlanders stated its actual profit was closer to 14% because most customers received discounts under various health plans. Stadtlanders claimed the profit from Crixivan would be much less because of the need to hire 400 additional employees to monitor its distribution. Nonetheless, AIDS activists were angered because non–health plan patients were required to pay full retail price. Merck's lawyers determined that negotiating a price with Stadtlanders, or pressuring it to lower prices, would be vertical price fixing because the producer and distributor involved in the sale negotiated its price. This is a *per se* violation of Section 1 of the Sherman Antitrust act, which deems every "contract, combination in the form of trust or otherwise, or conspiracy, in restraint of trade or commerce . . . illegal."[20]

Uncompensated Care Provisions

Merck's philosophy is that its business mission is to enhance health. Merck has stated an essential component of its corporate responsibility is to support charitable organizations that address critical health challenges.[21]

In keeping with this philosophy, Merck developed a program called SUPPORT™ that specifically assisted patients who needed Crixivan. The program provided free Crixivan to those unable to pay if certain conditions pertaining to third-party payers were met. Merck realized many patients had difficulty identifying and securing drug coverage and wanted to help them find resources to pay for Crixivan. Using a toll-free number, physicians and their patients could obtain assistance. SUPPORT™ assisted insured patients to obtain maximum reimbursement for Crixivan and assisted uninsured patients to locate and obtain insurance. Program counselors provided the following services:

- Answered questions regarding insurers' policies, regardless of whether someone had private insurance, was part of an HMO, or had insurance through public programs, such as Medicaid or AIDS Drug Assistance Programs (ADAPs)

- Assisted patients to identify and apply for insurance coverage for Crixivan

- Assisted physicians, patients, and patients' families with the application process for patient assistance

- Arranged for eligible patients to have Crixivan sent to the prescribing physician's office

- Assisted physicians with billing, claims form completion, and coding for Crixivan

- Worked with physicians or patients to resolve issues related to payment, reimbursement, or claims denials for Crixivan

For patients without insurance, the program could provide Crixivan at no cost when it was medically indicated and certain conditions were met, such as having an income of less than $20,000 per year. In addition, Merck planned to offer Crixivan free to those who had participated in most Phase II studies and one Phase III study.

There were, however, limitations to SUPPORT™. Merck's policy stated that if a state ADAP or private insurance company did not cover Crixivan, Merck would block all patients in that state's ADAP or insurance program from entering its patient assistance program, regardless of financial need. Merck predicted that otherwise payers would refuse to pay for Crixivan because Merck would pay for those who could not pay out-of-pocket.

The Public Outcry

Merck believed it had acted in good faith to assist Crixivan users and had developed a fair and comprehensive distribution plan. During the early years of Crixivan's development, Merck had established what it thought was a strong, positive relationship with AIDS activists. A community advisory board was created to keep the AIDS community informed as to the drug's development and, after receiving increasing pressure from the AIDS activist community, Merck created a compassionate use program to provide Crixivan to dying patients. In addition, Merck had cooperated with AIDS activists when they accused Merck of developing Crixivan too slowly. Merck responded by allowing an independent drug-manufacturing consultant to evaluate Merck's production efforts. The consultant reported to AIDS activists that Merck was doing all it could to make the drug ready for public consumption. Despite best efforts, Merck received a great deal of bad press.

Distribution and Pricing

Once Merck's plan to distribute Crixivan primarily through Stadtlanders became public, AIDS activists called for public protests against Merck and Stadtlanders. A spokesperson for a prominent AIDS activist group said that it made the restricted distribution of Crixivan a "target issue" in its meetings with legislators and with the Federal Trade Commission. The group sought to have a provision added to an FDA reform bill that required FDA-approved drugs to be available to all licensed pharmacies in the United States.[22] The group demanded review of Crixivan distribution and an investigation into why the FDA approved it and how Crixivan's approval was obtained so quickly.

The National Alliance for the Restoration of Democracy (NARD) called the decision to use a single distributor "anticompetitive," "ill-conceived," "ludicrous," and "cynical and preposterous." NARD's president asked Merck to dismantle the program and to immediately open the distribution of Crixivan to all community pharmacies that wished to dispense it.[23] NARD's president argued that if Merck wanted accountability, it could set out clinical guidelines as was done for other drugs that required limited distribution. Merck responded there was a critical difference between the two situations; in earlier cases of limited supply continuous treatment was not as crucial.

Furthermore, AIDS activists and pharmacists accused Stadtlanders of using its virtual monopoly to price-gouge AIDS patients. Kate Krauss, the former spokesperson for the AIDS activist group ACT UP Golden Gate, commented, "We want to send a message to Merck, Hoffmann La Roche, and Abbott that price gouging is unacceptable. . . . Boycotting Stadtlanders, which survives because of the goodwill of the AIDS community, would be easy for us to do."[24] The group accused Stadtlanders of imposing a 37% mark-up on the drug when the average profit on drugs sold in pharmacies is 15%. Moreover, local pharmacies felt that Stadtlanders had an unfair advantage because it had a mailing list of HIV-infected patients that it could use for direct marketing. As noted, Stadtlanders acknowledged Crixivan was marked up 37%, but added most patients would not pay full price because they had discounts under various health plans. In addition, Stadtlanders was incurring monitoring costs.

To a lesser extent, Merck was criticized for its decision to deny entry into its indigent-patient program if a person's insurance plan or state ADAP program would not pay for Crixivan. Opponents said it was unfair to block entry into the program on this basis regardless of a person's financial need. Many believed this policy prevented the vulnerable HIV-positive population from obtaining a drug that could extend their lives. Patients were caught between Merck and healthcare payer organizations that were disputing who should pay for treatment.

The accusation that the limited distribution system violated antitrust law seemed unfair to both Merck and Stadtlanders. Some AIDS activists agreed. Martin Delaney, founding director of the AIDS activist group, Project Inform, defended Merck: "People should understand that the reason they [Merck] did it this way was a patient-oriented one: to guarantee that no patient would be cut off. Everyone agrees there had to be some tracking method. I don't know if this was the only way to do it or not."[25] Merck received similar support from other AIDS activists who said the company was trying to be responsible.

Pharmacist/Patient Relationship

Merck was also accused of insensitivity to how much AIDS patients relied on local pharmacists to counsel them about their medications and to provide allowances for patients with financial problems. The editor and publisher of the *Journal of the International Association of Physicians in AIDS Care* stated that AIDS patients "rely on their pharmacists as much as they rely on their doctors. Merck wasn't sensitive to this at all."[26] Critics did not believe a single, mail-order pharmacy across the country could provide the same support neighborhood pharmacies provided. Merck considered that view untrue.

As to the accusation that Merck was not sensitive to the needs of AIDS patients for a relationship with their local pharmacists, none of the critics mentioned that Stadtlanders was unique in providing specialized support to customers. Although a mail-order pharmacy, Stadtlanders supported the needs of HIV/AIDS patients through clinical counseling and assistance with financial issues. Stadtlanders's mission was to be a partner in successful management of high-risk disease. AIDS activists felt, too, that not enough information was provided to the public about Crixivan and its dosage. This accusation was frustrating to Merck because its publications department had written the literature about Crixivan, but the documents were delayed by the FDA approval process. The literature gave instructions on accessing and using the drug.

Retail Pharmacy Industry

Retail pharmacists were fearful that pharmaceutical companies that grant exclusive distribution rights to one pharmacy could start a trend that threatens them. Pharmacists were particularly wary of pharmacies that obtain exclusive rights to AIDS drugs because the profit from an HIV-inhibiting drug is substantially greater than from most common drugs. In response to the limited distribution of Crixivan, pharmacy trade groups initiated a letter-writing campaign to federal regulators and lobbied Congress to prohibit pharmaceutical companies from restricting drug distribution. Lobbyists argued that exclusive distributorship agreements are unlawful if they decrease competition and do not include procompetitive justifications.

NEXT STEPS

Merck's mission and vision statements at the time seemed to prohibit the actions of which the company was accused. Its philosophy included:

- Merck's mission is to provide innovations and solutions that improve lives and satisfy customer needs.

- Merck is committed to the highest standards of ethics and integrity. "In discharging our responsibilities, we do not take professional or ethical shortcuts. Our interactions with all segments of society must reflect the high standards we profess."

- Merck has an expectation to make profits, but only from work that satisfies customer needs and benefits humanity.

Merck management and directors were nonplussed about the public outcry over a temporary measure that was necessary only until Merck could produce sufficient supplies of Crixivan to meet demand. The chair called an emergency meeting of the board to determine how to handle the situation.

ASSIGNMENT

The chair asked Merck's CEO to brief the board of directors by:

1. Summarizing the facts of the present situation, especially the public relations debacle

2. Recommending next steps in releasing Crixivan, with special attention to minimizing negative public relations for Merck.

In addition, the chair asked the CEO to prepare the following:

1. Identify and analyze likely public policy changes resulting from the Crixivan controversy, and how the changes will affect release of new drugs.

2. Propose changes (if any) in the decision process to be used when Merck releases new drugs that will be in short supply.

To assist in responding to the board chair, the CEO deems it prudent to gather information and opinion from those affected by Merck's decisions regarding Crixivan. The CEO assembles a focus group including:

*   Patient with HIV-AIDS who could benefit from Crixivan

*   Representative from an HIV-AIDS patient advocacy group

*   Representative from a patient safety organization

*   Representative from the trade association for community pharmacies

*   Member of the public randomly selected from a local civic association

ENDNOTES

1. Merck's corporate website. (2001, September 1). http://www.merck.com /about/mission.html
2. Merck's corporate website. Code of conduct. Retrieved March 25, 2016, from https://www.merck.com/about/code_of_conduct.pdf
3. Merck's Annual Report on Form 10K. Retrieved March 25, 2016, from http://phx.corporate-ir.net/External.File?item=UGFyZW50SUQ9MzI1Nz kwfENoaWxkSUQ9LTF8VHlwZT0z&t=1&cb=635923586331680523
4. MacPherson, K., and Silverman, E.R. (1996, February 27). Business makers chase profits in quest for AIDS drug. *The Plain Dealer*, 4C.
5. amfAR. Thirty years of HIV/AIDS: Snapshots of an epidemic. Retrieved March 30, 2016, from http://www.amfar.org/thirty-years-of-hiv/aids-snapshots-of-an-epidemic/
6. AIDS.gov. What is HIV/AIDS? Retrieved March 30, 2016, from https:// www.aids.gov/hiv-aids-basics/hiv-aids-101/what-is-hiv-aids/
7. AIDS.gov. Opportunistic infections. Retrieved March 30, 2016, from https:// www.aids.gov/hiv-aids-basics/staying-healthy-with-hiv-aids/potential -related-health-problems/opportunistic-infections/
8. Altman, L. (1996, November 28). U.N. Reports 3 million new H.I.V. cases worldwide for '96. *The New York Times*. Retrieved April 11, 2016, from http://www.nytimes.com/1996/11/28/world/un-reports-3-million-new-hiv -cases-worldwide-for-96.html

9. Womack, A. (1996, April 11). AIDS activists may boycott pharmacy over sale of Merck product. *Dow Jones News Service.*
10. Tanouye, E. (1997, November 5). Medicine: Success of AIDS drug has Merck fighting to keep up the pace. Online posting. The Pulitzer Board. Retrieved March 28, 2016, from http://archive.pulitzer.org/archives/6001
11. Tanouye, E., and Waldholz, M. (1996, May 7). Pharmaceuticals: Merck's marketing of an AIDS drug draws fire. *The Wall Street Journal,* B1.
12. Gottschalk, K. (1996). Protease inhibitors—the cost of AIDS drugs. *Consumer News,* 1.5. Retrieved September 1, 2001, from http:// cidronline .com/cnews/healthcare/9605.html
13. Company News; CVS to pay $124 million for pharmacy unit. *The New York Times,* July 6, 2000. Retrieved April 18, 2016, from http://www .nytimes.com/2000/07/06/business/company-news-cvs-to-pay-124-million -for-pharmacy-unit.html
14. Stadtlanders Pharmacy profile. The industry standard. Retrieved September 21, 2001, from http://www.thestandard.com/companies /dossier/0,1922,264504,00.html
15. AIDS Activists/Merck-2-: Stadtlanders main distributor. *Dow Jones News Service,* April 11, 1996.
16. Ibid.
17. Ibid.
18. Waldholz, M. (1996, March 15). Merck's newly approved AIDS drug is priced 30% below rival medicine. *The Wall Street Journal,* B5.
19. *Ibid*
20. Greenberg, W. (1998). *The Health Care Marketplace* NewYork: Springer-Verlag, 103.
21. Merck's corporate web site. Retrieved March 28, 2016, from https://www .merckresponsibility.com/our-givingcommunity/priorities-guidelines/
22. Breu, J. (1996). AIDS drug distribution eases—by a crack. *Drug Topics,* 140.9, 30.
23. Breu, J. R. (1996). Ph.s steamed over AIDS drug's limited distribution. *Drug Topics,* 140.8, 32.
24. AIDS Activists/Merck-2-: Stadtlanders main distributor. *Dow Jones News Service,* April 11, 1996.
25. AIDS Activists/Merck -4-: HMOs could negotiate lower cost. *Dow Jones News Service,* April 11, 1996.
26. Tanouye, et al., B1.

BIBLIOGRAPHY

AIDS Activists/Merck-4-: HMOs could negotiate lower cost. *Dow Jones News Service,* April 11, 1996.

AIDS Activists/Merck-2-: Stadtlanders main distributor. *Dow Jones News Service,* April 11, 1996.

A Program of Reimbursement Support and Patient Assistance Services. Retrieved September 1, 2001, from http://www.crixivan.com/indinavir_sulfate/crixivan /consumer/patient_ resources/support.jsp

Barnett, A. A. (1996). Protease inhibitors fly through FDA. *The Lancet, 347,* 678.

Breu, J. (1996). AIDS drug distribution eases—by a crack. *Drug Topics, 140*(9), 30.

Breu, J. (1996). R.Ph.s steamed over AIDS drug's limited distribution. *Drug Topics,140*(8), 32.

Gottschalk, K. (1996). Protease inhibitors—the cost of AIDS drugs. *Consumer News, 1*(5). Retrieved September 1, 2001, from http://cidronline.com/cnews_/healthcare/9605.html

James, J. S. (1996, April 5). Indinavir (Crixivan®) access and distribution. *AIDS Treat News 244,3.*

MacPherson, K., and Silverman, E.R. (1996, February 27). Business makers chase profits in quest for AIDS drug. *The Plain Dealer*, p. 4C.

Tanouye, E. (1997, November 5). Medicine: Success of AIDS drug has Merck fighting to keep up the pace. Retrieved from http://archive.pulitzer.org/archives/6001

Tanouye, E. and Waldholz, M. (1996, May 7). Pharmaceuticals: Merck's marketing of an AIDS drug draws fire. *The Wall Street Journal*, p. B1.

Walker, J. (2015, April 8). Gilead's $1000 pill is hard for states to swallow. *The Wall Street Journal.* Retrieved March 31, 2016, from http://www.wsj.com/articles/gileads-1-000-hep-c-pill-is-hard-for-states-to-swallow-1428525426

Womack, A. (1996, April 11). AIDS activists may boycott pharmacy over sale of Merck product. *Dow Jones News Service.*

4

Pineridge Quality Alliance

A Case Study in Clinical Integration and Population Health

Tracy J. Farnsworth
Idaho State University, Pocatello, ID

CASE HISTORY/BACKGROUND

Pineridge Quality Alliance is a study in clinical integration, accountable care organizations, and population health. The case study profiles the history, challenges, and opportunities related to development of a clinically integrated network and the sponsoring organization's quest to become an accountable care organization and engage in population health.

In June, 2012, Brent Priday arrived in Pocatello, Idaho, as the newly appointed CEO of the 187-bed Pineridge Medical Center (Pineridge), which had been established in 2002 following the consolidation of Pocatello's two regional hospitals. Priday had served previously as CEO of West Valley Medical Center in Harrisburg, Oregon, where his 120-bed hospital participated in a "coordinated care organization"[1]—a new state-sponsored healthcare delivery model that seeks to lower costs and improve quality for Oregon Medicaid patients. Priday is convinced that coordinated care organizations and their variants are the wave of the future, and that Pineridge had to get onboard.

Priday believes that passage of the Patient Protection and Affordable Care Act in 2010 (U.S. Department of Health and Human Services, 2016) is a catalyst for disruptive forces that are transforming the traditional healthcare business model, including reimbursement reductions, provider recapitalization and reconfiguration, and new payment models moving from a Curve 1 (volume-based) to Curve 2 (value-based) paradigm (Butts & Gursahaney, 2014).

Though the pace of change will vary by market, Priday believes the shift from Curve 1 to Curve 2 will happen irrespective of an organization's readiness. The question looming for Priday and the Pineridge board is Which of three common approaches should Pineridge take?

- *Wait and see:* Maximize fee-for-service opportunities until the market requires a shift or creates sufficient financial upside to do so.

- *Be an early adopter:* Create first-mover advantage by creating an accountable care organization/clinically integrated network to offset the impact of reduced reimbursement and utilization by increasing market share of covered lives and keeping more of the services delivered to those living within our network.

- *Hedge our bets:* Experiment with pay-for-performance contracts and manage our health system's employee populations until more drastic change is warranted (Butts & Gursahaney, 2014).

Since passage of the Affordable Care Act, over 750 accountable care organizations have been formed nationwide.[2] In advancing the concept of accountable care and the merits of clinical integration, Priday explained to Pineridge Medical Center's board of trustees that accountable care organizations are basically groups of doctors, hospitals, and other healthcare providers who organize voluntarily to give coordinated, high-quality care to Medicare and other patients. Coordinated care helps ensure that patients, especially the chronically ill, get the right care, in the right place, at the right time, with the goal of avoiding unnecessary duplication of services and preventing medical errors. Priday noted that when an accountable care organization succeeds in both delivering high-quality care and spending healthcare dollars more wisely, it will share the savings it achieves for the Medicare program (Center for Medicare and Medicaid Services: Accountable Care Organizations, 2016).

Priday knows his organization is not ready to form an accountable care organization per se and participate in accountable care organization programs with the Centers for Medicare & Medicaid Services. Nevertheless, he understands the different kinds and types of accountable care organizations and is preparing his organization for eventual participation. A sample of accountable care organization programs sponsored by the Centers for Medicare & Medicaid Services is outlined in Table 4.1.

Table 4.1. Centers for Medicare & Medicaid Services–sponsored accountable care organization types

Medicare ACO type	Launched	Description
Medicare Shared Savings Program (MSSP)	2012	Initial ACO model established by the Patient Protection and Affordable Care Act.
Pioneer ACO Model	2012	Designed specifically for organizations with experience offering coordinated, patient-centered care, and operating in ACO-like arrangements. More advanced and more flexible than MSSP.
Advance Payment ACO Model	2013	Provides advance, up-front payment to ACOs in MSSP model. Designed to provide support to organizations whose ability to achieve the three-part aim would be improved with additional access to capital, including rural and physician-owned organizations.
ACO Investment Model	2015	An ACO model of pre-paid shared savings that builds on the experience with the Advance Payment Model.
Next Generation ACO Model	2015	For HCOs experienced with ACOs—designed to assume more risk and reward.
Comprehensive End-Stage Renal Disease (ESRD)	2016	First disease-specific ACO model designed by CMS for Medicare beneficiaries with ESRD.

Source: Centers for Medicare & Medicaid Services (2016).

CLINICAL INTEGRATION: A PREREQUISITE TO ACCOUNTABLE CARE

From his experience in Oregon, Priday understands that development of a clinically integrated network is an essential precursor to establishment of an accountable care organization in southeast Idaho. Within days of his arrival at Pineridge, Priday advocated the merits of clinical integration and a Pineridge-sponsored clinically integrated network. With assistance from trusted advisers he developed a white paper on clinical integration that he shared with interested parties and potential stakeholders. The three-part paper addressed the questions: What is clinical integration? Who should clinically integrate? and Why should you clinically integrate? (See Appendix A.)

THE PINERIDGE QUALITY ALLIANCE

Priday and the Pineridge board decided that "being an early adopter" and "hedging our bets" were prudent choices. Ultimately, the Pineridge

Quality Alliance (PQA)—a clinically integrated network—was established in August 2013. PQA has the following mission:

> To be an innovative healthcare team dedicated to utilizing the medical resources of the community to bring higher quality medical care, enhanced medical value, improved medical outcomes, reduced medical costs, and increased collaboration between the men, women, and children of southeastern Idaho and their medical providers. (Adopted by the PQA Board, December 19, 2013)

Concurrent with its launch in late summer 2013, initial physician contracts were extended to clinicians initially in Bannock and Bingham counties (PQA's primary service area) with the goal of extending an invitation to hospitals and clinicians in seven adjacent counties over the next 12–36 months (Appendix B). PQA contract addressed the following key provisions: the need for transparency; joint contracting with insurance plans; compliance with PQA initiatives—including adherence to clinical benchmarks, participation in PQA-sponsored training programs, and adoption of efficient and high-quality clinical practices; and agreements to track and share quality performance measures and other data.

LEADERSHIP AND STRUCTURE

In the months leading up to and immediately following initiation of the PQA, the alliance was led by an external consultant. In September 2014, Karlyn Norton was hired as PQA's first full-time executive director. In August 2015, PQA hired Dr. David Bryan as its first full-time medical director. Bryan noted, "Pineridge Quality Alliance is the first and only clinically integrated network in eastern Idaho. It was founded and is operated by physicians in the interest of improving quality and controlling the cost of medical care using robust and accurate data. It is clearly the future of medical care."

Since its inception, PQA has been a physician-led organization, with a 9-person board of directors, 6 of whom are physicians (Table 4.2). In December 2013, the PQA governance structure was formed (Table 4.3).

By mid-2014 the foundational governance and operating structures for PQA were established (Table 4.3 and Figure. 4.1). Norton is especially pleased with the July, 2015, hiring of two full-time "care managers" who coordinate care for patients with high-risk or chronic conditions, or who simply need someone to help them navigate the complicated healthcare system.

Table 4.2. Pineridge Quality Alliance (PQA) board of directors

Member name	Specialty
Brock Bailey, MD (Chair)	Family medicine
Camila Wixom, MD	Cardiology
Donald Davis, MD	Pediatrics
Alexis Gomez, MD	Family medicine
Raymond Marriott, MD	Family medicine
Mia Wesley, MD	Orthopedics
Brent Priday	Pineridge Medical Center Administration (CEO)
Jake Abram	Pineridge Medical Center Administration (CFO)
Luciana Martinez	Pineridge Medical Center Foundation (CEO)

INSURANCE COMPANY/PAYER CONTRACTS INITIATIVES

In January 2014, Blue Cross ConnectedCare[3] became an offering on the Idaho Insurance Exchange.[4] Previously, PQA had formed a partnership with Blue Cross of Idaho to manage patients who reside in southeast Idaho. Concerning its partnership with Blue Cross of Idaho, Norton opined "this is an extremely important venture and, hopefully, the first of many partnerships with payers that allow PQA providers the opportunity to offer their patients a more guided and personalized healthcare experience. By referring patients to the highest quality PQA providers and

Table 4.3. Pineridge Quality Alliance governance structure: board and committee responsibilities

Board of Directors	Overall program oversight and decision-making authority; budget approval; committee participation approval
Network Participation Committee	Provider participation criteria; recruitment and oversight of provider participation agreements
Payer and Finance Committee	Oversight of contract terms, payer opportunities, employee benefit plan, and financial distributions
Quality, Utilization, and Health Information Technology (HIT) Committee	Creation of HIT infrastructure, reporting needs, and implementation plan; development of clinical performance measures for provider disease groups and provider participants; and establishing utilization management targets
Practice Administrators Advisory Council and Operations Committee	Feedback and recommendations on program decisions related to ambulatory and inpatient clinical operations

Note: The Pineridge Quality Alliance board and subcommittees of the board meet bimonthly to quarterly, or as needed.

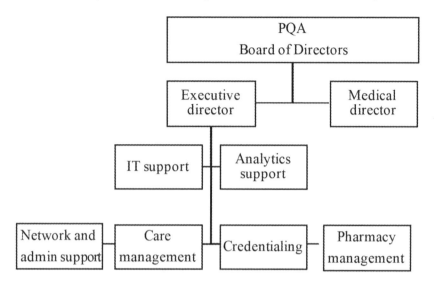

Figure 4.1.   Pineridge Quality Alliance, table of organization.

helping them navigate their services, PQA enables primary care providers the opportunity to more actively participate in their patients' downstream care. Only then will the alliance begin to coordinate care better, reduce unnecessary procedures, and improve overall health status of those they serve."

In July 2016, Norton explained that drastic changes were being made to the Blue Cross ConnectedCare benefit design and fee schedules to further incentivize patients to receive their care within the PQA network. Going forward, the added copay and deductibles to patients who opt out of PQA will be so significant that far fewer services will be sought outside the network. The shift in plan design will reinforce the importance of staying in the network and allowing PQA to manage care more effectively than could be done with traditional preferred provider organization[5] plans. In early 2015 PQA extended its relationship with Blue Cross of Idaho to support True Blue Medicare Advantage[6] members in southeast Idaho, thus enabling PQA to perform population health and care management activities for these more resource-intensive, difficult-to-manage Medicare patients.

In mid-2015 PQA contracted with Regence BlueShield of Idaho on that insurer's Total Cost of Care program[7] in southeast Idaho. Another population managed by PQA was Pineridge employees and their dependents (effective January 2015). This arrangement required an expansion from a physician-only network to one that included providers across the

Table 4.4. Population health contract initiatives

Date	Pineridge Quality Alliance partnership	Summary
Jan. 2014	Blue Cross of Idaho Connected Care	Commercial point of service.[1] Population estimate: 1,200 members
Jan. 2015	PMC Employee Health Plan through UMR[3]	Commercial third party administrator.[2] Population estimate: 2,300 members
Jan. 2015	Blue Cross of Idaho True Blue	Medicare Advantage health maintenance organization. Population estimate: 900 members
July 2015	Regence Blue Shield of Idaho Total Cost of Care	Commercial preferred provider organization. Population estimate: 700 members.

Note: Humana, PacificSource, and Aetna have expressed interest in partnering with Pineridge Quality Alliance.

1. A point-of-service plan (POS) is a type of managed care plan that is a hybrid of health maintenance organization (HMO) and preferred provider organization (PPO) plans. Like an HMO, participants designate an in-network physician to be their primary care provider. But like a PPO, patients may go outside of the provider network for healthcare services.

2. UMR is not a health-insurance provider in its own right but rather a third-party plan administrator. Founded in 1983 as United Medical Resources, UMR provides administrative services for self-funded health-insurance plans.

3. A third-party administrator (TPA) is an organization that processes insurance claims or certain aspects of employee benefit plans for a separate entity.

entire continuum of care, including allied and ancillary professionals/ providers (see Table 4.4), thus allowing the provider network to support the employee health plan's third-party administrator (UMR [United Medical Resources]). Norton said the hospital is interested in using its new clinically integrated network to prove it could deliver better quality care for employees at lower overall cost. A summary of these population health-related contracting initiatives is provided in Table 4.4.

NETWORK DEVELOPMENT AND GROWTH

Two years following inception, PQA included 580 clinicians from 71 provider groups representing not-for-profit, for-profit, public, private, urban, and rural-based domains—all working toward a common goal of clinical transformation and collaboration consistent with the Institute for Healthcare Improvement Triple Aim.[8]

By fall 2016, PQA included representation from over 30 medical and allied health specialties (Table 4.5). The PQA network growth by selected specialties is outlined in Table 4.6.

Table 4.5. Pineridge Quality Alliance network and specialty composition

Anesthesia	Home health	Otorhinolaryngology
Ambulatory surgery center	Hospice	Pediatrics
Behavioral health	Independent lab	Physical/occupational/ speech therapy
Cardiology	Internal medicine	Podiatry
Chiropractic	Nephrology	Psychiatry
Durable medical equipment	Neurology	Psychology
Endocrinology	Obstetrics/gynecology	Pulmonology
Family practice	Ophthalmology	Radiology
Gastroenterology	Optometry	Skilled nursing facility/long-term acute care unit
General surgery	Orthopedics	Urgent care
		Urology

The PQA was relatively successful in recruiting participation from physicians and allied health professionals in Bannock County, but by early 2016 the alliance had been unable to secure contracts with surrounding critical access hospitals and clinicians in southeast Idaho (Appendix B, District 6). Norton explains that these rural, independent hospitals and their local physicians do not feel any urgency to change. She also believes

Table 4.6. Pineridge Quality Alliance network growth by selected specialties

Provider types	2014	2015	2016
Family practice	185	213	240
Internal medicine	12	13	17
Pediatrics	8	9	9
Obstetrics/gynecology	12	12	12
Orthopedics	14	16	16
Cardiology	16	25	25
General surgery	7	7	7
Behavioral health	33	44	45
Chiropractic	1	4	5
Physical/occupational/speech therapy	111	133	135
Home health/hospice	9	16	16
Other	408	492	527

they don't fully understand the purpose and importance of participating in a clinically integrated network. Some balk at paying a 5% tax (5% off the PQA fee schedule) to care for patients they already see independent of PQA–insurance company contracts. Norton notes, however, that some critical access hospitals in the region are showing a more active interest in PQA; she understands that without a broader network of providers PQA will be limited in its ability to fully realize the benefits of a clinically integrated network (see Appendix A: Why should you clinically integrate?).

CLINICAL INTEGRATION TOOLS–PROGRAMS–SERVICES

Not surprisingly, the more than 70 organizations that made up the PQA by early 2014 employed many kinds and types of medical records and practice management systems. To facilitate realization of the benefits of a truly clinically integrated delivery system, in mid-2014 PQA purchased a set of tools known as Crimson from the Advisory Board Company, a consulting firm (Advisory Board Company, 2016). PQA board member Dr. Donald Davis explains that Crimson "will allow us to start collecting data and observing quality measures from all providers in the network. Once we have meaningful data we can decide where there is variation, why outliers exist, and how we can implement strategies to improve our individual and collective outcomes." The three modules that make up Crimson Clinical Advantage are outlined in Table 4.7.

Table 4.7. Crimson Clinical Advantage

Crimson Continuum of Care
Helps hospitals achieve the physician alignment needed to advance quality goals and secure cost savings. Places credible performance profiles in the hands of physicians, enabling them to better meet healthcare organization cost and quality goals.
Crimson Population Risk Management
Helps hospitals manage total cost and quality for defined populations—including self-insured employee plans—and inform risk-based contract negotiations with payers. Combines insight on health system strategy with a robust benchmarking database and clinical algorithms; physicians get a 360-degree view of patient care, including an evaluation of the organization's strengths and liabilities, and more.
Crimson Care Management
Helps hospitals create and run effective, collaborative care management programs by providing intelligent workflows and integrating complex data sources to customize care programs and drive compliance. Generates data that will unlock actionable insights that help care managers work smarter and maximize impact.

Davis explains that one important benefit to a clinically integrated network—with access to powerful data—is that "we start to pay more attention to our patients' overall health, no matter where they receive their care, because we now have visible data. And, because we are now working together as a collective team to provide the highest quality care, we want the entire network of PQA providers to do well, not just ourselves."

Concerning Crimson Care Management, Norton notes that Crimson analyzes data fast enough to provide real-time updates to patient care teams. Crimson generates to-do tasks, alerts, and reminders in response to patient admission, discharge, or care program data. It then routes action requests to the appropriate care team members for prompt intervention, as needed. The Crimson Population Risk Management tool can easily track member, population, and provider progress toward organizational and contractual goals. In elaborating the merits of clinical integration and the need for population health and care management, Norton often uses Figure 4.2 as an example of how the Crimson software categorizes populations into high-risk, rising-risk, and low-risk care categories. Once the population is risk stratified, providers can focus on persons who need the most help. Norton further explains that Crimson software integrates data from patient registries, electronic health records, and other practice management systems to improve coordination of care delivery between and among primary and special practices and hospitals.

Since 2014, PQA has implemented the capabilities of Crimson Continuum of Care at each physician site, enabling these providers to

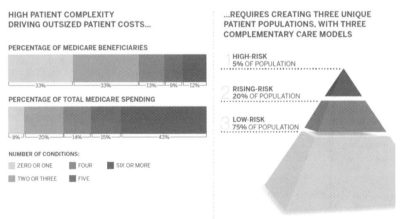

Meet Your Three Patient Populations

HIGH PATIENT COMPLEXITY
DRIVING OUTSIZED PATIENT COSTS...

...REQUIRES CREATING THREE UNIQUE
PATIENT POPULATIONS, WITH THREE
COMPLEMENTARY CARE MODELS

PERCENTAGE OF MEDICARE BENEFICIARIES

33%   33%   13%   9%   12%

HIGH-RISK
5% OF POPULATION

PERCENTAGE OF TOTAL MEDICARE SPENDING

8%   20%   14%   15%   43%

RISING-RISK
20% OF POPULATION

LOW-RISK
75% OF POPULATION

NUMBER OF CONDITIONS:

ZERO OR ONE   FOUR   SIX OR MORE
TWO OR THREE   FIVE

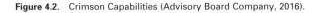

Figure 4.2. Crimson Capabilities (Advisory Board Company, 2016).

track both aggregate and patient-specific clinical and financial data. Additionally, PQA staff provides aggregate and practice-specific reports to practices and selected PQA committees. Provider and patient-specific problems represent opportunities for improvement. Sample reports are provided in Appendix C.

CLINICAL AND OPERATIONAL MEASURES

In conformance with the PQA Participating Provider Agreement, PQA providers agree to actively and meaningfully participate in the alliance's performance improvement and data-sharing initiatives—to share data contained in medical records, billing, claims, practice management, or other systems, electronic, or otherwise. In fall 2014, the PQA Quality, Utilization, and HIT committee, with approval of the PQA board, selected 15 measures to begin tracking and analyzing. Donald Davis, a pediatrician on the board, explains "These are Physician Quality Reporting System[9] and National Quality Forum[10] measurements and represent a great starting point" (Appendix D). In 2015, PQA legal counsel recommended the alliance add 48 more measures: 5–10 per major provider type for a total of 63 measures.

EDUCATION AND TRAINING

In November 2014, PQA leaders announced it would collaborate with Optum[11] to provide a series of educational opportunities focused on the Medicare Advantage Risk Adjusted Program[12] and the Medicare Access and CHIP Reauthorization Act of 2015.[13] Norton reported the following:

> Optum works with healthcare professionals and health plans to help them attain improved health outcomes. With relevant tools and support, Optum can help healthcare providers in the early detection, ongoing assessment, and accurate reporting of chronic conditions. . . . Optum has technology and health intelligence solutions that help providers accurately document and code conditions while improving the overall quality of care. . . . The investment in technology, education, and training is key to PQA's ability to achieve the noted "Triple Aim."

Buck Ridley, PQA's information technology specialist, observed "in the first year (following implementation of the Crimson and Optum initiatives) "we will be able to see, individually and collectively as an alliance, where the opportunities for improvement are. By year 5, we will use the information in a sophisticated manner to improve the overall cost, quality, and utilization of care we deliver."

LOOKING BACK—LOOKING AHEAD

Reminiscing three years following its inception, Pineridge CEO Priday observed, "We wanted to create a purposeful change in the way we deliver patient care that will directly affect the health of our community. At a time in which our industry has been turned on its head and stressed past it limits, we have instituted a transformation that will require even more from us than has already been demanded."

Three years following its launch, PQA has invested roughly $2.5 million in legal and consulting fees, staffing, information technology, and marketing; administrators and clinicians have invested well in excess of 20,000 hours in planning and implementation-related activities. The future includes many methods of expansion, such as broadening existing payer partnerships, working with Humana[14] regarding opportunities for their Medicare Advantage members, partnering with Aetna on their commercial group members, and fostering relationships with larger employer groups in the community to improve quality and reduce costs of care for their employees. Additional quality measures, clinical pathways, and care management programs represent other opportunities for developing improvement.

At the June 2016, PQA board retreat Priday addressed the following challenges common to the industry:

- Succeeding in population health requires more than completing a Medicare Shared Savings Program application and creating a Federal Trade Commission–compliant structure.

- Creating an effective and scalable population health/clinical integration infrastructure requires a significant investment of capital, time, and resources.

- It is extremely difficult to align providers across the care continuum in a way that drives quality and sufficient cost savings to create meaningful shared savings dollars.

- The financial benefits of shared savings programs are directed at primary care physicians and are inherently short term unless they incorporate bundled payments as a means to engage specialists and focus on reducing spending on high-cost procedures.

- Payers are often unwilling to structure mutually beneficial contracts with networks that offer sufficient upside potential to offset losses in fee-for-service revenue because the networks have unproven track records or lack sufficient geographic reach to meet access requirements.

- Not all networks are capable of contracting directly with employers, either due to their insufficient payer capabilities or limited geographic coverage for a broad employee base.

In the context of these industry-wide issues, Norton discussed a handful of challenges specific to PQA:

- PQA has unique challenges compared with clinically integrated networks in other parts of the county due to mountainous topography and rurality.

- We don't have the span of providers and specialties that larger markets have. Thus it's critical for us to align with independent providers in our community to form lasting and collaborative partnerships that will allow our patient populations to access the high-value services they need without leaving the area.

- The geographic, rural, and relatively sparsely populated nature of our provider community means we must strive for excellence in cost and quality—and to have an accurate measure of what the healthcare consumer perceives as "value" because their definition may be quite different from ours. As consumers become more savvy, we must ensure that what we offer meets their expectations.

- Although PQA board members publicly affirm their commitment to the clinically integrated network, getting those leaders and other physician network members fully engaged in using Crimson data to improve their practices is difficult. One prominent board member privately stated, "Honestly, I'm not sure I get it. Crimson is complex and I'm still not using the data to change or improve my practice." Even though the PQA medical director is talented and committed to the cause, he is stretched too thin and unable to meet with network physicians and clinicians to teach, motivate, or monitor their performance.

In frustration, Norton occasionally reaches out to a seasoned and accomplished mentor from across the state. "Look" the mentor said, "your network is new and small, but look at what you have accomplished . . . be patient, learn to fail 'as fast and inexpensively as possible' . . . and just keep moving forward!"

Priday and Norton say their observations/conclusions should not lead PQA to abandon its clinically integrated network and eventual accountable care organization strategy because pressure from employers to reduce premiums and the government's expansion of value-based programs will continue, regardless. Rather, they contend, "If we are going to be paid differently, we must organize and deliver care in a way that leads to different results. Developing our clinically integrated network is a way for us to respond to these changes, overcome the above challenges, and achieve the requisite level of transformation to secure sustainable contracts and successfully navigate the transition from Curve 1 to Curve 2" (Butts & Gursahaney, 2014).

Following vigorous and sometime contentious discussion, the PQA board agreed to the following broadly stated goals for 2017–2019:

1. Increase provider network participation.

2. Design and expand the PQA information technology platform to make data fully accessible and actionable.

3. Develop full transparency and integration of data across the continuum of care.

4. Expand the PQA care management structure.

5. Achieve better management of high-risk patients.

6. Establish clinical practice guidelines and related metrics for headache/migraine and hypertension patients.

7. Connect PQA patients to nonclinical community resources.

8. Improve engagement of patients and caregivers in care planning.

9. Optimize deployment of staff.

10. Establish additional payer contracts based on value and shared savings opportunities, including preparing an application for the Medicare Shared Savings Program.

CASE STUDY QUESTIONS

1. Briefly explain the forces that led Pineridge Medical Center to launch PQA.

2. List and evaluate the structures and tools PQA employs to improve patient quality and increase provider accountability.

3. What evidence shows that PQA follows best practices?

4. Explain why more hospitals in southeast Idaho have not joined PQA.

5. How would you recruit more hospitals and clinicians in southeast Idaho, and how would you market PQA to them and other stakeholders?

6. Develop a timeline showing PQA's key accomplishments.

7. How would you prioritize and operationalize PQA's proposed 2017–2019 goals?

8. You have been assigned by the PQA board to analyze the network's readiness to participate in Centers for Medicare & Medicaid Services–sponsored accountable care organization programs. What criteria can be used to determine its readiness?

APPENDIX A[15]

What Is Clinical Integration?

Clinical integration describes the integration of clinical information and healthcare delivery services from distinct entities. The Institute for Healthcare Improvement has defined the key elements for improving healthcare value through its "Triple Aim": improving the health of the population, reducing per capita costs, and improving the experience of care. In a clinically integrated network, the participating providers share clinical and financial information to encourage improved coordination of care and adherence to evidence-based care protocols. It is also responsive to payers' interest in rewarding outcomes consistent with the Triple Aim. Incentives shift from maximizing the *volume* of services to rewarding better-quality outcomes, improved patient access to services, and more efficient use of healthcare resources. Primary care and specialty physicians, hospitals, and providers, including pharmacists, social workers, post–acute care providers, and other clinicians work together in developing policies and procedures to improve care delivery. Tools are introduced that track providers' clinical performance, outcomes, and utilization of evidence-based care protocols. Care plans are reviewed and compared to care path guidelines to identify opportunities to improve adherence to protocols.

Clinical integration maintains a focus on quality, value, and population health management. Through risk stratification, the most chronically ill, frail, and high-risk patients are targeted and referred to case management or disease management programs in which their condition is monitored. Health information is made available to providers within a clinically integrated network through development of a clinical data repository to ensure collection of all relevant patient data; a robust health information exchange enhances communication among providers, encouraging frequent collaboration with the intent of reducing inadequate handoffs or transitions of care. It does not require all providers to use the same electronic medical record system. As a clinically integrated network continues to develop and grow, continuous evaluation of metrics and performance is necessary to modify clinical protocols or guidelines and foster collaboration among providers.

Who Should Clinically Integrate?

The decision to clinically integrate can be difficult. Clinical integration requires buy-in from senior leaders in the organization, particularly physician leaders, who are championing the necessary care delivery redesign. It also requires significant investment in resources to ensure all providers are aligned, engaged, and educated. Historically, clinical integration has been developed among independent physician practices to enhance the ability of physicians practicing in a variety of practice settings and with various electronic medical record systems to work together to respond to payers' "pay for performance" initiatives to financially reward improved outcomes (quality and cost). Currently, many clinically integrated networks choose to become "accountable care organizations," taking responsibility for the quality and total cost of care for a population of patients. Medicare's Shared Savings Program authorized by the Affordable Care Act is one such example. Some commercial payers and self-insured employers are pursuing similar arrangements with providers. Clinically integrated networks and accountable care organizations must be physician led and are not hospital centric; healthcare providers or entities across the continuum can participate in clinical integration, including medical groups, health plans, pharmacies, retail clinics, skilled nursing facilities, and home health agencies, among many others. So every healthcare delivery entity should consider its role in a clinically integrated network: organizer or participant. This decision becomes the cornerstone of the entity's strategic plan and future role in the healthcare marketplace.

Why Should You Clinically Integrate?

The healthcare delivery system, as we know it, is evolving. Employers as well as the federal and state governments who fund the majority of healthcare expenditures are demanding lower costs and more consistent quality. Measures of patient satisfaction, quality, and clinical outcomes are now tracked and reported; transparency of these reports, as well as pricing, will increase. Evolving reimbursement structures put both physicians and hospitals under pressure to deliver higher-quality care, while reducing unnecessary admissions, tests, and procedures. Sharing information, a fundamental element of clinical integration, reduces waste and focuses providers on improving the health of a population. Organizing providers in clinically integrated networks allows these entities to work with payers to achieve the goals of The Institute for Healthcare Improvement's Triple Aim; separately, it is difficult for providers to either work effectively with payers or achieve these objectives. The fragmented, fee-for-service structure that has historically existed neither encourages care coordination nor rewards high-quality care. Clinical integration affords providers relevancy during the transition of the healthcare environment; it improves the chance for success since it aligns incentives and provides real financial rewards through new relationships with payers. Not to be missed, it also focuses efforts to improve the health of the population and enhances the consumers' experience of interacting with the healthcare system.

APPENDIX B

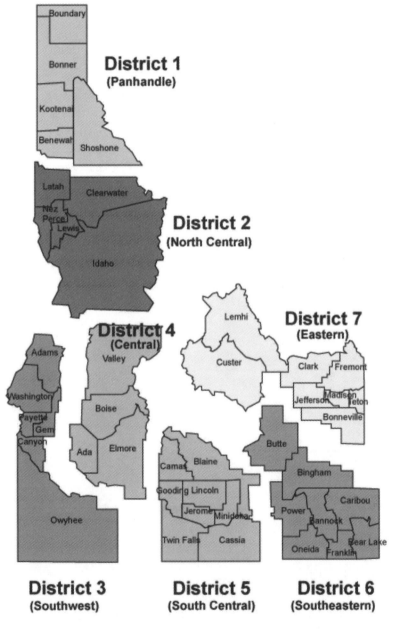

Figure 4.B.1. State of Idaho health planning districts.

APPENDIX C

Sample Crimson Reports

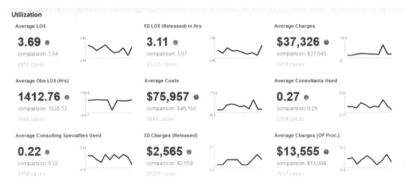

Figure 4.C.1.   Hospital report card (utilization).

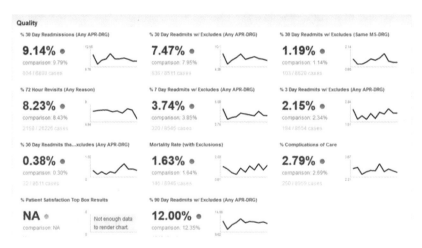

Figure 4.C.2.   Hospital report card (quality).

Overview of Top 100 ED Users

TOTAL COST	AVG COST PER PATIENT	AVG ED COST (TREND)
$4.42M	$44.2K	
	comparison: $29.5K	

$0.00 ——————————————————————————————

JAN 2015   DEC 2015

Top 100 ED Users

PATIENT	ED VISITS ▾	TOTAL VISITS	ED COST	LATEST ED DIAGNOSIS
Patient Name Hidden	75	78	$0.00	Contusion Of Chest Wall
Patient Name Hidden	45	45	$0.00	Chest Pain Nec
Patient Name Hidden	39	39	$0.00	Acute Uri Nos
Patient Name Hidden	36	37	$0.00	Constipation Nos
Patient Name Hidden	34	37	$0.00	Headache
Patient Name Hidden	31	31	$0.00	Foreign Body Hand
Patient Name Hidden	29	31	$0.00	Pain In Limb
Patient Name Hidden	27	27	$0.00	Headache

Average ED Visits

1.00 visits

16.4 visits
comparison: 1.64
indv. outliers: high 75.0 | low 11.0

Average LOS

ED	INPATIENT
2.75 hours	**3.85 days**
100 patients	42.0 of 100 patients

Average Time Between Visits

5.60 days

14.4 days
comparison: 47.4
indv. outliers: high 159 | low 0.00

% of Patients W/O an Office Visit

13.0%

% of Total ED Volumes

VISITS	COSTS
6.24%	**0.00%**
1.64K of 26.2K visits	$0.00 of $0.00

% 72 Hour Revisits

ED	INPATIENT
24.1%	**1.10%**
394 of 1.64K visits	18.0 of 1.64K visits

Figure 4.C.3. Hospital report card (ED users).

Performance Summary

OVERALL PMPM

$**304**
benchmark: $312.34

MEDICAL PMPM
$**244**
benchmark: $275.18

DRUG PMPM
$**60**
benchmark: $37.16

Top Savings Opportunities (Total Potential Savings: $219K)

MEASURE	ACTUAL	TARGET	OPPORTUNITY
Generic Utilization	$1.5M	$1.3M	$172K
Avoidable Admissions	$30.4K	$0	$30.4K
ED	$223K	$206K	$16.9K

Utilization Summary

Admissions per 1K benchmark: 57	57
ED Visits per 1K benchmark: 94	158
Office Visits per 1K benchmark: 3120	2916
Generic Utilization	89%

Top Chronic Diseases

DISEASE	ACTUAL	BENCHMARK	DIFFERENCE
Other mental health/substance abuse	$575K	$208K	$367K
Diabetes without CAD	$622K	$469K	$153K
Dermatologic disorders	$98.2K	$29.9K	$68.2K
Unhealthy newborns and preemies	$280K	$238K	$41.4K
Neurologic disorders	$427K	$397K	$29.4K

Quality Summary

EBM Compliance	65%
30-day Readmission Rate	7%
Avoidable Admissions	1%

Figure 4.C.4.   Population dashboard.

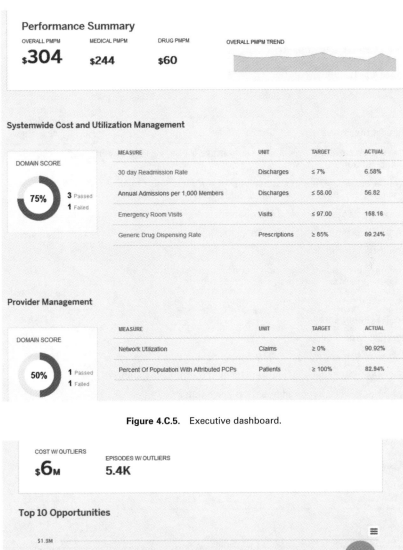

Figure 4.C.5. Executive dashboard.

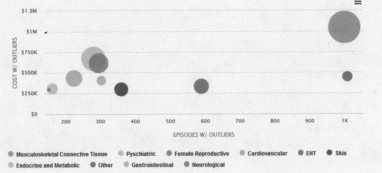

Figure 4.C.6. Episode explorer.

APPENDIX D

Initial PQA Clinical and Operational Measures Reported

Table 4.D.1.   Initial Pineridge Quality Alliance clinical and operational measures reported

Clinical measures	Number of clinicians reporting
Preventive care and screening: body mass index (BMI) screening and follow-up	298
Weight assessment and counseling for nutrition and physical activity for children and adolescents	298
Diabetes: hemoglobin A1c poor control	298
Controlling high blood pressure	320
Childhood immunization status	298
Preventive care and screening: tobacco use: screening and cessation intervention	310
Colorectal cancer screening	320
Breast cancer screening	320
Cervical cancer screening	298
Coronary artery disease (CAD): lipid control	310
Diabetes: low density lipoprotein (LDL-C) control ($<$ 100 mg/dL)	310
Pneumonia vaccination status for older adults	300
Appropriate treatment for children with upper respiratory infection (URI)	298
Heart failure (HF): angiotensin- converting enzyme (ACE) inhibitor or angiotensin receptor blocker (ARB) Therapy for left ventricular systolic dysfunction (LVSD)	310
Perioperative care: timing of prophylactic antibiotic—administering physician	153

ENDNOTES

1. In 2012, the Oregon legislature enacted its plan to transform the Oregon Health Plan system through coordinated care organizations. The Oregon Health Authority defines coordinated care organizations as "networks of all types of healthcare providers who have agreed to work together in their local communities" for Oregon Health Plan (Medicaid) recipients. CareOregon is engaged in building coordinated care organization partnerships with healthcare providers in multiple counties across Oregon.

2. According to a Leavitt Partners report, the number of accountable care organizations was 782 by December 2015, covering 23 million lives.

3. ConnectedCare is a group of managed care health insurance plans that are supported by select provider networks in southwestern and eastern Idaho.

4. The Idaho Health Insurance Exchange, Your Health Idaho is the official Idaho state marketplace for health insurance under the Affordable Care Act.

5. A preferred provider organization is a type of health insurance arrangement that allows plan participants relative freedom to choose the doctors and hospitals they want to visit.

6. True Blue HMO is a Medicare Advantage health maintenance organization plan offered by Blue Cross of Idaho. True Blue HMO provides comprehensive coverage with affordable premiums and predictable costs. The plan offers an all-around approach to good health with healthcare services from local providers.

7. Total cost of care (TCOC) programs are designed to support affordability initiatives, to identify instances of overuse and inefficiency, and to highlight cost-saving opportunities. Many organizations have experimented with TCOC models in recent years.

8. The IHI Triple Aim is a framework developed by the Institute for Healthcare Improvement (IHI) to optimize health system performance. It is IHI's position that new designs must be developed to simultaneously pursue three dimensions—the "Triple Aim": (1) improving the patient experience of care (including quality and satisfaction), (2) improving the health of the population, and (3) reducing the per capita cost of healthcare.

9. The Physician Quality Reporting System (PQRS) is a quality reporting program that encourages individual eligible professionals and group practices to report information on the quality of care to Medicare. PQRS gives participating eligible professionals and group practices the opportunity to assess the quality of care they provide, helping to ensure that patients get the right care at the right time.

10. National Quality Forum (NQF) is the only consensus-based healthcare organization in the nation as defined by the federal Office of Management and Budget. This status allows the federal government to rely on NQF-defined measures or healthcare practices as the best, evidence-based approaches to improving care.

11. Optum is a health services and innovation company dedicated to making the health system work better for everyone.

12. Risk adjustment is the process by which the Centers for Medicare & Medicaid Services reimburses Medicare Advantage Plans, such as Excellus BlueCross BlueShield, based on the health status of their members. Risk adjustment was implemented to pay Medicare Advantage Plans more accurately for the predicted health cost expenditures of members by adjusting payments based on demographics (age and gender), as well as health status.

13. The federal Medicare Access and CHIP Reauthorization Act of 2015 (MACRA)—passed with bipartisan support—is expected to fundamentally change the way the United States evaluates and pays for healthcare.
14. Humana Inc. (Humana), incorporated on July 27, 1964, is a health and well-being company. The company's medical and specialty insurance products allow members to access healthcare services primarily through its networks of healthcare providers. The company's segments include retail, group, healthcare services, and other businesses.
15. This summary on clinical integration is provided by GE Healthcare Camden Group, 2016a–c.

5

Hawaii Health Systems Corporation

The Politics of Public Health Systems Governance

Earl G. Greenia
Colorado State University–Global Campus,
Greenwood Village, CO

CASE HISTORY/BACKGROUND

For nearly two decades, healthcare managers and researchers have witnessed numerous mergers and acquisitions of hospitals and related healthcare providers. Efforts to consolidate the industry generally resulted in new holding companies and corporations, and reduction in power (e.g., relegating local boards to serve in an advisory capacity, or outright elimination of local governing boards). While most healthcare systems were strengthening the powers of corporate boards, efforts were initiated in 2007 to decentralize governance of the Hawaii Health Systems Corporation (HHSC). This case examines legislative mandates between 2007 and 2013 in which the HHSC system changed from centralized governance (single corporate board with strong oversight) to decentralized governance (five community-based regional boards and near-elimination of corporate office oversight).

THE HAWAII HEALTH SYSTEMS CORPORATION

The HHSC is one of the largest public healthcare systems in the country and the largest provider in Hawaii, except for the islands of Oahu and Molokai.

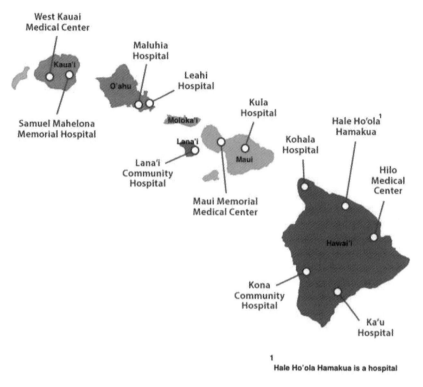

Figure 5.1. Hawaii Health System Corporation Hospitals

In addition, HHSC's facilities are the only provider of acute care services on the islands of Maui and Lanai. Currently, HHSC operates 1,275 beds in facilities[1] on five islands (Figure 5.1). In a typical fiscal year, the HHSC hospitals admit over 20,000 acute-care patients, serve 1,300 long-term care patients, deliver 3,500 babies, and have over 110,000 emergency room visits. Most of HHSC's $650 million annual operating budget is derived from operations. However, it is dependent on state appropriations for approximately 15% of its operating budget (Hawaii Health Systems Corporation, 2016).

INTRODUCTION

When Dr. George Elliott joined the HHSC in 2006, the governance and management structure of this large public hospital system were typical. There was a corporate office and a system CEO. There were five geographically based regional systems, each headed by a CEO; each had a local management advisory committee. The regional CEOs reported to the HHSC system CEO; regional operating and capital budgets were established and controlled by the HHSC system leadership (Figure 5.2—Before Act 182). During his

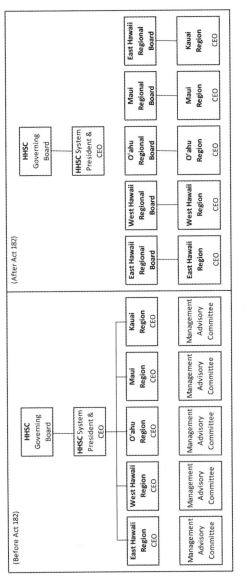

Figure 5.2. HHSC Reporting Structure

tenure, Elliott witnessed the effect of new laws that changed both system and regional governance and management structure: Hawaii Act 290 in 2007, and Hawaii Act 182 in 2009 (Figure 5.2—After Act 182).

In July 2009, Elliott sat at his desk pondering the potential impact of Hawaii Act 182 (2009), which had just been enacted. As one of five regional chief executive officers, he immediately recognized the problem with the shifting role of the corporate office. No longer would he, or his regional CEO peers, be required to gain corporate approval for major capital or human resources decisions. While important decisions could be made locally, the economies of scale of this large hospital system could be lost. For example, the purchase of one type of electronic medical record system for all 13 facilities might come with a significant discount and operational efficiencies. He also pondered the fate of the system president and CEO—a leader whom had become his friend and mentor over the past 3 years.

THE PAST IS PROLOGUE

The evolution of the HHSC predates statehood (1959) when the major economic activities of the "neighbor islands" (a term used to refer to all islands except Oahu) were based on sugar and pineapple plantations. These plantations were self-contained communities with schools, stores, housing, and medical services. While some plantations had small hospitals, care was usually provided through plantation dispensaries (Goodell, 1995). During this period, the public sector was not actively involved in the provision of healthcare services, although several counties built tuberculosis sanitariums. As Hawaii's economy evolved, many plantations reduced production or closed and the health services they provided ended. In response, the counties assumed control and ownership of the private healthcare facilities.

Between 1950 and 1965, cost of care increased to levels that could not be supported by county government. Legislative action began in 1965 (Figure 5.3), which expanded the state's role in providing "safety-net" healthcare services (a term used to refer to facilities that serve those needing medical care, regardless of ability to pay). Such facilities are often the only provider in a geographic area.

In 1965, the county public hospitals became a state responsibility; however, the counties continued to operate the facilities with limited state control. Two years later, the state department of health transitioned management control from the counties to the state (see Figure 5.3). At this time, state government leaders recognized that the increasing cost was becoming a significant financial burden on Hawaii's general fund.

Pre 1959: Major activities of the neighbor islands centered around the sugar and pineapple plantations, which were responsible for providing medical care to their employees

1965: State government assumed financial responsibility for public hospitals; with most operational responsibility retained by counties

1967: State transitioned operational control of public hospitals from the county to the state

1996: Act 262 created the Hawaii Health System Corporation (a special State / public entity)

1998: HHSC internally reorganized into 5 geographic regions (no act noted).

2003: Act 290 returned most governance and management responsibilities from the HHSC board and management to the 5 regions.

2009: Act 182 changed the composition of the HHSC board and allowed regions to adopt different sponsorship (ownership) arrangements.

2011: Act 126 increased state oversight over regional boards.

2013: Act 278 HHSC board restructured; five regional chief executive officers status on corporate board changed to nonvoting

2015: Act 103 provided specific statutory authority for regions to form alternative organizational forms including partnerships or devolved operating responsibilities to a 3rd party

Figure 5.3.   Major legislative acts and their impact

Over the years, numerous studies were conducted; nearly all concluded that operational efficiency and efficacy would only be possible via significant organizational and structural reform.

In 1994, the governor appointed a task force charged with creating a new agency (a public benefit corporation) to reorganize the public hospitals. One significant recommendation of the task force included establishment of five decentralized regional system boards of directors. However, during the 1996 committee hearings, the regional board concept was replaced with regional management advisory committees, which provided community input but had no governance oversight. Following these hearings, the legislature passed Act 262 (1996), which formally created the HHSC (see Figure 5.2).

The law established a 13-member corporate board of directors appointed by the governor, which was responsible for creating the committees, policies, and procedures needed to plan, operate, and manage the hospitals. The purpose of Act 262 (1996) was to free the community hospital system from state regulations; the legislation exempted the HHSC from many laws applied to other government agencies. When Act 262 (1996) passed, there were 12 hospitals—most located in remote, rural, and sparsely populated areas with insufficient resources to meet operating expenses (see Figure 5.1). As a result, it was understood and generally accepted that their operation required state funding support. In 1998 the hospital system was reorganized into five geographic regions (Kauai, Oahu, East Hawaii, West Hawaii, and Maui) in the belief that this would provide each region with shared-services support for the hospitals and thus improve operational efficiencies.

SEEDS OF DISCONTENT AND NEW LEGISLATION

Some regional CEOs felt their authority and budgets were subject to close oversight and control by corporate management and their governing body. For example, year after year, regional requests for additional funding to create new or expand existing service lines were denied. While most understood the denials reflected constrained budgets and a general reluctance of the legislature and governor to increase the state appropriation, some believed there was favoritism in allocating capital. By 2007, the discontent and frustration of some regional management teams reached a boiling point. As a result, some regional CEOs, with support from their local management advisory committees, lobbied the state legislators from their districts to change the governance and management structure.

Senate Bill 1792 was introduced on January 24, 2007. Following numerous public hearings, conference committee meetings, and revisions, the legislature passed Act 290 (Hawaii State Legislature, 2007). The law cited rapid changes in the healthcare industry and noted the need to change the structure of the HHSC to provide the flexibility and autonomy to compete and remain viable while responding to the needs of their communities. The bill became law without Governor Linda Lingle's (R) signature even though she recognized the importance of "improving the access of local communities in decision-making regarding their health" (Lingle, 2007). When implemented, the act would shift numerous governance and management responsibilities from the corporate board and system leadership to the regions.

Prior to passage of Act 290 (2003), the governor appointed 12 of 13 members of the corporate board with little legislative direction. The new law increased the board size to 15, with 10 appointed by the governor. Act 290 removed all sitting members of the corporate board, which resulted in loss of shared experience and knowledge. The act also established five regional governance systems and specified requirements for the size and composition of regional system boards. To provide corporate–regional linkage, the corporation board chair also served ex officio (without vote) on all five regional system boards.

Act 290 (2003) phased in the changes over 18 months. Following establishment of each regional system board, governance, operations, and administration of delivery of services would transition to the regional level. The new law gave regional boards and management the ability to decide which services and functions the corporation would provide and establish means to fund those services and functions. It also gave regional chief executive officers authority to hire employees without corporate approval. Perhaps more significant was the provision to allow the regions to issue revenue bonds to $100 million with corporate board and legislative approval.

The act exempted the corporation and each regional system's operating and capital improvement budgets from review and approval by the governor and state agencies. However, a consolidated budget for the five regions and the corporate office would be submitted to the legislature each year because all HHSC facilities remained dependent on the state to cover operating deficits and pay for high-cost capital projects. In addition, regional systems had to give the legislature notice of any planned reduction or elimination of direct patient care services. Such notifications would result in legislature-sponsored public hearings. Thus the legislature, and to some degree, the governor, retained considerable control.

Elliott and his CEO peers welcomed this change. The law, however, failed to address an expensive and politically sensitive issue faced by HHSC as a quasi-state agency: civil service protections for staff. When HHSC was created, staff became state civil service employees. It was estimated the generous retirement program, health benefits, and paid time-off policies inflated HHSC labor costs by 20% compared to the private sector. Given the state's liberal social policies and powerful position of its two public-service unions, privatizing the HHSC workforce seemed unlikely.

For Elliott, who had spent the last twenty years in private-sector hospitals, the most unusual part of the law was the change in reporting relationships for the five regional chief executive officers and chief financial officers from the system CEO to the regional boards. The regional boards could now hire, fire, and determine compensation for the regional CEO and CFO, subject to review by the regional system board and the corporation board. Elliott was also concerned that corporate office functions, such as human resources, legal services, information management/technology, and contracting, would change drastically as his peers voiced their frustration with these services. Regional CEOs could now create these functions at the regional level. While doing so could reduce the need for retaining these functions at the corporate level the shift in cost would be felt at the regional level. Perhaps more important, Elliott was concerned about his ability to find qualified staff to fill these positions given the shallow pool of applicants in his rural region.

SHAKING IT UP AGAIN

No region requested full control before the 2009 legislative session in January, yet the new structure caused discontent among regional executives and some influential legislators. Many legislators hoped the reduced bureaucracy of the new system would provide greater managerial efficiency and effectiveness and result in cost savings and reduced reliance on the state for deficit funding. Savings did not materialize, however.

On January 28, 2009, Senate bill (SB) 1673 was introduced. Like SB 1792, there were numerous hearings, revisions, and public comment before SB 1673 became law as Act 182 (2009). Although the governor reiterated her support for reforms to strengthen the network of state hospitals, once again she allowed the bill to become law without her signature (Lingle, 2009). Act 182 changed the composition of the board and reduced the size from 15 to 12. The state's director of health (a governor appointee) remained on the board ex officio, without vote. The five regional boards selected six members with two selected from the Maui region. The remaining appointments were made by the five regional CEOs, which created a new dynamic in which a health system CEO reported to a board whose membership included individuals who were once their direct reports. By year's end the long-serving corporate CEO would submit his letter of resignation.

Act 182 (2009) allowed regional systems or individual facilities to transition to new legal entities, including not-for-profit corporations, for-profit corporations, municipal facilities, or public-benefit corporations. Such changes had to be approved by the regional system board. Proceeds from the sale, lease, or transfer of assets had to be used for healthcare services in the respective regional system or facility. Act 182 stated that if a regional system or facility became a new legal entity all liabilities of the former organization were the responsibility of the state (Hawaii State Legislature, 2009). It was thought this incentive would improve the likelihood that a region could be acquired or merge and leave the state system.

Again, the new law (Act 182) did not address the status of HHSC employees. This oversight caused several potential partners to express concern that the state and civil service unions would take the position that employees remained in the state civil service system, thus limiting operational flexibility. Only one public–private joint venture (an ambulatory surgery center) was created after passage of Act 182. Several regions found no partners for a full "take-over" of their hospitals.

TRANSFORMATION WITHOUT END

In 2011, Governor Neil Abercrombie (D) signed Act 126 (2011), a law that changed the size of the corporate board once again. This law restored the voting rights of the state director of health "to increase the input of the [State] administration and further the implementation of public health policies" (Hawaii State Legislature, 2011). To avoid tie votes, the size of the board increased from 12 to 13. The 13th member would be an at-large, voting member appointed by the governor.

In 2013, the size of the corporate board was changed once again by Act 278 (2013). Five members were added to the 13-member board for a total of 18. The five regional chief executive officers would continue to serve as ex officio members, but now without vote. The legislature felt it was "appropriate to shift the voting powers of the five regional chief executive officers on the board to the community members from each of the regional systems" (Hawaii State Legislature, 2013).

Between 2008 and 2013, one region contacted more than 20 companies to explore joint ventures and submitted confidential information to several potential partners describing the operational and financial condition of its physical plant. HHSC regional managers found most potential partners hesitant to evaluate partnership opportunities without enabling legislation addressing structural issues related to such a transaction. Indeed, one potential partner withdrew when enabling legislation was not adopted (Hawaii State Legislature, 2015). In 2015, Act 103 included the necessary provisions. The law authorized the Maui regional system of HHSC, "in collaboration with a private entity, to transition any one or more of its facilities to management and operation [for a fixed term by lease] by a new private nonprofit entity" (Hawaii State Legislature, 2015).

MAKING SENSE OF THE CHANGES

Elliott understood that this legislation allows his peers to do what is best for their local communities, but he feared the largest region (Maui) would find a partner and leave the system. If this were to happen and the regions were unable to find their own partners, the allocation of corporate costs would increase significantly, adding to their financial challenges. Elliott estimated his region's allocation of overhead costs would double. Eager to understand the changes and to offer his regional board and leadership team insights into the potential opportunities of the situation, Elliott considered using elements of the McKinsey 7-S Framework (Waterman, Peters, & Phillips, 1980) and Bolman and Deal's Four Frame Model (Bolman & Deal, 1991) as a starting point for discussions at the board meeting and with his management team. While the future was uncertain, Elliott recognized the importance of considering various scenarios because the board was eager to craft its first strategic plan (Kaplan, 2005).

ASSIGNMENT

Develop a presentation that Dr. George Elliot could use to brief his board and senior executives in understanding the changes that occurred and options for responding to them. In developing your presentation, consider the following questions:

1. How might Elliot use the McKinsey 7-S or Bolman & Deal's Four-Frame model to explore the issues and help his regional board understand the governance and structural changes and their impact on the region and the HHSC system?

2. How might the changes affect the region's management structure and ability to deliver high-quality, cost-effective care to the local community? What are the advantages, disadvantages, and new opportunities?

REFERENCES

Bolman, L., & Deal, T. (1991). Leadership and management effectiveness: A multi-frame, multi-sector analysis. *Human Resource Management, 30*(4), 509–534.

Goodell, L. M. (1995). Plantation medicine in Hawaii 1840 to 1964: A patient's perspective. *Hawaii Medical Journal, 54,* 786–790.

Hawaii Health Systems Corporation. History of HHSC. Retrieved March 1, 2016, from http://www.hhsc.org/about-us/history/11280/content.aspx

Hawaii State Legislature. (2007). Act 290 (SB1792 SD3 HD3 CD2) relating to the Hawaii Health Systems Corporation. Retrieved from http://www.capitol.hawaii .gov/session2007/bills/GM1088_.PDF

Hawaii State Legislature. (2009). Act 182 (SB1673 SD2 HD2 CD1) Relating to the Hawaii health systems corporation. Retrieved from http://www.capitol .hawaii.gov/session2009/bills/GM853_.PDF

Hawaii State Legislature. (2011). Act 126 (SB1300 SD2 HD2) relating to the Hawaii Health Systems Corporation. Retrieved from http://www.capitol.hawaii .gov/session2011/bills/GM1229_.PDF

Hawaii State Legislature. (2013). Act 128 (HB 1130 HD1 SD 1) relating to the Hawaii Health Systems Corporation. Retrieved from http://www.capitol.hawaii .gov/session2013/bills/HB1130_SD1_.HTM

Hawaii State Legislature. (2015). Act 103 (HB1075 SD2) relating to health. Retrieved from http://www.capitol.hawaii.gov/session2015/bills/HB1075 _SD2_PROPOSED_.htm

Kaplan, R. S. (2005). How the balanced scorecard complements the McKinsey 7-S Model. *Strategy & Leadership, 33*(3), 41–46.

Lingle, L. (2007). Letter to Colleen Hanabusa, President, and members of the Senate, Re: Senate Bill No. 1792 SD3 HD3 CD 2, dated July 11, 2007. Retrieved from http://www.capitol.hawaii.gov/session2007/bills/GM1088_.PDF

Lingle, L. (2009). Letter to Colleen Hanabusa, President, and members of the Senate, Re: Senate Bill SB1673 SD2 HD2 CD1, dated July 16, 2009. Retrieved from http://www.capitol.hawaii.gov/session2009/bills/GM853_.PDF

Waterman, R. H., Peters, T. J., & Phillips, J. R. (1980). Structure is not organization. *Business Horizons, 23*(3), 14–26.

ENDNOTE

1. HHSC used the term *facilities* when referring to these hospitals.

PART II

Strategic Management

6

Riviera Medical Center

Michael J. King
Tenet Healthcare Corporation, Dallas, TX

Robert C. Myrtle
University of Southern California, Los Angeles, CA

CASE HISTORY/BACKGROUND

Alex Harrington joined Riviera Medical Center as CEO 18 months ago. Riviera Medical Center is a 350-bed acute care hospital located in Northern California. It is part of a nonprofit chain of hospitals that has had financial challenges over the past several years that have redirected some of Riviera Medical Center's earnings to support capital investment at other locations. As a result, Riviera Medical Center has not had adequate funds available to reinvest in facilities and equipment.

In addition, approximately 5 years ago Riviera Medical Center entered into a contract with the county to provide services to medically indigent adult patients who are the responsibility of the county. The county contract and inadequate reinvestment have damaged Riviera Medical Center's image in the region.

Harrington is aggressively looking for ways to improve the hospital's image in the community without making significant capital investment. He believes the opportunity to partner with employers to help control the cost increases associated with employee health benefits is a way to align more closely with employers and improve the hospital's image with that constituency. He knows that when employers select the health plans for their companies, cost is a central component in their decision making.

During recent months, Harrington has led efforts to develop a workplace wellness program, which he calls Riviera Wellness Services. He is considering whether it is time to present the concept to the Riviera Medical Center board of directors and seek their approval of the new program. His consideration includes one more review of the business plan developed for Riviera Wellness Services and another opportunity to think about how Riviera Medical Center came to develop the plan for Riviera Wellness Services. He settles into his office on a Saturday morning and begins his review, starting with some of the history of Riviera Medical Center.

RIVIERA MEDICAL CENTER HISTORY

Through the 1980s and much of the 1990s, Riviera Medical Center grew to become the hospital of choice and technological leader in its region. It developed itself as a cardiac specialty center, and was the dominant women and children's hospital in the region. The facilities were the best in the area, the equipment was state of the art, the nursing staff was highly trained, and the medical staff was on the cutting edge. The hospital was also financially very successful.

There was only one primary competitor in Riviera Medical Center's region—Northern Valley Medical Center. That competitor had started a strategy focused on developing a foundation model medical group practice as a way to develop a referral base. Northern Valley Medical Center reinvested its hospital earnings into the development of its medical group practice rather than its facilities. In contrast, Riviera Medical Center focused on the independent physicians who were entrepreneurial and were attracted to the high-quality technology leadership offered by Riviera Medical Center.

When Riviera Medical Center negotiated the contract with Riviera County to purchase and close the old County Hospital, the action prevented the county from selling the hospital to another party and increased Riviera Medical Center's census, which used some of its excess capacity. The addition of the uninsured or underinsured population, however, created a risk of changing the hospital's demographics. The administration had determined that the benefits of adding the volume outweighed the risk associated with patient demographics; however, the changes that took place over the next several years proved that management grossly underestimated the impact of the changing patient demographics. The contract with Riviera County remains in place through 2018.

One of the most immediate impacts of the county contract was the growth in emergency department activity. The emergency department was built in the early 1990s for a capacity of around 40,000 visits annually. By 1998, the department added about 15,000 visits and was seeing a total of about 55,000 visits annually. Most of the growth was in uninsured patients or patients covered by the Medicaid program. The emergency department was quickly overloaded, and many insured patients felt uncomfortable around the newly added clientele.

The medical staff was extremely upset with the change, and many doctors looked to shifting some or all of their practices to Northern Valley Medical Center. That hospital had established a strong foundation medical group and was in fact attracting private physicians who had been loyal to Riviera Medical Center, resulting in a shift of insured business to Northern Valley Medical Center. This shift permitted Northern Valley Medical Center to begin a construction campaign to modernize its facilities and expand capacity.

In addition, during the decade of the 1990s, Western Health System aggressively marketed in the Riviera service area and expanded its membership to cover approximately 20% of the population. Western is a fully integrated health system that insures its members and provides physician services and hospital services to its population of enrollees. In 2005, Western commenced construction of a new 200-bed hospital, which opened in late 2008.

Following the county contract, the demographics in the community got worse as far as Riviera Medical Center was concerned, with the uninsured population exceeding 25% by 2007. Riviera Medical Center required significant increases in managed care rates to offset the increased cost of care for uninsured or underinsured patients. Northern Valley Medical Center more aggressively increased rates to finance several hundred million dollars in new facilities, making employers in the region unhappy with the rate of increase in healthcare costs. Much of their dissatisfaction was directed toward the hospitals. The more sophisticated employers, however, saw that the costs associated with Northern Valley Medical Center were higher than with Riviera Medical Center.

Riviera Medical Center lost profitability, and the system it was a part of had other priorities for the funds it was generating. Capital reinvestment ran at approximately 50% of depreciation during the most recent decade. Competing hospitals made significant investments during the same period.

Riviera Medical Center has followed a strategy focused on quality of care and has achieved notably higher quality scores on publicly reported data than competitors in the region. Harrington thought that this was an important advantage for Riviera Medical Center. This accomplishment was recognized by others, as the hospital achieved numerous quality awards, including from the American Heart Association, health plans, and other organizations. Harrington was especially pleased that Riviera Medical Center had received trauma certification as a level II trauma center from the American College of Surgeons. He felt strongly that from a quality standpoint Riviera Medical Center occupied a leadership position. He also told himself that, although quality is important to health plans and employer groups, it is often not well understood or fully appreciated by the general consumer. Harrington concluded that, although Riviera Medical Center does not have the newest hospital, it does have a reputation with employers as being a good alternative for quality and cost.

His thoughts turned to a point of considerable concern. Over the past decade Riviera Medical Center has gone from the premier institution in the region to third in image with patients. Still, in Harrington's view Riviera Medical Center has the opportunity to be identified as the hospital of choice by working with employers. He reminded himself that Riviera Medical Center has plans for building replacement hospital beds to create modern facilities that can compete with the other two hospitals in the immediate area, but turned his thoughts to another potentially important strategic step—the plan he is reviewing to introduce a worksite wellness program to help employers lower their healthcare costs while improving the overall health and well-being of their workforces.

PLANS FOR RIVIERA MEDICAL CENTER'S WORKSITE WELLNESS PROGRAM

Harrington thought about the importance of his vision for the hospital to be a partner with the community, and especially to develop relationships with local employers in the hospital's service area. As a part of this effort, Riviera Medical Center has worked with the California Health Collaborative, an organization representing mostly union health and welfare funds that are primarily self-funded for health insurance. California Health Collaborative's goal is to improve health and lower costs for its members and their employees. With approximately 3 million Californians represented by California Health Collaborative, Harrington had, in his view, wisely sought involvement with the organization.

An important accomplishment from working closely with California Health Collaborative was the development of a model direct contract between the hospital and those employer and payer groups represented by California Health Collaborative. The contract covers inpatient and outpatient services provided by the hospital, and there is an annual pay-for-quality component of the contract. Riviera Medical Center has significantly higher quality scores than other hospitals in the area, which California Health Collaborative members benefit from. California Health Collaborative and their members have recognized that improved quality translates into fewer complications and ultimately lower costs.

Harrington believes Riviera Wellness Services will build on and extend the past accomplishments made possible by working with California Health Collaborative. In his view, Riviera Wellness Services will allow increased direct interaction with employers and employees at their place of business, which is a powerful opportunity for Riviera Medical Center to establish itself as a partner in health for the community.

He concluded that the combination of high-quality healthcare services and a position as a partner for wellness for the community should translate into an improved image in the community and ultimately increased market share. Harrington believes these efforts are part of an overall value proposition that Riviera Medical Center brings to the community.

Harrington mentally reviewed how far his plans for Riviera Wellness Services had come, acknowledging that some aspects of the plans are still under way. Initial plans call for Riviera Wellness Services to send a team of healthcare professionals to an employer's worksite to conduct comprehensive screenings of employees. A personal wellness profile will be prepared for each employee who chooses to participate in the screening process. An aggregate wellness profile will be prepared for the employer to summarize the state of wellness for those employees who participate in the screenings.

The Riviera Wellness Services team will help employees and employers to establish individual and aggregate wellness improvement plans. Employees deemed at high risk of developing a chronic disease will be referred to their physician or to a participating Riviera Medical Center physician. To protect employee privacy rights, individual information will not be available to employers.

Riviera Medical Center's administration shares Harrington's view that the hospital needs to develop and implement strategies to help the hospital be seen as an attractive partner for the employers in Riviera County. They are convinced that Riviera Wellness Services will provide one such strategic advantage in the hospital's service area, especially because it will be the first program of its kind in the region.

As he reviewed the status of Riviera Wellness Services, Harrington's thoughts turned to some of the larger influences in the healthcare industry that have brought Riviera Medical Center to the point of presenting plans for Riviera Wellness Services to the governing board.

THE INDUSTRY

Riviera Medical Center's administration has identified the renewed awareness of healthy living and wellness as an opportunity to work with employers throughout California and to develop programs designed to improve the health of their workforces and reduce their insurance cost through health improvements. There is a significant increased awareness of how healthy behaviors can improve the quality of life through increased energy and reduced health complications.

Harrington remembered that he was especially influenced by release of an important study by the Partnership for Prevention, a nonprofit, nonpartisan organization that develops evidence-based solutions to major national health challenges. The study, Leading by Example, evaluates numerous CEOs' views on the business case for worksite health promotion. The study pointed out that the primary driver of soaring health costs is inadequate investment in health through primary prevention, health risk reduction, and disease management. It further noted, "Some forward-thinking organizations are integrating employee health as a business strategy that enables them to manage costs effectively, while investing in the potential of their human capital." Harrington concluded that this information is highly supportive of plans for Riviera Wellness Services.

THE SERVICE

In reviewing the business plan for Riviera Wellness Services, Harrington recalled that the essence of the service is to provide health assessments for employees with a focus on risks for chronic disease, and to establish programs to help employees minimize the risks associated with such chronic diseases. The initial phase of the program is planned to be a series of medical screenings conducted at various stations staffed by experts in the respective medical or clinical areas involved. Prior to conducting such screenings, the employees will be required to provide blood for laboratory tests that will be reviewed the following day as a part of the screening process. Separate stations will be set up for (1) cardiac care, (2) oncology, (3) orthopedics/bone density (4) exercise and conditioning, (5) nutrition and diet, (6) sleep and respiratory, (7) diabetes, and (8) women's health.

Based on the results of the screenings, a tailored healthy lifestyle program will be established for each employee. Chronic conditions, such as diabetes and obesity, will be addressed through education in group settings, such as weight management and diabetes classes or support groups. For employees who need more in-depth attention, Riviera Medical Center will use its certified diabetes clinic and Cardiac Center of Excellence. These specific resources can be used where appropriate to help prevent further deterioration of the chronic conditions identified in people who are screened. Other areas of concern will be addressed on an individual basis or by referral to a primary care physician.

Riviera Wellness Services' screening results will be accumulated and a health rating determined for each employee at the beginning and the end of the year. The data will be aggregated for the participants in an employer's workforce and an aggregate average score established for its workforce. The employers will be able to present their aggregate data to managed care companies when negotiating annual health insurance rates; measured improvements should lower health insurance costs.

Recognizing that individual health is a highly confidential topic and subject to the privacy provisions of the Health Insurance Portability and Accountability Act, Harrington was satisfied that Riviera Medical Center's plans for individual health information to be maintained anonymously with access available only to those developing and implementing the individually tailored wellness programs as well as the physician overseeing the program were consistent with the Health Insurance Portability and Accountability Act. He had made certain that the intent of the program is to help employees of participating companies improve their health through lifestyle changes, and not to create a health record that is available to their employers.

Riviera Medical Center administrators are convinced that their work-site wellness program will be unique, with tailored health improvement plans for each employee and oversight by a uniquely qualified team of professionals headed by a primary care physician. They also plan for specially trained local primary care physicians to be available for consultation for employees who require special attention. In addition, the measures used to rate employee health are supported by evidence that they are primary indicators of individual health and wellness.

KEY ASPECTS OF RIVIERA WELLNESS SERVICES

Harrington reviewed several of the key aspects of Riviera Wellness Services that he and other Riviera Medical Center administrators had developed during their planning, including the following:

Organizational Mission: Coordinate efforts with employers to improve the wellness of their workforce. This will be accomplished through easily accessible health screenings and development of tailored health improvement plans for individual employees.

Vision Statement: Our vision is to establish the standard for employers and employees to make health improvement and wellness continuous priorities.

Objectives: Objectives of the worksite wellness program are (1) to limit the increase in health insurance cost to 5% or less by year 3 for self- funded employers that participate in the program; and (2) to reduce absenteeism due to illness by 3% during year 2 for employers that participate in the program.

Culture: The desired organizational culture for Riviera Wellness Services includes the following: (1) Riviera Wellness Services' employees will have an enthusiasm for wellness, (2) employees will present an image of a professional and well-coordinated healthcare team, (3) employers will have a service orientation and will go out of their way to make the service convenient and user-friendly, and (4) employees will be active participants in community events and organizations focused on health and wellness.

Entry and Growth Strategy: A team of specialists representing each of the eight focus areas will be available to begin screenings at client sites by January, year 1. The teams will consist of registered nurses and will be aided by a phlebotomist who will assist with blood drawing for laboratory work. As demand for the service grows, the number of teams available for the screenings will be increased. The initial targeted population is the self-funded preferred provider organization employer groups. To the extent that major health reform plans include incentives and possibly funding for wellness improvement among the lower-income populations in California, demand for services should substantially increase, perhaps far in excess of Riviera Medical Center's initial expectations.

Once the program is launched in Riviera County, it can quickly be expanded to surrounding counties. Riviera County has more than 450,000 residents. There are more than 1 million people in the Riviera Medical Center extended service area, which is within 30 miles of the hospital. Growth of the service will be more controlled by the desire to have manageable growth than by maximizing potential growth. In order to be successful in the long term, the service must be delivered with quality. Riviera Medical Center's administration believes that controlled growth of the service is the most certain way to ensure excellence.

Being first to market in the local service area is strategically important. Riviera Medical Center's administrators plan to market to key employers immediately, and strive to bring wellness to the workplace in a more focused way than has previously been experienced in the community.

Once this initiative has been rolled out, it can be duplicated by Riviera Medical Center's competition within a period of about 6 months. By developing the foothold as the hospital bringing wellness to employers and employees, Riviera Medical Center's administrators believe that the hospital will be in a position to have a competitive advantage for delivering the service over the next several years. First to market can erect barriers to entry and may deter other hospitals from offering similar services.

MARKET RESEARCH AND ANALYSIS

Customers

Harrington recalled that initial target clients will be members of the California Health Collaborative. He remains convinced that, because they are determined to reduce health costs and improve quality without degrading benefits, Riviera Wellness Services is a close fit with California Health Collaborative's objectives.

Harrington also recalled that additional potential customers include employers or employer groups with self-funded health insurance plans. These groups typically see the direct correlation between the improved health of their members and lower health costs. Another group of potential customers is the health maintenance organization populations within employer groups. Well-documented health status of a workforce will be a selling point to health maintenance organizations.

Competition and Competitive Edge

Nationally, Comprehensive Health Services and Ceridian Corporation are the two largest players in the area of workforce health assessment and health management programs. Comprehensive Health Services is based in Vienna, Virginia, and Ceridian Corporation is based in Minnesota. Neither organization has an office in California. There are wellness plans developed by many larger employers. However, in Harrington's thinking, there is significant opportunity to provide these services to employers with fewer than 1,000 employees.

There appears to be minimum competition in communities throughout California with populations below 500,000 and for companies between 100 and 1,000 employees. This will give Riviera Wellness Services a competitive edge in those initial target markets.

Estimated Market Share and Sales

In Harrington's view, market share will start on a small scale and grow as the service gains a positive reputation, as evaluation teams are developed, and as marketing and sales efforts take hold. Riviera Medical Center's administrators believe that the initial target, California Health Collaborative, can generate approximately $300,000, $500,000, and $700,000 in revenue for years 1 through 3, respectively. (See Tables 6.1–6.4.)

Table 6.1. Riviera Wellness Services, financial projections

	Year				
	One	Two	Three	Four	Five
Employee screenings	1,500	2,500	3,500	4,500	7,500
Revenue	$ 300,000	500,000	700,000	900,000	1,500,000
Direct screening costs	108,928	176,640	247,296	317,952	529,920
Admin salaries	189,000	194,666	201,483	208,535	215,834
Supplies and forms	34,500	47,864	87,500	112,500	187,500
Sales and marketing	40,000	30,000	25,000	25,000	25,000
Other admin	24,000	24,000	24,000	24,000	24,000
Total costs	396,428	473,170	585,279	687,987	982,254
EBITDA	$ −96,428	26,830	114,721	212,013	517,746
Percent	−32.14%	5.36%	16.39%	23.56%	34.52%

Note: EBITDA, earnings before interest, taxes, depreciation, and amortization.

Table 6.2. Riviera Wellness Services, financial projections (with cash flow)

Year one					Month								Year
	One	Two	Three	Four	Five	Six	Seven	Eight	Nine	Ten	Eleven	Twelve	
Employee screenings	80	80	120	120	120	120	120	120	124	164	164	168	1,500
Revenue	$ 16,000	16,000	24,000	24,000	24,000	24,000	24,000	24,000	24,800	32,800	32,800	33,600	300,000
Direct screening costs 8 RN per diems (40 to 44 screenings/day)	5,888	5,888	8,832	8,832	8,832	8,832	8,832	8,832	8,832	11,776	11,776	11,776	108,928
Admin salaries	15,750	15,750	15,750	15,750	15,750	15,750	15,750	15,750	15,750	15,750	15,750	15,750	189,000
Supplies and forms	1,840	1,840	2,760	2,760	2,760	2,760	2,760	2,760	2,852	3,772	3,772	3,864	34,500
Sales and marketing	4,000	4,000	4,000	4,000	3,000	3,000	3,000	3,000	3,000	3,000	3,000	3,000	40,000
Other admin	2,000	2,000	2,000	2,000	2,000	2,000	2,000	2,000	2,000	2,000	2,000	2,000	24,000
Total costs	29,478	29,478	33,342	33,342	32,342	32,342	32,342	32,342	32,434	36,298	36,298	36,390	396,428
EBITDA	−13,478	−13,478	−9,342	−9,342	−8,342	−8,342	−8,342	−8,342	−7,634	−3,498	−3,498	−2,790	−96,428
Increase in A/R	−16,000												−16,000
Increase in A/P													
Free cash flow	−29,478	−13,478	−9,342	−9,342	−8,342	−8,342	−8,342	−8,342	−7,634	−3,498	−3,498	−2,790	−112,428
Capital expenditures	−40,000												−40,000
Interest													
Debt service													
Net operating cash flow	−69,478	−13,478	−9,342	−9,342	−8,342	−8,342	−8,342	−8,342	−7,634	−3,498	−3,498	−2,790	−152,428
Cash from hospital	100,000		50,000					25,000					175,000
Cash from borrowing													
Cash balance	$ 30,522	17,044	57,702	48,360	40,018	31,676	23,334	39,992	32,358	28,860	25,362	22,572	22,572

Note: A/P, accounts payable; A/R, accounts receivable; EBITDA, earnings before interest, taxes, depreciation, and amortization.

Table 6.3. Riviera Wellness Services, financial projections (with cash flow)

Year two

							Month						
	One	Two	Three	Four	Five	Six	Seven	Eight	Nine	Ten	Eleven	Twelve	Year
Employee screenings	168	168	210	210	210	210	210	210	210	210	242	242	2,500
Revenue	$ 33,600	33,600	42,000	42,000	42,000	42,000	42,000	42,000	42,000	42,000	48,400	48,400	500,000
Direct screening costs	11,776	11,776	14,720	14,720	14,720	14,720	14,720	14,720	14,720	14,720	17,664	17,664	176,640
Admin salaries	16,223	16,223	16,222	16,222	16,222	16,222	16,222	16,222	16,222	16,222	16,222	16,222	194,666
Supplies and forms	3,864	4,000	4,000	4,000	4,000	4,000	4,000	4,000	4,000	4,000	4,000	4,000	47,864
Sales and marketing	2,500	2,500	2,500	2,500	2,500	2,500	2,500	2,500	2,500	2,500	2,500	2,500	30,000
Other admin	2,000	2,000	2,000	2,000	2,000	2,000	2,000	2,000	2,000	2,000	2,000	2,000	24,000
Total costs	36,363	36,499	39,442	39,442	39,442	39,442	39,442	39,442	39,442	39,442	42,386	42,386	473,170
EBITDA	−2,763	−2,899	2,558	2,558	2,558	2,558	2,558	2,558	2,558	2,558	6,014	6,014	26,830
Increase in A/R Increase in A/P			−10,000										−10,000
Free cash flow	−2,763	−2,899	−7,443	2,558	2,558	2,558	2,558	2,558	2,558	2,558	6,014	6,014	16,830
Capital expenditures													
Interest													
Debt service													
Net operating cash flow	−2,763	−2,899	−7,443	2,558	2,558	2,558	2,558	2,558	2,558	2,558	6,014	6,014	16,830
Cash from hospital													
Cash from borrowing													
Cash balance	$ 19,809	16,910	9,467	12,025	14,583	17,141	19,699	22,257	24,815	27,373	33,387	39,401	39,401

Note: A/P, accounts payable; A/R, accounts receivable; EBITDA, earnings before interest, taxes, depreciation, and amortization.

Table 6.4.   Riviera Wellness Services, daily revenue and variable cost detail

	No. of employees per day	Rate per employee	Per day amount	No. of days annually	Actual totals
Revenue	40	$200	$8,000	38	$304,000
Cost	Hours	Rate per hour	Per day amount		
Oncology screen cardiac	8	$46	$368		
Testing diabetes screening	8	$46	$368		
Nutrition evaluation	8	$46	$368		
Weight management	8	$46	$368		
Ortho screening	8	$46	$368		
Sleep and respiratory	8	$46	$368		
Woman's health	8	$46	$368		
Total cost			$2,944	38	$111,872
Contribution margin			$5,056		$192,128
Percentage			63.20%		63.20%

ECONOMICS AND BUSINESS

Harrington quickly reviewed some of the key business variables in the plans for Riviera Wellness Services, including the following:

Gross and Operating Margins: Employee health assessment and wellness program development are the primary initial markets to be pursued by Riviera Wellness Services. Contribution margin percent is expected to be more than 60% from the primary activities. Years 2 through 5 of operations are expected to generate progressively improving earnings before interest, taxes, depreciation, and amortization (EBITDA) margins ranging from 5% to 34%.

Profit Potential and Durability: Riviera Medical Center administrators project achieving EBITDA of $500,000 in year 5, while serving only 1% of the target market. This model will have highly sustainable profits so long as Riviera Wellness Services can demonstrate that the healthcare cost savings its clients are achieving are a result of healthier lifestyles and reduction of chronic diseases.

Fixed and Variable Costs: Variable costs primarily consist of the service delivery teams that provide the screening services to groups of employees. Each service delivery team consists of eight professionals. It is anticipated that this team screens 48 employees during an

8-hour day. The service teams cost $2,900 per day to conduct the screenings. Other variable costs relate to health risk–appraisal packages, which cost $12 per screening, and lab testing, which costs $11 per screening. Fixed costs relate primarily to administrative services and marketing costs.

Months to Breakeven: Riviera Medical Center's administrators project achieving breakeven status by month 16. The service teams will develop slowly and gain productivity as sales efforts start to take hold.

MARKETING PLAN

Harrington's thoughts next turned to marketing Riviera Wellness Services and to some of the critical components of the marketing plan being developed for the service.

Overall Marketing Strategy

Riviera Wellness Services' service is directly tailored to help employees change their lifestyles and achieve health cost savings and incentives for themselves and their employers. The sales and marketing focus will be directed to employers with self-funded health insurance plans. These employers will see immediate and direct savings and should be eager to hear how Riviera Wellness Services can help improve the health of their workforce.

Initial target employers will have between 100 and 1,000 employees and will be identified through coordination with California Health Collaborative or through local chambers of commerce. The program manager will identify key markets and prospective customers.

Pricing

In Harrington's view, there is little competition that is directly comparable to Riviera Wellness Services. The initial pricing is based on a full-day screening of 40 employees per day per team, and a margin of approximately 50% based on direct cost of services. A price of $200 per employee for the screening service achieves the margin objective, allows for support of the administrative functions, and provides for marketing costs. The cost considers the need to involve expensive medical professionals in the screening process. The pricing is expected to be at a level that Riviera Medical Center can ultimately demonstrate a return on investment of at least 500% through the combination of reduced healthcare costs and reduced absenteeism. It is possible the return to employers could be much higher than the initial estimate.

Advertising and Promotion

Riviera Medical Center's administrators plan for advertising and promotion to be designed to support the sales team's efforts. A professionally designed brochure will describe the service to be provided, the employee health scorecard, and the aggregate employee health report. This will also demonstrate anticipated savings in health costs attributable to the improved health of the workforce. As an example, Safeway Stores, a large grocery store chain with $45 billion in revenue and 197,000 employees, has implemented a wellness program to reward healthy choices and activities. The program was estimated to decrease total healthcare costs by 30% over a 2-year period. Results will also be tracked from Riviera Wellness Services' clients and will be used in ongoing sales brochures.

IMPLEMENTATION

In his review of how implementation of Riviera Wellness Services was to unfold, Harrington thought about several aspects of implementation that he and his administrative colleagues had focused on, beginning with the tools they planned to use in implementing Riviera Wellness Services.

Reporting Tools

Riviera Medical Center will purchase the software and services of Wellsource, Inc., to provide reporting to clients. Wellsource, a wellness company, offers software and Internet services that generate individual wellness profiles and aggregate wellness reports. Their Personal Wellness Profile Software will allow the Riviera Wellness Services team to present health risks, target risk groups, track progress, and evaluate cost–benefit performance. The software is a proactive tool to manage the wellness of individuals and groups. It considers lifestyle, health factors, and measurements of health risk, including personal and family medical history, nutrition, stress, and biometrics. Assessment scores and recommendations are based on optimal health factors rather than risk of death.

The Wellsource tools also include a weight and health profile, a coronary risk profile, a diabetes risk profile, and a HealthStyle Index, which is a comprehensive lifestyle and health assessment.

Service Delivery

Riviera Wellness Services will start with a single-service delivery team, which will include a few individuals formally trained in using the Wellsource tools. Once the sales team engages a customer for the screening and health-scoring services, a date or dates will be set for the screening services, and scheduling will be based on customer preference first and availability second. The individual wellness profile is a detailed report of health and wellness and will be made available to each employee who has a screening. Aggregate reports are prepared and presented to clients to identify health risks in their organization. Trend reports can also be prepared over time after follow-up visits to demonstrate progress within the organization.

Intervention plans can be designed to establish one-to-one coaching for those who desire such structured interaction. Also, classroom instruction and self-study can be made available to those who prefer such intervention methods. Interventions can be tailored to the needs and desires of the individual and can also be coordinated with the employer in an effort to help address the needs of the workforce.

Screenings and interventions will be conducted at the employer's worksite whenever possible. If the employer does not have adequate facilities, screenings and interventions can be performed at the hospital. If space is a limiting factor to selling the service, Riviera Medical Center will invest in a mobile unit for future use.

There will also be tools available to help motivate individuals and employees, such as e-mail notices and reminders. There are also wellness challenges that can be issued to help keep target groups focused on their goals.

Tools can also be made available to track health activity. A personal health diary is available for participants to log health, exercise, and nutrition practices. These tools make it easy to track individual and organization progress. Rewards and recognition programs can be introduced to motivate individuals and organizations as they accomplish their goals.

The Wellsource software allows clients to track changes and improvements. Employers should also track trends and savings in productivity, work-loss time, and healthcare expenses.

All of these efforts should help employers to modify their corporate culture to promote a healthy work environment and healthy lifestyles.

Development Plan

A key component of the health assessment is the process for health screening and development of the health report card. The reporting will be a combination of the data from the Wellsource software and some proprietary reporting. The Riviera Wellness Services administration will work with patent and trademark counsel to ensure that proprietary processes and documents are adequately protected. The process for such assessment and patent and trademark filings must be completed before Riviera Wellness Services becomes operational.

The health assessment team qualifications have been identified and Riviera Medical Center's administrators are in the early phases of locating qualified candidates for such positions. It is anticipated that the first screenings will not take place until the first quarter of year 1.

A marketing brochure is a key component of the sales team's effort. The brochure is being developed with the assistance of a professional public relations and marketing firm. This brochure will be available at the beginning of year 1.

Organization

Riviera Wellness Services will be a division of Riviera Medical Center. The clinical staff will be recruited out of the Riviera Medical Center workforce, which currently stands at about 2,000 individuals. A program manager will be hired to oversee all aspects of operations of the program. This individual will likely have a background and training in wellness. Candidates include exercise physiologists with training in nutrition. This individual will also be supported by a program coordinator, a sales manager, and an administrative assistant.

Harrington is comfortable that Riviera Wellness Services will have joint reporting to Debbie Pike, Riviera Medical Center's director of public relations and marketing, and John Morse, chief operating officer. This joint reporting was decided on because of the emphasis on having Riviera Wellness Services benefit the community, which is part of Harrington's larger strategy for the hospital.

HARRINGTON'S CONCLUSIONS AND THOUGHTS

Following his review of the business plan for Riviera Wellness Services and his more general thinking about the environment facing Riviera Medical Center, Alex Harrington concluded that it is indeed time to share plans for Riviera Wellness Services with the board of directors and to ask for their approval of the plan. His rationale includes a conviction, based on the significant planning that has gone into development of Riviera Wellness Services, that this is a service opportunity that will be in strong demand in the current environment. He believes that the fact that there is little immediate competition helps make this an attractive business prospect for Riviera Medical Center. Riviera Wellness Services complements the Riviera Medical Center's hospital strategy and provides value to the community, employers, and their employees. The opportunity to provide a roadmap to improved health to numerous individuals will be widely valued. Along with Riviera Medical Center's leading quality of care, which is publicly reported by numerous sources, the Riviera Wellness Services initiative will help Riviera Medical Center achieve its objective of being the hospital of choice for employers in Riviera County.

Although Harrington feels the proposed program is ready to present to the board of directors, he wonders how the board will react. Specifically, he wonders if they will see the wellness service as merely viable or as a significant strategic advance for the hospital. He also wonders if the business community will be pleased by Riviera Wellness Services's availability.

ENDNOTE

This case is based on actual events. The organization, its location, and the names of people have been disguised.

7

Edgewood Lake Hospital

Leadership in a Rural Healthcare Facility during Challenging Economic Times

Brent C. Pottenger
Johns Hopkins School of Medicine, Baltimore, MD

Douglas Archer
Sutter Memorial Hospital–Los Banos, Tracy, CA

Stephen Cheung
School of Dentistry, University of Michigan,
Ann Arbor, MI

Robert C. Myrtle
University of Southern California, Los Angeles, CA

CASE HISTORY/BACKGROUND

After 8 months of searching nationwide, the Edgewood Lake Hospital's board has just hired a new CEO, Shannon Johnson. She recently served as CFO of Rocky Hills Valley Hospital, a critical access facility in rural northern California. The previous CEO, Richard Fuchs, failed to make Edgewood Lake Hospital profitable and made several missteps by engaging in high-cost capital projects, including an elaborate wellness center that did not deliver expected profits. During the last 8 months, the interim CEO, Jenny Mayview, did little to rectify the situation.

Located in northern California, Edgewood Lake Hospital is a 30-bed, independent, not-for-profit hospital. It provides inpatient and outpatient services for a close-knit, small community in a rural, forested, lakeside setting. Given challenging economic times, both inside and outside the nation's healthcare system, the incoming CEO (Johnson) must provide strong leadership while determining how to make Edgewood Lake Hospital profitable in 2 years (by 2018). Having experienced losses from 2013 to 2016, the board gave Johnson the challenge when hiring her. Finally, while solving the current fiscal situation and developing a plan to ensure fiscal health, Johnson must also address the hospital's glaring physician recruitment problems, particularly in general surgery and primary care. If successful, the board hopes Johnson can stabilize the hospital's executive leadership team and inspire increased staff productivity and performance.

EDGEWOOD LAKE HOSPITAL HISTORY

Despite operating with financial losses since 2013, Edgewood Lake Hospital has established itself as the rural region's leader for quality care. Members of the community hold the hospital in high regard. Special recognition is given its exemplary team of experienced nurses who play active roles in the community and serve as leaders of multiple volunteer and religious organizations. Edgewood Lake Hospital opened in 1945 as the Edgewood Community Hospital, a 30-bed not-for-profit facility. In order to capitalize on the hospital's beautiful lakeside setting, its board renamed the facility Edgewood Lake Hospital in 1985.

In 2010, then CEO Fuchs pursued a strategy of focusing on wellness and prevention instead of treatment and intervention. He initiated an enormous capital campaign to fund a state-of-the-art wellness facility on the hospital's property. When presenting this plan to the hospital's board, Fuchs said the following:

> Healthcare in the 21st century will revolve around keeping people healthy, not reacting to illness and treating disease. With access to a healthy community space that provides nutrition classes, gym memberships, physical activity programs, and other social interactions, the Edgewood County community members will lead longer, healthier, and happier lives. As a healthcare facility, Edgewood Lake Hospital has a responsibility to the community to provide preventive and wellness services to people, while continuing to provide high-quality, traditional medical care.

After receiving board approval for a $1.2 million wellness center, Fuchs raised $120,000 in community donations to help fund the wellness center construction project. With so much community support behind this new venture, he expected the center to serve the community profitably for many years, especially as the population aged, retired, and spent more time (and money) focusing on health maintenance.

In 2013, Fuchs proudly opened the Edgewood Lake Wellness Center at a well-attended ribbon-cutting ceremony. "Edgewood Lake Wellness Center will provide the entire Edgewood County community with a place to be well, feel well, and get well," proclaimed Fuchs during his opening ceremony speech. Two years later, in summer 2015, the board voted to dismiss Fuchs after Edgewood Lake Hospital posted large losses in both 2014 and 2015. Fuchs had mobilized the community behind his wellness idea; however, the wellness center's operation was never profitable. Fuchs also failed to address the hospital's core operational problems of (1) poor financial performance, including extensive losses on Medicare patients; (2) low physician recruitment, especially in general surgery and primary care; and (3) strong community competition from Creekside Trails, a 45-bed, for-profit hospital 35 miles away across Lake Edgewood that opened in 1995 with an emphasis on cardiology care.

CURRENT STATE OF RURAL HOSPITALS

Rural hospitals are often the sole provider of healthcare services for residents in rural communities. However, rural hospitals must overcome the complex public policies that often benefit larger, metropolitan hospitals. They must also surmount the effects of local economies and shortages of health professionals.

The current state of rural hospitals is dismal. Although about 19% of Americans live in rural areas (U.S. Census Bureau, 2015), only about 11% of physicians practice in rural areas (Fordyce, Chen, Doescher, & Hart, 2007). Citizens in rural areas have longer travel times to a hospital and, consequently, have difficulty accessing hospital services. This leads to residents delaying routine visits, which may exacerbate their illnesses.

DEMOGRAPHICS AND POPULATION DATA

Rural residents tend to have lower household incomes than the national average. In Edgewood County, the estimated median household income in 2014 was $44,238 (California Department of Finance, 2014), compared to $53,367 nationally (U.S. Census Bureau, 2015). Residents of rural areas tend to be older. In Edgewood County, the median age is 40.8 years, whereas the national average is 37.6 years (U.S. Census Bureau, 2015). The demographics in Edgewood County reflect other rural areas.

The population of Edgewood County is 6,386. With a larger percentage of older residents, the need for timely, efficient, and comprehensive medical care for chronic conditions is paramount. However, this small county is similar to others across the nation and lacks specialty physicians. As a result, primary care providers must often provide care that is beyond their training, beyond their comfort level, or both. Moreover, rural hospitals may not be able to provide the same level of services. This necessitates referring some patients to other facilities. This increases travel time for patients. To alleviate longer travel times and difficulties accessing care for elderly patients, Edgewood Lake Hospital created the mobile health service unit, a large vehicle that serves residents throughout Edgewood County. Equipped with basic equipment to perform physical assessments and other primary care services, this mobile unit solves the problem of geographic limitations for many of Edgewood Lake Hospital's most needy patients.

NATIONAL HEALTHCARE POLICY

Small size means rural hospitals are affected disproportionately by changes in public policy. For example, Edgewood Lake Hospital is a 30-bed facility. If a new public policy dictates that hospitals increase their fixed nursing ratio, Edgewood Lake Hospital will be challenged to attract qualified providers. Other public policies and accreditation agencies are increasing oversight of quality, privacy, efficiency, costs, and services. These actions affect hospitals nationwide. Larger hospitals, however, can more easily meet new requirements because they have more resources. In addition, hospital systems can affect their environment by lobbying government and leveraging their economies of scale.

GOVERNMENT REIMBURSEMENT

Government reimbursement is declining, while demands for quality and compliance regulations are increasing. This is a challenging combination for management. Hospitals must bill Medicare correctly by having knowledgeable staff, as well as by implementing ongoing training programs and extensive information technology software to facilitate accurate coding and record keeping. Large hospital systems are more likely to have the resources to keep up with increasing quality and compliance demands from Medicare. Small rural hospitals have fewer coders and internal auditors than large hospitals. With the demands on rural hospitals, they may not be able to allocate the resources to maintain compliance with Medicare's standards. The result is more fines and denied claims for rural hospitals. In response to these pressures, many rural facilities have secured the designation critical access hospital to receive higher reimbursement from Medicare. A critical access hospital designation changes hospital reimbursement from diagnosis-related groups to cost-based reimbursement, which provides rural facilities with financial stability. To qualify as a critical access hospital, hospitals must be located at least 35 miles from the nearest hospital, operate fewer than 25 beds, have an average length of stay under 96 hours, and offer emergency services 24 hours a day, 7 days a week. Currently, Edgewood Lake Hospital is not a critical access hospital.

QUALITY

As demand for quality services grows, costs will initially rise as hospitals increase staffing, refine procedures, and create new workflows and introduce best practices. Edgewood Lake Hospital's focus on quality has had an impact. For instance, Edgewood Lake Hospital scored 100% for delivering discharge instructions and 100% for providing smoking cessation counseling for congestive heart failure patients, compared with U.S. averages of 69% and 89%, respectively (VanSuch, Naessens, Stroebel, Huddleston, & Williams, 2006; Williams et al., 2005).

NATIONAL HEALTHCARE OBJECTIVES

There is increasing pressure from Medicare to ensure that hospitals and physicians' offices are connected by electronic medical records. Furthermore, the tenth edition of the World Health Organization's International Statistical Classification of Diseases and Related Health Problems (ICD-10) coding will require new computer programs to process the coding. Rural hospitals will continue to struggle with financing large electronic medical record systems. Given their small size and relative simplicity compared to large hospitals, the benefits of electronic medical records may not outweigh the costs. Small hospitals and single-physician or small group practices will have to invest in ICD-10 coding software and learn new rules and regulations. Many do not have the profit margins to support this investment. In addition, learning new billing requirements will take a heavy toll on staff.

AN ORGANIZATION IN TRANSITION

Shannon Johnson's experience at Rocky Hills Valley Hospital—a 24-bed rural facility like Edgewood Lake Hospital—gave her some perspective regarding the main issues affecting Edgewood Lake Hospital's operations, including (1) the current state of rural hospitals, (2) demographics and population dynamics, (3) implementation of the Affordable Care Act, (4) government reimbursement, and (5) quality care. In addition, she understands that many rural hospitals have survived by joining healthcare systems.

Edgewood Lake Hospital's financial situation is bleak. The last 2 years have resulted in significant losses. Over half of patients in the community are Medicare beneficiaries. Since the Balanced Budget Act of 1997, government-sponsored healthcare programs, such as Medicare, have drastically reduced reimbursement rates (Edgewood Lake Hospital's payer mix is shown in Figure 7.1). In addition to challenges with payer mix, Edgewood Lake Hospital is experiencing a rise in uncompensated care because of the socioeconomic demographics in Edgewood County, which are consistently below average relative to the rest of California.

Staffing inefficiencies have increased operating costs and exacerbated Edgewood Lake Hospital's financial problems. Currently, Edgewood Lake Hospital has nearly 8 full-time equivalents per occupied bed, which is 40% higher than the industry benchmark of 5.2 full-time equivalents. In addition, the new collective bargaining agreement with the Hospital Workers Union Local 189 resulted in higher salaries for the registered nurse job class. Physician staffing has increased costs too. Vacancies on the medical staff have forced the hospital to employ locum tenens physicians, at significant cost. In addition to declining reimbursement, a challenging payer mix, and increasing operating costs, which are relatively uncontrollable elements, poor executive management is the most disappointing contributor to failures at Edgewood Lake Hospital. The 2016 budget in relation to the actual figures for 2016 illustrate this management shortcoming (see Table 7.1). Projected net income for 2015

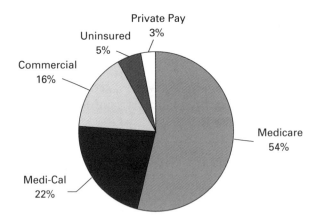

Figure 7.1. Edgewood Lake Hospital payer mix.

Table 7.1. Edgewood Lake Hospital financials

	2014 Actual	2015 Actual	2016 Actual	2016 Budget
Inpatient revenue	$86,968,734.00	$81,401,833.48	$76,694,069.00	$89,822,682.00
Outpatient revenue	$90,024,084.00	$106,483,479.44	$101,733,548.00	$89,889,713.00
Gross patient revenue	$176,992,818.00	$187,885,312.92	$178,427,617.00	$179,712,395.00
Revenue from wellness center	$698,435.00	$841,862.57	$704,532.00	$732,997.00
Revenue deductions	−$109,167,181.00	−$116,818,105.41	−$109,552,632.00	−$107,407,333.00
Charity care	−$3,020,986.00	−$3,104,415.57	−$2,863,373.00	−$1,440,001.00
Other revenue from operations	$1,438,726.00	$1,149,310.67	$1,116,269.00	$1,188,552.00
Net operating revenue	$66,941,812.00	$69,953,965.18	$67,832,413.00	$72,786,610.00
Salary expense	$25,083,781.00	$27,824,871.73	$26,596,301.00	$24,970,955.00
Employee benefits	$8,650,023.00	$9,251,729.66	$6,925,576.00	$10,016,599.00
Physician fees	$3,812,265.00	$5,067,416.09	$5,242,532.00	$3,732,940.00
Professional fees	$2,641,380.00	$2,742,964.13	$2,572,612.00	$2,897,930.00
Supplies	$7,185,118.00	$7,503,717.04	$7,104,929.00	$7,457,775.00
Purchased services	$5,508,030.00	$7,652,252.60	$7,337,465.00	$6,543,781.00
Insurance	$745,358.00	$846,496.13	$798,446.00	$772,193.00
Utilities	$1,287,189.00	$1,682,912.79	$1,403,369.00	$1,345,270.00
Rentals	$359,438.00	$385,136.19	$405,820.00	$352,479.00
Depreciation	$3,510,991.00	$4,004,516.25	$3,906,404.00	$3,648,059.00
Interest expense	$1,260,038.00	$1,675,614.30	$1,515,552.00	$1,439,000.00
Management fee	$3,018,165.00	$3,816,865.51	$3,723,525.00	$3,391,489.00

Continued

Table 7.1. Edgewood Lake Hospital financials *(Continued)*

	2014 Actual	2015 Actual	2016 Actual	2016 Budget
Licenses and taxes	$116,276.00	$208,449.01	$186,340.00	$112,256.00
Bad debt	$2,872,678.00	$3,758,728.68	$4,106,819.00	$3,221,136.00
Other operating expense	$2,148,975.00	$1,645,783.12	$1,551,847.00	$2,113,982.00
Total operating expense	$68,199,705.00	$77,307,853.23	$72,887,542.00	$72,015,844.00
Non-operating income	$388,403.00	$463,309.58	$239,333.00	$369,444.00
Net income	–$869,490.00	–$6,890,578.47	–$4,815,796.00	$1,140,210.00
Pt days (excluding nursery)	9,937.00	7,923.05	7,380.00	10,300.00
IP revenue per patient day	$8,752.01	$10,274.05	$10,392.15	$8,720.65
Average daily census	27.2	20.6	20.16	28.2
Net operating revenue per patient day	$3,275.63	$3,779.23	$3,909.73	$3,496.44
Discharges (excluding nursery)	2,591.00	1,159.00	2,360.00	2,641.00
Net revenue per discharge	$12,562.69	$12,244.18	$12,226.18	$13,636.26
Salaries cost per patient day	$3,275.63	$3,779.23	$3,909.73	$3,496.44
Supplies cost per patient day	$188.51	$277.10	$305.34	$181.14
Length of stay	3.8	3.2	3.13	3.9
FTEs per occupied bed	6.56	7.74	7.8	6.21
Other visits	99,548.00	110,656.84	105,006.00	101,040.00
Surgeries	3,611.00	1,672.00	3,309.00	2,587.00
Emergency room visits	17,849.00	18,850.74	17,597.00	18,328.00

Note: FTEs, full-time equivalents; IP, inpatient.

shows hospital leadership was "asleep at the switch." Instead of a surplus over $1 million, the facility lost nearly $5 million. This is a tremendous discrepancy for a hospital with roughly $70 million in operating revenue. On the positive side, Edgewood Lake Hospital enjoys strong community support and a regional reputation for superior quality. The competitor hospital, Creekside Trails, is an aggressive for-profit hospital known in the community for performing excessive numbers of cardiac procedures. Creekside Trails is newer than Edgewood Lake Hospital (it is 15 years old) and, as a result, its facilities are superior to Edgewood Lake Hospital's. Creekside Trails and Edgewood Lake Hospital are located 35 miles apart at opposite ends of the lake, and they serve distinct patient populations. Because Creekside Trails offers more specialty services, Edgewood Lake Hospital has noticed increased competition for patients in recent years.

For Edgewood Lake Hospital to survive, new sources of revenue must be found. One solution is to recruit additional medical staff members to alleviate locum tenens costs and increase inpatient volumes. Physician recruitment has not been easy. The rural environment is not appealing to most physicians, and the lack of a medical foundation, or large medical group that offers an employment relationship, forces new physicians to bear the financial risk of starting a practice in a sparsely populated area. In California, hospitals are not allowed to employ physicians directly, and, although a hospital can offer an income guarantee for 1–3 years, it is illegal to directly employ a physician. Edgewood Lake Hospital's payer mix also affects physicians and this, combined with the risk of startup, makes recruitment nearly impossible.

Edgewood Lake Hospital has a large, loyal customer base. Outmigration data show the hospital captures 84% of patients who need the services offered by Edgewood Lake Hospital; only 16% of patients seek care elsewhere. Each year, the hospital organizes a health and wellness fair, and the recent addition of the wellness center has enhanced the community image of the facility. The wellness center provides classes in weight management and nutrition, aerobics, and yoga, as well as a workout center. In preparation for designing and opening the new facility, the hospital launched a capital campaign to raise funds for renovating the existing office complex that would be the future site of the wellness center. This campaign resulted in $120,000 in donations, further illustrating local support for and interest in the success of Edgewood Lake Hospital.

The hospital has very low annual employee turnover—6% in 2015—which is important because of the difficulty of recruiting nursing and other skilled personnel. In 2015, the hospital participated in an employee satisfaction survey and achieved scores that placed it in the 96th percentile of similar-sized organizations. Luckily, the facility has a capable middle management team with significant tenure that is responsible for maintaining morale and commitment to patient care despite challenging times and lack of effective executive leadership. However, a tide of uncertainty is rising as the employees and the medical staff attempt to understand how the hospital came to such a dire financial position. The management style of the interim CEO demolished morale, and staff productivity dropped precipitously as a result. The entire community is anxious for new leadership to turn the Edgewood Lake Hospital around.

THE LEADERSHIP CHALLENGE

At Edgewood Lake Hospital's most recent board meeting, the senior management team and board members all agreed that Johnson, the new CEO, is the right fit for the facility and the community. A graduate of a major university and a CPA, Johnson is bright and personable with a strong, diverse financial background. Figure 7.2 is an organization chart of Edgewood Lake Hospital.

In an interview with the local Edgewood County newspaper, *The Edge*, Johnson discussed why she felt ready for this new challenge and step in her career:

> Working in a rural setting taught me so many things about managing the operations of small hospitals. I had my hands in everything from engineering to nursing management to human resources. I look forward to combining my extensive financial background with my improved operational management skills to provide strong leadership at Edgewood Lake Hospital.

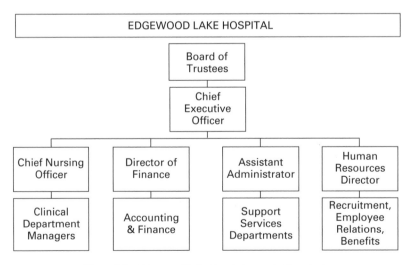

Figure 7.2. Edgewood Lake Hospital organization chart.

After 5 years as CFO at Rocky Hills Valley Hospital, Johnson feels she is prepared to excel as CEO of Edgewood Lake Hospital. However, after interviewing the interim CEO, Jenny Mayview, meeting with board members, and enjoying brief conversations with hospital physicians, nurses, and staff, Johnson is not quite sure how to turn the tide at Edgewood Lake Hospital. What can she do to the address the hospital's bleeding financials and challenging payer mix? Should she reduce the wellness center budget? Should she shut down the wellness center to use the space for more profitable services? If either option were pursued, how would the community react after investing so much money and energy into the wellness center? What can she do to recruit and retain physicians? These questions swirled through Johnson's mind as she ran on a treadmill in the Edgewood Lake Wellness Center after her first day as CEO. When questioned about physician recruitment during a senior management team "huddle" earlier in the day, Johnson said that she had tackled these challenges in her previous position:

> Luckily, at Rocky Hills Valley Hospital, I managed and led our hospital's efforts to recruit physicians in general surgery, as well as in primary care. It takes a special type of doctor to work in a small, rural setting; but, with some years under my belt, I feel confident that I can help improve the recruitment situation here at Edgewood Lake Hospital. But, I do recognize that Edgewood County is a new region for me, so I am actively reflecting, talking to people, and searching for effective ways to build a more sustainable physician staff at our facility.

Clearly, challenges lie ahead for her. Using her hands-on experience, Johnson has tried to transition effectively into her CEO role through collaboration, openness, transparency, and creativity. She wants to find new solutions to old problems. She also wants to understand what her predecessor, Fuchs, did wrong.

DISCUSSION QUESTIONS

1. What should Johnson do?

2. How should Johnson prioritize her action items?

3. What solutions could Johnson use to turn Edgewood Lake Hospital around that previous executives had not tried?

4. How does Johnson not "rock the boat" too much and achieve balance between instituting change and respecting existing relationships and cultural dynamics in the organization?

5. The wellness center has not yet proved to be economically viable even though there appeared to have been community support for it.

Given the hospital's fiscal condition, is this a sustainable activity or are there other options to consider?

6. Finally, the hospital has launched a capital campaign to replace the existing medical offices. Where does this fit into the overall strategy to improve the fiscal health of the hospital and to respond to the challenges presented by its major competitor?

Operating in difficult economic times, Johnson faces a major leadership test; however, with the right decisions, she has the opportunity to make a lasting positive impact on her organization and in the community it serves.

ENDNOTE

This case is based on actual events. The organization, its location, and the names of people have been disguised.

REFERENCES

California Department of Finance. (2014).

Fordyce, M. A., Chen, F. M., Doescher, M. P., & Hart, L. G. (2007). 2005 physician supply and distribution in rural areas of the United States. *Final Report, 116.*

U.S. Census Bureau. (2015). Retrieved from https://www.census.gov/geo/reference/ua/urban-rural-2010.html

VanSuch, M., Naessens, J. M., Stroebel, R. J., Huddleston, J. M., & Williams, A. R. (2006). Effect of discharge instructions on readmission of hospitalised patients with heart failure: Do all of the Joint Commission on Accreditation of Healthcare Organizations heart failure core measures reflect better care? *Quality and Safety in Health Care, 15*(6), 414–417.

Williams, S. C., Morton, D. J., Jay, K. N., Koss, R. G., Loeb, J. M., & Schroeder, S. A. (2005). Smoking cessation counseling in U.S. hospitals: A comparison of high and low performers. *Journal of Clinical Outcomes Management, 12*(7), 345–352.

8

Klamath Care

Targeting and Managing Growth and
Company-Wide Development

Tracy J. Farnsworth
Idaho State University, Pocatello, ID

Leigh W. Cellucci
East Carolina University, Greenville, NC

Carla Wiggins
Weber State University, North Ogden, UT

CASE HISTORY/BACKGROUND

Robert Patterson, Chief Executive Officer of Klamath Care, slouched easily in his chair, his feet comfortably outstretched across his paper strewn desk. It was late Friday afternoon, and he returned to his office having just reviewed the loan applications required to fund his anticipated expansion into Pocatello—a moderately sized college town in southeast Idaho. Nearly 13 years previously, Klamath Care welcomed patients to its first urgent care facility in the family-oriented community of Idaho Falls, Idaho. As Patterson sat quietly, he reflected on the well-managed growth his company had achieved since his arrival 10 years ago. And now, this one-time start-up organization had grown to five (perhaps soon to be six) locations with over 100,000 patient encounters per year (Appendix A).

What was the impetus for this steady and sustained growth? And what was Patterson's role in instigating, facilitating, and directing it?

After opening three new clinics in only five years, was this latest venture into a relatively saturated and highly competitive market the best thing for Klamath Care? Would such an expansion represent a needed service for the people of Pocatello? If so, would the foray into Pocatello be Patterson's last for the next few years, or were other ventures forthcoming? Was the company well positioned strategically, financially, and operationally to expand into additional markets or service lines?

COMPANY OVERVIEW (2002–2015)

Established in 2002, Klamath Care's four founding physicians envisioned a walk-in medical facility with short waiting times and friendly staff. From its beginning, Klamath's mission was to provide high-quality, cost-effective urgent care. The company's vision is to be the preeminent urgent care provider in each of its markets. Klamath's core values—articulated at a company strategic planning retreat in 2009—address the principles of choice, convenience, competence, customer service, fairness, and integrity (Appendix B).

After the successful 2002 opening of its first urgent care facility in Idaho Falls, Klamath followed three years later (2005) with a second facility in Rexburg, a small but growing college town of 17,000 about 20 miles northeast of Idaho Falls. This venture expanded an established, well-understood service into a new, but less understood market. Moreover, this was the company's first joint venture with a new physician partner—one who had sought out Klamath Care.

In 2009, with increasing experience, confidence, and growing public support, Patterson and his colleagues added a third facility in Rigby, a town of 3,000 located between Rexburg and Idaho Falls. As with Klamath's second venture, this third expansion was initiated by a physician seeking a partnership with Klamath Care. This physician owned land and had architectural plans approved by the City of Rigby. However, he lacked urgent care experience and other needed resources. Because of Rigby's small population, many of whom lacked healthcare insurance, the need for an efficient and low-cost operation was apparent. Happily, within six months the partnership was thriving; growth was sufficient, operations were efficient, and the facility was profitable.

One year later (2010) and 8 years after opening its first urgent care clinic, Klamath's board was approached by two competing physicians from Idaho Falls, who lamented "you're eating our lunch . . . it's time for us to partner." Negotiations followed and in late 2010 Klamath assumed ownership and operation of Dr. David Bryan's and Dr. Edward Norton's two Idaho Falls–based urgent care facilities.

From 2002 through 2015 Klamath Care had not only seen steady and consistent growth in its practice locations and company-wide volumes, but the organization's scope of services had evolved from basic urgent care to a comprehensive range of services, including the following:

Patient services:

- Acute illness

- Acute injuries

- Physical examinations

- Wellness care

- Minor surgery

- Lab screening tests/full-service labs

- Free blood pressure checks

Employer services:

- Workers' compensation and care management

- Physicals/consultations

- Drug screening

Klamath Care's company profile is summarized in Table 8.1. (A complete list of Klamath Care's patient and employer services is found in Appendix C.)

Local and Regional Competition and Demographics

Just as the public embraced urgent care, competition to provide it increased steadily. According to Patterson, industry experts recommend about one urgent care facility per 10,000 population (assuming primary care is offered in addition to urgent care). Generally speaking, an urgent care–only model would require about 25,000 population per facility. By 2011, the population per urgent care facility in Klamath Care's current (and projected) service areas ranged from 1,499 in Rigby, to 34,469 in Twin Falls (Table 8.2). Frequent users of urgent care centers include families with children and older adults. Urgent care centers accept all or most forms of medical insurance. Patients without insurance pay cash or agree to a payment plan. Key demographics in Klamath Care's established and potential markets are outlined in Table 8.3.

In early 2011, Patterson concluded the time was right to introduce its operation to the community of Pocatello, Idaho, a college town of 50,000 located 50 miles south of Idaho Falls. A long-established urgent

Table 8.1. Klamath Care company profile (2015)

Selected statistics	
Number of urgent care facilities	5
Number of full- and part-time providers (MD, PA, NP)	31
Visits per provider per hour	5
Number of full- and part-time employees	136
Number of annual visits	152,000
Average daily visits per facility	52
Number of lab tests performed in-house	155,000
Total annual revenues	$16.1 million
Average charge per patient visit	$125.00
Net collections	70%
Annual operating and other expenses	$12.8 million
Annual net income	$425,000
Administrative overhead as a percent of total expenses	5%
Years in business	13

Note: MD, medical doctor; PA, physician assistant; NP, nurse practitioner.

care provider, Doctors Instant Care, was considering opening its second Pocatello-based clinic too. Meanwhile, the local community hospital relocated, expanded, and renamed its community-based urgent care clinic. That same hospital also maintained a "fast track/urgent care" component to its hospital-based emergency department. In addition,

Table 8.2. Total population per urgent care facility in 2011 select markets in various mountain west communities

Community	Approx. population	Number of urgent care facilities/Klamath Care and (total)*	Total population per urgent care facility
Idaho Falls, ID	60,730	3 / (8)**	7,591
Rexburg, ID	17,257	1 / (2)	8,628
Rigby, ID	2,998	1 / (2)	1,499
Pocatello, ID	51,466	0 / (4)**	12,866
Twin Falls, ID	34,469	0 / (1)	34,469
Jackson, WY	8,647	0 / (1)	8,647

Notes: *First number in column is number of Klamath care facilities followed by (total) facilities in the community.

**Number includes hospital-based urgent care facilities.

Table 8.3. Key demographics in Klamath Care's established and potential future markets (2011)

Community	% Pop. growth: 2008–2012	% of persons under age 18	% of persons 65 and over	Est. % w/o medical insurance	Median household income
Idaho Falls, ID	3.8	30.3	11.1	12.0	$40,512
Rexburg, ID	22.0	19.3	9.4	11.0	$36,232
Rigby, ID	4.3	26.3	12.3	16.0	$31,934
Pocatello, ID	4.7	16.6	10.4	18.0	$34,326
Twin Falls, ID	15.9	26.5	15.0	13.0	$32,600
Jackson, WY	5.2	20.8	5.8	6.0	$97,456
U.S.–average	6.0	24.3	12.8	15.0	$50,740

"fast track/urgent care" centers in Pocatello were operated by a private physician, and another by a large investor-owned hospital in Idaho Falls. These facilities' data are summarized in Table 8.2.

Understandably, many citizens in Pocatello, Idaho Falls, and elsewhere did not differentiate community-based urgent care centers from hospital-based emergency departments. Consequently, the patient mix at hospital emergency departments in Pocatello and Idaho Falls followed the national trends shown in Table 8.4.

With effective marketing, Patterson was confident that customers who frequented Pocatello's hospital or community-based urgent care facilities would favor Klamath Care. By fall 2011, the competition in Pocatello and the surrounding region had increased. Klamath Care's urgent care market share is estimated in Table 8.5.

Notwithstanding increasing competition from local healthcare providers, by 2011 Klamath Care would confront the competitive threat of Walmart, the world's largest retailer. Generally, the urgent care industry did not regard "retail clinics" as credible; nonetheless, their presence was a threat. To complicate matters, Klamath Care's attempt to become Walmart's in-store provider at two local sites was rebuffed because of a personal and professional relationship between the local hospital CEO (whose facility won the contract) and Walmart's local general manager.

Table 8.4. Patient mix by acuity in U.S. emergency departments

Immediate	Emergent	Urgent	Semiurgent	Nonurgent	Unknown
5.5%	9.8%	33.3%	20.7%	13.0%	16.7%

Source: Sultz and Young, 2011. See also Urgent Care Industry Information Kit, Urgent Care Association of America, 2013.

Table 8.5. Klamath Care's urgent care business market share

	2004 (%)	2008 (%)	2011 (%)	2016 (est. %)
Idaho Falls, ID	90	90	80	70
Pocatello, ID	0	0	0	0
Rexburg, ID	0	100	100	90
Rigby, ID	0	0	100	75
Twin Falls, ID	0	0	0	0
Jackson, WY	0	0	0	0

By 2010, part of Klamath's intermediate and longer-range growth plans included potentially entering the Twin Falls and Jackson markets. Twin Falls had one urgent care provider and a hospital emergency department. This meant the Twin Falls community of 35,000 was underserved. Jackson, Wyoming, a resort town with world-class snow skiing and an outdoorsman's paradise in summer, is a more competitive environment than Twin Falls. Even though Jackson's relatively small and seasonal population is presently served by one urgent care provider, the reimbursement rates from Blue Cross and others were customarily 50% higher than rates in Idaho Falls, Twin Falls, or Pocatello. Furthermore, by early 2011, Jackson's established urgent care provider indicated a willingness to sell.

Growth, Diversity, Innovation, and Organizational Development

Almost from inception, the founders of Klamath Care had a vision of pushing the boundaries of growth and innovation to provide better care to its customers. The company's initial plan was to build and grow from the site of its founding. Prior to entering the Pocatello market, Patterson's forays into new markets had been invited by physicians already in those markets and who would become Klamath's partners. Pocatello was different. Indeed, if pursued, Klamath's uninvited entry into Pocatello would represent one of Patterson's boldest moves and greatest challenges in the company's 13-year history.

Delivery of urgent care was the company's core business, but new lines would include services for employers, including medical care covered by workers' compensation. By early 2008, workers' compensation was approximately 19% of Klamath revenues (Table 8.6.) In addition, more and more customers asked Patterson why he didn't offer a mini-health plan, or whether he had considered developing loyalty cards. In 2008, Klamath introduced loyalty cards that extended credit and other incentives to customers.

Klamath Care's commitment to innovation gave it national recognition from CNN Headline News and other media outlets. Notably, it

Table 8.6. Klamath Care's service portfolio, by revenue and percent by payer (in thousands)

Product/service	2005	2008	2012	2016
Total revenue/(%) from walk-in clinic operations	$869/(90%)	$2,100/(81%)	$5,900/(80%)	$9,500/(76%)
Total revenue/(%) from workers' compensation	$96/(10%)	$500/(19%)	$1,500/(20%)	$3,000/(24%)
Total revenue	$965	$2,600	$7,400	$12,500

used cell phones to notify patients to return to the clinic when a provider could see them, thus allowing them to undertake other tasks. Perceived waiting times declined, and public response was positive. In addition to CNN Headline News, CKLW Detroit and two local affiliates carried the story. Patterson was mindful of the important contributions the Klamath Care staff made to this success, and he made certain the staff shared and celebrated its recognition.

By 2008 (according to a local market study cited by Patterson), Klamath's name recognition in its markets was second only to that of Walmart. Its steady and fervent commitment to supporting community events brought added recognition. In recent years, Klamath Care's clinic system had become the provider of choice for some of the largest employers in Idaho. For five consecutive years (2010–2014), the people of Idaho Falls have shown their support for Klamath Care by naming it the clinic with the shortest wait time (People's choice awards, *Idaho Falls Post Register*).

Meanwhile, the company had strengthened internal operations by consolidating billing and receivables management, information technology, planning, marketing, human resources, group purchasing, and corporate finance. Executive management, including a full-time, company-wide medical director, was also well established. Moreover, Klamath Care's growing reputation and volume of business strengthened its relationships and negotiating position with business partners, including pharmaceutical and medical suppliers. With improved operations and a healthy financial outlook, was it again time to build, to reach, to grow?

CHALLENGES AND NEXT STEPS

In its 13th year, Patterson and Klamath Care's owners and senior executives had reason to be pleased. With five facilities in four markets offering a comprehensive array of traditional urgent care and employer health-related services, Klamath seemed well positioned for the future.

Notwithstanding the increasing competition Klamath Care faced, opportunities to explore new markets—as well as creative new business arrangements—continued to capture Patterson's attention. Opportunities in Twin Falls and Jackson were especially enticing. The implementation of new technologies, including electronic medical records, demanded attention. The development of an innovative "patient preferred card-network" and exploring creative new business partnerships with specialty physician groups were other opportunities needing decisions. Enhancing a marketing campaign to increase business from "walk-ins" and workers' compensation also required attention.

Other initiatives facing Klamath as it considered expansion to Pocatello included (1) enter and grow the Pocatello market share from roughly 25% in its first year of operation to 65% by 2018; (2) expand into additional markets—notably the resort town of Jackson, approximately 88 miles east of Idaho Falls, and/or Twin Falls, a community 115 miles west of Pocatello; (3) initiate increased cost management and operations improvement, including potential facility consolidations in Idaho Falls due to serious and increasing market/economic forces; (4) leverage the company's positive name recognition to gain and improve market share—notably in Pocatello; and (5) evaluate and implement new technologies to improve clinical and financial performance.

For Klamath Care, the past has been good and the future looks bright. There is also much to do! With a sluggish economy and increasing competition, how should Klamath move forward?

DISCUSSION QUESTIONS

1. Identify and analyze the characteristics and competencies that made Patterson an excellent leader/entrepreneur for Klamath Care.

2. Using Porter's Five Force Analysis technique, conduct a strategic evaluation of Klamath Care's plan to open a new clinic in Pocatello.

3. Conduct a SWOT analysis of Klamath Care's plan to open a new clinic site (Pocatello, Twin Falls, and Jackson). Clearly identify the information you use that is found in the case, and the information you want and need that is not provided in the case to conduct an appropriate SWOT analysis.

4. What, if any, is the strategic importance of Klamath Care's historic joint ventures?

5. Consider the role of a strategic partner.

6. In addition to a joint venture partnership, what other strategic market entry strategies should Patterson consider (e.g., acquisition, alliance with local hospital, or going it alone)?

7. Recommend a course of action for Klamath Care.

REFERENCES

Sultz, H.A., & Young, K. M. (2011). *Health care USA: Understanding its organization and delivery* (7th ed.). Sudbury, MA: Jones and Bartlett Publishers.
Urgent Care Association of America. (2013). Urgent care industry information kit, 2013. Retrieved July 21, 2016, from https://c.ymcdn.com/sites/ucaoa.siteym. com/resource/resmgr/Files/UrgentCareMediaKit_2013.pdf

APPENDIX A

Klamath Care Facilities Locations—Current and Projected

Table 8.A.1. Klamath Care facilities locations—current and projected

Community	Date Klamath Care operations established	Location/comments
Idaho Falls, ID	2002 (1st facility); 2010 (4th and 5th facility)	Eastern Idaho
Rexburg, ID	2005 (2nd facility)	Eastern Idaho
Rigby, ID	2009 (3rd facility)	Eastern Idaho
Pocatello, ID	Potential expansion (2015+)	Southeastern Idaho
Twin Falls, ID	Potential expansion (2015+)	Southern Idaho (115 miles west of Pocatello; 90-minute drive)
Jackson, WY	Potential expansion (2015+)	Western Wyoming (88 miles east of Idaho Falls; 110-minute drive)

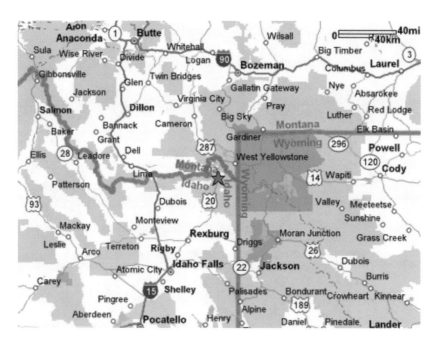

Figure 8.A.1. Map of eastern Idaho and western Wyoming.

APPENDIX B

Klamath Care Values Statement

- *We believe in choice.* We promise to provide a quality alternative urgent care facility that meets patients' immediate medical needs.

- *We believe in convenience.* We promise to deliver timely medical services in a comfortable, inviting atmosphere.

- *We believe in competence.* We promise that our service providers will have the education and experience necessary to assure our patients the best medical treatment with state-of-the-art diagnostic procedures.

- *We believe in providing comprehensive care.* We promise to provide an essential link in the continuum of care through assessment, intervention, and when needed, referral to specialized services.

- *We believe in customer service.* We promise to remember that our job is to meet the needs of our patients in a professional, friendly, and responsive manner.

- *We believe in fairness.* We promise to provide the highest-quality medical services at a reasonable cost and to make billing procedures convenient and fair.

- *We believe in education.* We promise to empower our patients by providing them with the knowledge to take responsibility for their physical and mental health.

- *We believe in people.* We promise to provide the staff at Klamath Care with a rich and rewarding work environment that enables them to achieve their full professional potential.

- *We believe in integrity.* We promise to operate professionally, ethically, and in a manner consistent with our organizational values.

APPENDIX C

Klamath Care Patient and Employer Services

Table 8.C.1. Klamath Care patient and employer services

Patient services		
Acute illness	**Physicals**	**Minor surgeries**
• Sore throats	• Sports	• Moles
• Coughs and flu	• School	• Ingrown toenails
• Infections	• Premarital	• Cysts
• Rashes	• Missionary	• Abscesses
• Allergic reactions	• College	• Warts
• Eye injuries	• Camp	• Other
• Abdominal pain	• Other	
• Vomiting and diarrhea		
Acute injuries	**Ongoing healthcare**	**Lab screening**
• Minor fractures	• Mild hypertension	• Cholesterol
• Sprains	• Acne	• Blood sugar
• Lacerations	• Allergies	• PSA
• Bruises	• Mild depression	• TB testing
• Burns	• Smoking cessation	• Other
• Bites	• Other	
• Back pain		
Other		
• Free blood pressure medication refills (when primary physician unavailable)		
Services to employer		
Workers' compensation	**Physicals/consultations**	**Drug screening**
• Treatment (effective return to work program)	• Preemployment exams	• Preemployment exams
• Tracking—12-hour employer turnaround	• Fitness for duty exams	• NIDA-DOT, random, for cause, etc.
• Case management (on-site working with patient and employer)	• DOT/HAZMAT exams	• Medical review officer
	• Hearing/screening/ certification	• Alcohol abuse testing
	• Respiratory exams	

Note: DOT, Department of Transportation; HAZMAT, hazardous materials; NIDA, National Institute on Drug Abuse; PSA, prostate-specific antigen.

9

Hospital Consolidation

Idaho State University, Pocatello, ID

CASE HISTORY/BACKGROUND

Healthcare providers have a dynamic relationship with their local and regional markets that requires them to balance organization and community interests when making decisions that affect the healthcare marketplace.

Strategic initiatives have long-term impacts on healthcare organizations and their stakeholders, including patients, physicians, payers, and the public—and stakeholders' expectations must be considered in connection with these decisions. This case discusses important healthcare industry issues and trends, including forces that shape a healthcare organization's mission, vision, and market-based strategies for growth and development.

INTRODUCTION

In many ways, the 2014 holiday season was no different than any other, and, thankfully, Dallin Burnham enjoyed the traditional music, decorations, and seemingly endless social gatherings that accentuated this time of year. Yet this year is different, and Burnham—chief executive officer (CEO) of Kimball Hospital—is anxious. Three months earlier, Burnham's Rocky Mountain–based healthcare system—The Great

133

Western Hospital Corporation (Great Western)—initiated discussions with his hospital's chief rival—Tanner Medical Center (Tanner Medical), a county-owned, freestanding, not-for-profit hospital. The purpose of these discussions is to decide if the two hospitals should form a joint venture to offer services, or if they should consolidate or merge; acquisition is another possibility. The December 31st deadline to initiate formal discussions or "walk away" is looming. Burnham understands that his personal recommendation to his corporate supervisors and community-based board could greatly influence their decision to proceed with discussions and, perhaps, negotiations. The alternative is to continue the more than 40+ year history of offering competing and often duplicative healthcare services to the community. Burnham's recommendation and the ultimate decision regarding joint ventures, acquisition, consolidation, and/or merger could be the most important local healthcare market decision in a generation, or more. The results would affect the lives of healthcare professionals and the nature and quality of healthcare services for years to come.

MERGER, ACQUISITION, AND CONSOLIDATION TRENDS

In many ways, the local market mirrors the healthcare issues and challenges observed nationally, including an increasing trend toward affiliations, hospital mergers, acquisitions, joint operating agreements, and other organizational forms that is accelerated by healthcare reform and myriad organizational and market forces (Cuellar & Gentler, 2003; Dixon Hughes Goodman LLP, 2013; Gamble & Sachs, 2015; GE Camden Group, 2016). Similarly, in the decade preceding the deliberations between Great Western and Tanner Medical, the hospital industry had undergone a wave of acquisitions, mergers, and consolidations that transformed the hospital marketplace. By 2005, the rate of such activity had increased nearly tenfold over the rate five years previously (Strode, 2015; Vogt & Town, 2006). From his research, Burnham understood that hospital mergers and acquisitions take many forms (Table 9.1). He also noted that the more important advantages to hospital mergers, acquisitions, or consolidations include access to capital, avoidance of non-value-added duplication of expensive healthcare services, and leverage when contracting with insurers, suppliers, and employers.

Mindful that such organizational actions are rarely a panacea, Burnham identified concerns or potential disadvantages, including increased costs and prices, and decreased quality following reduced

Table 9.1. Hospital consolidation: types and forms

Affiliation	Joint venture	Joint operating agreement	Merger	Acquisition
Most flexible form of consolidation, though option of a weak vs. strong affiliation exists	A mildly flexible arrangement used to create something new (limited inpatient or outpatient activity, service, purpose) that may be overwhelming to do alone	Virtual mergers, where assets may separate, but services are coordinated	Mutual decision of two companies to combine	Purchase of one hospital by another
Utilized to increase footprint, gain economies of scale, create referrals, supplement an already successful set of services, exchange best practices	Shared governance between two hospitals	New overarching governing board is created, but hospitals maintain independent boards	Leadership may be a combination of the two hospitals, or from an outside source	Usually, smaller acquired by larger, but not always
Do not necessarily change management or governance	Contains some form of profit and risk sharing	May borrow for capital investment as one organization	Hospitals absorb each other's assets and debts	Goals: increase market share, footprint, acquire additional services, financial stability
		Similar to joint venture, but larger. Extends beyond specific service or activity	Goal is to increase economy of scale, improve quality, increase market share	Hospitals may continue to function semi-independently or make transformational changes to match buying hospital

Source: Dixon, Hughes, and Goodman (2013).

competition (Vogt & Town, 2006). The difficulty of merging long-standing cultures and operating systems is another major concern.

As he reflected on potential strategic actions to facilitate hospital, corporate, and community needs, Burnham reasoned that Tanner Medical cannot merge with Great Western because their sizes are so disparate. Tanner Medical cannot merge with Kimball because Kimball is owned by

Great Western and is not an independent facility. Isn't acquisition the only course? Once acquired, either hospital could be merged or absorbed into the other since both are part of the same corporate entity. After that, clinical programs as well as ancillary and support services could be rationalized.

LOCAL MARKET AND DEMOGRAPHICS

Prattville's high desert community of 60,000 has supported two competing hospitals for over 70 years. Approximately 75 percent of clinical programs and services are duplicative; nearly $40 million per year in potential hospital-based services are lost due to physician referrals or patient self-referrals to other medical centers 50 to 150 miles distant.

In early 2012, and continuing through mid-2014, changes in leadership and governance at Prattville's hospitals set the stage for the negotiations that followed. These changes included new hospital board chairs, hospital administrator/CEOs, Blade County commissioners (Tanner Medical), and regional and system-wide leadership at Great Western. Moreover, each hospital's plans to introduce or expand duplicative services have caused Burnham to ask himself three questions: Is our hospital's mission focused on what is right and best for our service area, or Great Western? Would an acquisition, merger, or consolidation involving Kimball Hospital and Tanner Medical improve access and quality and reduce cost of healthcare to Prattville's service area? Should some form of acquisition or consolidation of hospital operations occur, is Kimball Hospital (Great Western) or county-owned Tanner Medical better positioned to assume ownership and management of the community's consolidated healthcare system?

Mindful of the changes in local and central office leadership, and troubled that each hospital's strategic plan calls for more and more duplication of hospital services—including OB/GYN, imaging, clinical laboratory, cardiology, surgery, and pediatrics—Burnham contacted his supervisor at corporate and suggested they revisit the idea of hospital cooperation—including reviewing the merits of a potential merger, acquisition, or joint venture of selected clinical programs. Talks regarding acquisition, merger, or consolidation failed in 1993; hospital leaders and their community boards—including corporate executives at Great Western—considered those options again in 2000 without success. The 1993 talks failed primarily because both hospitals were performing reasonably well financially. In 2000, lack of trust and goodwill between local boards, dislike and distrust between the hospital administrators, and physicians' desire to pit one hospital against the other doomed any hope for success.

When similar discussions began in 2014, Great Western was mindful of its long-standing and public commitment to the community, including

Kimball Hospital's employees. In recent years, corporate leaders emphatically restated that, notwithstanding Kimball's poor financial performance, Great Western is in Prattville for the indefinite future. Yet Great Western's leaders are cognizant of important political and marketplace realities. Table 9.2 summarizes key ownership, market, financial, operating, and political aspects of the Prattville hospital and healthcare community.

Table 9.2. Selected financial, operating, and other indicators: Kimball Hospital and Tanner Medical Center (fiscal year 2014)

	Kimball Hospital	Tanner Medical Center
Hospital ownership and control	GWHC	Blade County
Ownership type	501(c)(3) corporation	County government
Licensed beds	110	150
Total patient days—trend (2012–2013–2014)	10,150–10,925–12,775	24,240–25,380–23,725
Average daily census	35 (40% of bed capacity)	68 (55% of bed capacity)
Annual gross patient services revenue	$49 million	$97 million
Annual net patient services revenue	$31.5 million	$54.6 million
Market share	26%	52%
Annual marketing/ advertising budget	$141,000	$310,000
Net operating income per- cent for 2012–2013–2014	(3%)*–(5%*)–(2%)*	2%–4%–6%
Total debt	N/A (consolidated w/GWHC)	$73 million
Financial reserves (savings)	N/A (consolidated w/GWHC)	$9 million
Employed physicians	8	0
Percent of local physi- cians who primarily admit to this hospital	35%	65%
Service lines unique to hospital in service area	Cardiology, acute rehabilitation	Pediatrics, neonatal level II, cancer
Percent of physicians who favor hospital merger or consolidation	80% (fall 2014 Kimball/Tanner medical staff surveys)	
Public preference for local (versus out-of-area) ownership and control	68% (spring 2014 Kimball Hospital community telephone survey)	

Note: (3%), (5%), and (2%) are negative numbers.

OTHER PROVIDER AND COMMUNITY CONSIDERATIONS

Since being formed in 1985, Great Western has established a 20+ hospital system in three contiguous states with sophisticated central office support services, including health information technology, central purchasing, laboratory, laundry, marketing and advertising, physician recruitment, and quality and risk management. The system's focus on evidence-based medicine has resulted in reduced costs and improved quality and has received national recognition for its work.

Local ownership and control allow staff and supporters of Tanner Medical to tout the hospital's ability to chart its own course—independent of "out-of-state" executives who may not share the community's healthcare goals. Tanner Medical enjoys a measure of "system" support through its affiliation with Voluntary Hospitals of America, the nation's largest not-for-profit hospital association. Importantly, and for various reasons, local physicians generally favor and support Tanner Medical over Kimball. This is reflected in the nearly 2:1 ratio of annual admissions to Tanner Medical over Kimball. It is theorized that, despite Kimball/Great Western's reputation as a high-quality, low-cost provider, area physicians resist the corporation's centralized and system-wide approach to planning and delivering care. Indeed, many physicians had relocated to Prattville because of its laissez-faire approach to medicine, including the relative nonexistence of "managed care," or insurance mechanisms that limit physician autonomy and reimbursement.

A TIME FOR DECISION

As chief executive, Burnham is also the chief market manager and promoter for his hospital. Positioning his organization for immediate and long-term growth and financial success is an ever-present and demanding mandate; orchestrating a well-balanced, integrated community-wide healthcare system to improve access, cost, and quality of care to the entire Prattville service area is no less important. Burnham understands these two imperatives are inherently in conflict, which adds complexity to the decision-making process. Burnham believes the time is right to combine the community's two competing hospitals. He also believes the leadership, financial resources, and other strengths of Great Western make Kimball Hospital and Great Western the best choice to own and manage the new entity. Yet Burnham understands his community's preference for local ownership and control and the physician community's long-standing reluctance to embrace Great Western's philosophy and approach to organizing and delivering care. Great Western executives and Kimball Hospital community board members are experienced and capable executives and community leaders, but they are looking to Burnham for guidance in this matter.

DISCUSSION QUESTIONS

1. What key organizational and marketplace issues likely reopened the door to a potential hospital merger, acquisition, consolidation, or joint venture between Great Western/Kimball Hospital and Tanner Medical?

2. Can Burnham balance the interests of his community with the interests of his employer? Suggest ways Burnham might achieve this balance.

3. From a patient and community perspective, what are some pros and cons to acquisition and consolidation of Prattville's community hospitals?

4. Use this case to identify and describe the forces that shape a hospital's mission and vision. Describe the forces that shape a healthcare organization's growth and development.

5. Who are the key decision makers and other stakeholders (individuals and groups) in this case? Identify their concerns regarding merger, acquisition, and/or consolidation. What are their relative positions of power and influence in effecting a decision to merge, acquire, or consolidate?

6. Do you recommend acquisition and consolidation of Prattville's two community hospitals? Why, or why not? What options short of acquisition and consolidation should the hospitals consider?

7. If you recommend acquisition/consolidation, which organization should assume ownership/control? Why? What are the strategic implications of your decision?

ENDNOTE

This case describes an actual situation. Fictitious names, settings, and data are used to preserve anonymity.

REFERENCES

Cuellar, A. E., & Gentler, P. J. (2003). Trends in hospital consolidation: The formation of local systems. *Health Affairs*, *22*(6), 77–87.

Dixon Hughes Goodman LLP. (2013). What hospital executives should be considering in hospital mergers and acquisitions. Retrieved July 22, 2016, from http://www2.dhgllp.com/res_pubs/Hospital-Mergers-and-Acquisitions.pdf

Gamble, M., & Sachs, B. (2015). 60 statistics and thoughts on healthcare, hospital and physician practice M&A. Retrieved June 13, 2016, from http://www.beckershospitalreview.com/hospital-transactions-and-valuation/60-statistics-and-thoughts-on-healthcare-hospital-and-physician-practice-m-a.html

GE Camden Group. (2016). 10 Forecasts: What will influence healthcare most in 2016? Retrieved June 13, 2016, from http://www.beckershospitalreview.com/hospital-management-administration/10-forecasts-what-will-influence-healthcare-most-in-2016.html

Strode, R. (2015). M&A and strategic partnerships: Looking ahead is past prologue? *Becker's Hospital Review*. Retrieved June 13, 2016, from http://www.beckershospitalreview.com/hospital-management-administration/m-a-and-strategic-partnerships-looking-ahead-is-past-prologue.html

Vogt, W. B., & Town, R. (2006). How has hospital consolidation affected the price and quality of hospital care? Research synthesis report no. 9. Robert Wood Johnson Foundation. Retrieved May 8, 2012, from https://folio.iupui.edu/bitstream/handle/10244/520/no9researchreport.pdf?sequence=2

10

Service Area Management

Tracy J. Farnsworth
Idaho State University, Pocatello, ID

CASE HISTORY/BACKGROUND

Twenty-seven-year-old Rachel McKee completed her graduate degree in healthcare administration with an emphasis in planning and marketing. To her delight she was offered, and she accepted, the position of assistant director of strategic planning and marketing at Community Medical Centers (Community Medical), a large healthcare organization in central California. McKee is ambitious and eager to make an impact early in her career. She was pleased that her new boss and mentor, Lindsey Chadwick—a seasoned healthcare executive with 25 years of leadership experience—seemed confident in her ability to process complex information and to assume increasingly important responsibilities.

Chadwick understood the complexities of Community Medical and the local healthcare market. Her supervisor had asked her to update the organization's strategic marketing plan in response to changes in the primary service area/market and national healthcare trends.

Chadwick assigned McKee the important task of performing an environmental assessment, the results of which would allow Chadwick, McKee, and members of the Community Medical senior leadership team to complete a strengths, weaknesses, opportunities, and threats analysis, followed by a summary of the organization's proposed strategic initiatives. Chadwick and McKee can update Community Medical's strategic marketing plan using these documents.

At the outset, Chadwick advised McKee to gather and assess relevant market information from various sources, including leading health industry publications and organization, statewide, and other publicly available data bases, and to conduct interviews with hospital and health system executives, physician groups, insurance company executives, regulators, and other stakeholders to help provide the framework and justification for Community Medical's marketing plan. A broad but detailed understanding of the public at large and the political dynamics between and among the provider community was also vital. Finally, an overview of key industry trends was needed. After four months of diligent study, interviews, networking, and thoughtful analysis, McKee presented her environmental assessment to Chadwick. The highlights are outlined here.

FRESNO MARKET/SERVICE AREA BACKGROUND

Community Medical's primary market or service area comprises Fresno County (Figure 10.1). With a population approaching 1 million people, Fresno County has had strong growth over the last decade—up 16.4%

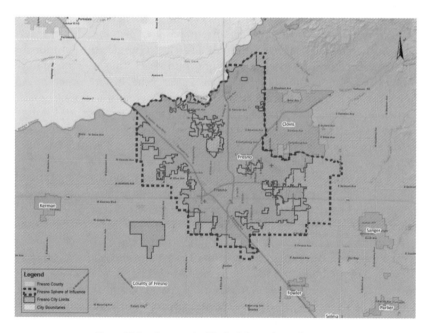

Figure 10.1. Community Medical Center's service area.

Table 10.1. Population statistics

Metro area	2000 population	2010 population	Gross difference	Percent change
California	33,871,648	37,253,956	3,382,308	10.0%
Fresno County	799,407	930,450	131,043	16.4%
City of Fresno	427,652	494,665	67,013	15.7%

compared to 10% statewide (Table 10.1). From 1980 to 2010, the county population grew 78%. From 2010 to 2040, the population is expected to grow by 283,000 (30% growth). Future population gains are projected to be half that rate.

Fresno County is among the poorest counties in California; half its families have an income below 200% of the federal poverty level. Educational attainment is also below the state average; only 22% of adults hold a college degree. Approximately 50% of the county's population is Latino; 37.5% are Caucasian. Roughly 20% of Community Medical's primary service area population is foreign born. The overall health status of service area residents is marginal. About 20% self-report fair or poor health status, and over 27% have asthma and/or diabetes. The service area unemployment rate is high and rising: 15.5% are currently unemployed. Agriculture is vital to the local and regional economy. The public sector is the largest employer in the service area, and two major healthcare systems, Community Medical and St. Agnes Hospital, are among the service area's largest private employers.

HOSPITAL PROVIDERS

Most hospitals in Fresno County and the counties adjacent to it are not-for-profit or government tax district hospitals (Appendix A). Fresno County has an acute-care bed capacity of 173 per 100,000 (slightly less than the statewide average of 182), and an occupancy rate of 68% compared to the statewide average of 59%. Major hospitals are near capacity at certain times of the year. Major hospitals in Fresno County include Community Medical—(3 hospitals with 900 total beds); 400-bed St. Agnes Hospital; and 165-bed Kaiser Permanente Medical Center. These hospital providers have approximately 53, 27, and 10% of the inpatient market, respectively (Table 10.2).

Community Medical and St. Agnes serve a large geographic area that includes Fresno County and a referral base from contiguous counties (Appendix A). Historically, the relationship between Community Medical

Table 10.2. Market share of major hospitals in Fresno County

Hospital system	Beds	Fresno County market share
Community medical centers		
Community Regional Medical Center (CMC)	600	
Clovis Community Hospital (CMC)	232	
Fresno Heart and Surgical Hospital (CMC)	68	
CMC system total	900	53%
St. Agnes Hospital (part of Trinity Health System)	400	27%
Kaiser Permanente Fresno Medical Center	165	10%

and St. Agnes has been characterized by little collaboration and intense, long-standing competition bordering on animosity. St. Agnes is located in more affluent north Fresno and is often described as the "cash cow" of its 40-hospital parent corporation, Trinity Health. Community Medical's 600-bed flagship facility, Community Regional Medical Center–Fresno, is located in the heart of Fresno and with its nine outpatient clinics is Fresno County's primary safety net provider. Financial losses at the Community Medical flagship are offset by profits from two sister hospitals located in affluent communities to the north and northeast. In recent years, Community Medical's financial performance improved, and it became modestly profitable.

Reports from the California Office of Statewide Health Planning and Development show an increasingly unfavorable payer mix for all Fresno County hospitals—an indication of the community's high levels of poverty, lack of private insurance, and Medi-Cal (California Medicaid) coverage compared with the community's commercial insurance payer base. The St. Agnes payer base is approximately 25% Medi-Cal. Community Medical—with a 30+ year contract with Fresno County to care for the medically indigent—reports nearly 40% of its patients are covered by Medi-Cal. A major initiative at Community Medical is opening 160 new beds (including 56 neonatal intensive care unit beds) at its downtown, flagship hospital. After opening a new patient tower recently, St. Agnes plans to add 36 neurosurgery and critical care beds. New hospital construction has been a response to capacity issues and an effort to comply with state seismic (earthquake) standards. New service lines have been a response to the exodus of patients to out-of-service-area providers. Additional financial, operational, demographic, and market share data about Community Medical and its competitors are available from the California Office of Statewide Health Planning and Development website.

Respondents' characterizations of the quality of care at hospitals in Fresno County range from poor to good, with many opting to leave the county when they get "really sick." In fact, a recent study showed nearly $500 million of medical care leaves Fresno County annually when patients seek care elsewhere because of long wait times, physician availability, and concerns about quality. In recent years, the region's hospitals have affiliated with academic teaching programs to support clinical and medical training programs, improve quality of care, enhance hospital reputation, and recruit physicians. Affiliations include Community Medical with the University of California, San Francisco, and St. Agnes's affiliation with Stanford for cardiac surgery and neurosciences.

St. Agnes is widely regarded as the premier hospital in the county, but recent, highly publicized outbreaks of methicillin-resistant *Staphylococcus aureus* infections and Legionnaires' disease have raised questions about quality of care. Selected case mix, volume, and quality/outcomes data about Community Medical and its primary competitors are provided in Appendixes B, C, and D.

PHYSICIAN AND ALLIED HEALTH COMMUNITY

Fresno County has a notable shortage of primary care and specialist physicians. There are 45 primary care physicians per 100,000 residents, compared with 59 statewide; and 118 physicians overall per 100,000 residents, compared with 174 statewide. Specialists in short supply include areas of neurosurgery, general surgery, cardiology, gastroenterology, oncology, otolaryngology, ophthalmology, and psychiatry. Nurses and other allied health personnel are also in short supply. This caused the federal government to classify Fresno County as a health professional shortage area. Physician shortages result in long wait times for appointments. A dermatology appointment, for example, requires nine to 12 months. Such delays are causing many insured patients to seek medical care outside the county. An aging physician workforce suggests shortages will worsen.

Recruiting new physicians to Fresno County is challenging because of poor payer mix, low reimbursement, hospital call coverage obligations, and quality-of-life considerations. Although many physicians are overworked, many of these same doctors have little interest in recruiting more help. The physician shortage in Fresno county would be more acute were it not for the many non-U.S.-trained physicians who practice there.

There are few large physician practices in Fresno County. Most primary care physicians are solo practitioners or practice in groups smaller than five. Specialists tend to practice in single-specialty rather than multispecialty groups. Although physicians across the city and county often maintain admitting and practice privileges at several hospitals, they generally admit primarily at one. For years, emergency room call coverage has been a source of friction between area hospitals and physicians; hospitals must pay stipends to physicians for call coverage.

Unlike many markets in California, Fresno County has limited formal integration, such as physician–hospital organizations, between physicians and hospitals. Generally, hospital–physician relationships have been marked by distrust. In recent years, Community Medical's relationship with the physician community has improved, whereas physician relations at St. Agnes have deteriorated. Hospitals' efforts to court and align primary service area physicians have focused on joint ventures, many of which failed.

Generally, physicians in Fresno County have a lack of loyalty to area hospitals. This is evidenced by long-standing and extensive shifts in referral patterns away from hospitals and toward physician-owned facilities that offer ancillary services, such as imaging and endoscopy, and specialty services, such as orthopedics and cosmetic surgery. Many reports suggest physicians' historical and ongoing dissatisfaction with area hospitals is the basis for this change. Shifts in referral patterns have likely also been driven by Medicare and private insurance reductions in reimbursement to physicians.

PAYER/INSURANCE COMMUNITY

In contrast to other California markets, Fresno County has been tentative in adopting managed care. Even at their peak in the mid-1990s, health maintenance organizations or their variants never achieved dominance in the Fresno area, and their market share decreased from 30% in 2000 to 25% in 2015. According to one report, absence of significant health maintenance organization or managed care penetration means that features common elsewhere, such as formation of large multispecialty physician groups, hospital–physician alignment, provider familiarity with performance measures and reporting, and aggressive care and utilization management, are not found in Fresno County.

Only 46% of Fresno County residents (compared to 59% of residents statewide) have private health insurance. Sixteen percent are uninsured. Medi-Cal enrollment is high in Fresno County, with just over 30% of residents enrolled. Fresno County's safety net appears to be weak, fragmented, and inadequate for population needs. Indeed, health appears to be a low priority for Fresno as well as surrounding county governments. Anthem Blue Cross and Blue Shield of California are the leading not-for-profit health insurers in Fresno County. As in other regional markets, health plans face strong pressure to moderate premium increases, which is challenging in the face of escalating hospital costs. Because hospitals such as St. Agnes and Community Medical's Clovis Community Hospital are considered "must haves" by employer purchasers, they are in a strong negotiating position with area health plans.

THE FUTURE OF HEALTHCARE: KEY INDUSTRY TRENDS

As a dynamic and ever-changing industry, the future of healthcare is difficult to predict. A summary of key trends that will define healthcare's future for the next five years includes the following (Masters & Valentine, 2015):

1. *Physician Engagement: Partners with Aligned Incentives:* New care models and payment methodologies associated with healthcare reform, clinical integration, and population health management will require alignment of hospital and physician financial and clinical incentives. To achieve and sustain clinical and financial success these initiatives must be led by physicians. The trend to employ physicians will continue in most hospitals and health systems (some estimates are that 70 to 80% of physicians could be employed by hospitals, medical groups, health plans, or other healthcare entities by 2020.

2. *Revenues, Operating Costs, and Financial Sustainability:* Despite a somewhat improved economic situation in 2015 versus 2008, rating agencies have determined the outlook for the not-for-profit healthcare sector is negative. Contributing factors include weak hospital top-line growth, projections of static inpatient volume, declining operating margins, and decreased revenue because of healthcare reform.

3. *Care Model Redesign and Clinical Integration:* Delivering high-quality, cost-efficient healthcare is the primary objective of redesigning care models and integrating clinical providers. Some healthcare leaders view an inpatient admission as a failure of outpatient care until proven otherwise. This philosophy is a framework for deploying processes, people, and resources to achieve quality outcomes in the most cost-effective setting. In the near future more organizations (hospitals, medical groups, and others) will create or join accountable care organizations and integrated clinical networks.

4. *Employer Exchanges and Health Plans:* Employers will try to moderate the effects of increasing healthcare costs. Options for self-insured employers will include direct contracting with providers, shared savings models, spending threshold guarantees, reference pricing for

costly procedures (e.g., cardiac, orthopedics, cancer treatment), and private exchange plans. Enrollment in public and private insurance exchanges will increase as people and businesses explore new options for health insurance. Employers will continue to shift costs to employees by offering plans with higher copayments and deductibles, and by moving from defined benefit to defined contribution models.

5. *Competitive Positioning: Consolidations, Affiliations, and Partnerships:* There will be further consolidation for hospitals and healthcare systems, medical groups, ancillary services, health plans, and post–acute care providers. Most consolidations will be driven by the need to achieve greater economies of scale, filling gaps in the continuum of services, streamlining transitions in care, and expanding geographic coverage. Some arrangements will be opportunistic to create financial, operational, and clinical synergies; others will be necessary to ensure survival. "Affiliations without merger" relationships are being developed between large systems. Many affiliations are clinically integrated networks of hospitals or systems that align to share financial risk and clinical programs. They affiliate to design care models and processes that improve quality of care, reduce costs, standardize care based on best practices, and aggregate data to improve outcomes.

6. *Information Technology: Supporting New Care Models:* Between 2015 and 2025 hospitals and physicians will embrace a new platform to use technology in the healthcare delivery. The technology emphasizes mobile devices and applications, social media, predictive analytics, and mHealth personal toolkits to connect patients to providers in direct, streamlined ways. The future will see significant investment in information technology to achieve interoperability across electronic health records systems and data warehouses to support new care and payment models. Significant investment will be required to create data warehouses and health information exchanges to support clinical integration and population health management. Competitive advantage will come to information technology systems and big data if they can securely connect providers to one another and to their patients anytime, anywhere, on any device, with subsecond response times.

7. *Transparency and Accountability:* There will be a push for quality and price transparency as consumers, employers, and others want to know what services will cost to compare quality and price among providers. The Centers for Medicare and Medicaid Services (CMS) is providing charge, payment (price), and quality information to consumers using its Medicare Provider Utilization and Payment Data files and Hospital Compare and Physician Compare Websites. CMS's release

of charge and payment data provides price transparency. Many states are implementing all payer claims databases, which will significantly boost price transparency and consumerism for healthcare services. This, linked with proliferation of high-deductible health plans, puts healthcare into the "retail" space as never before—price does matter. Price transparency must be inextricably connected with quality clinical outcomes as key variables in the value equation.

8. *Workforce/Culture of Accountability:* The near future will see layoffs and right-sizing, especially among nonclinical staff to reduce operating costs. The effects of the baby boom will be felt as more clinicians retire. Provider plans for their replacement must include balancing skills mix, cost constraints, staffing ratios, and flat volumes. The next few years will bring unionization efforts, labor strife, and workforce actions. Mergers and acquisitions will result in eliminating areas of duplication. To preserve smooth operations and bolster morale among remaining staff, change must be managed effectively. Culture and accountability planning and management will be essential to successful mergers and affiliations in all types of organizations.

9. *Population Health Management:* One of the three basic elements of the Institute for Healthcare Improvement *Triple Aim* (Institute for Healthcare Improvement, 2016)[1] is to improve population health. Strategic plans must include at least one strategy related to managing population health. Organizations that focus on population health will invest in infrastructure, such as information technology, data warehousing, predictive analytics, care models, care teams, and risk-based payment structures that align financial and clinical incentives for stakeholders. To be successful, physician leaders must champion population health initiatives. Patient engagement strategies must create shared accountability for wellness, compliance, and maintenance of personal health.

10. *Governance:* By 2017 and beyond many organizations will be grappling with board structure and governance issues. These issues arise when organizations merge, align, form joint ventures, and create new enterprises with multiple members or owners. Boards must become more streamlined, strategically focused, and composed of individuals with specific knowledge, experience, and bases for representation. Health systems must avoid the tendency to form numerous boards or add board members for each new venture or acquisition. Too many boards and boards that are too large create a cumbersome, ineffective structure for decision making and accountability. Allowing additional board seats for each acquisition furthers a culture of governance that

rewards decisions based on individual interests rather than decisions that benefit the enterprise. An effective, enterprise-specific board will be a competitive advantage as hospitals, health systems, accountable care organizations, clinically integrated networks, and other entities are formed to provide consumers with preferred healthcare services.

NEXT STEPS

Chadwick is pleased with the substance and quality of McKee's environmental assessment. The task of analyzing, synthesizing, and prioritizing these findings—including developing a summary of strategic issues and market plans—lies ahead.

DISCUSSION QUESTIONS

1. Using McKee's environmental assessment, what are Community Medical's most important strengths, weaknesses, opportunities, and threats (SWOT analysis)?

2. Identify and analyze Community Medical's most important strategic issues.

3. In what ways should Community Medical's strategic issues determine its strategic marketing plan?

4. What key issues should McKee and her teammates emphasize to position Community Medical and promote it to service area physicians, patients, payers, and the general public?

5. After completing the environmental assessment—including the SWOT analysis and summary of strategic issues—Chadwick, McKee, and Community Medical leadership must develop business and operating plans to advance the organization's strategic initiatives. Identify the elements of an effective marketing plan.

APPENDIX A

Greater Fresno Area Hospitals

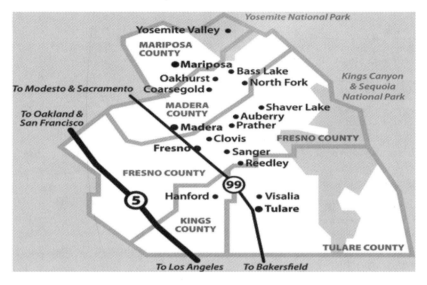

Figure 10.A.1. Greater Fresno area map.

- Adventist Medical Center–Reedley*
- Adventist Medical Center–Selma*
- Clovis Community Medical Center–Clovis*
- Coalinga Regional Medical Center–Coalinga*
- Community Behavioral Health Center–Fresno
- Community Regional Medical Center–Fresno*
- Community Subacute and Transitional Care Center–Fresno
- Crestwood Psychiatric Health Facility–Fresno
- Coalinga State Hospital–Coalinga
- Fresno Heart and Surgical Hospital–Fresno*
- Fresno Surgical Hospital–Fresno
- Kaiser Foundation Hospital–Fresno*
- San Joaquin Valley Rehabilitation Hospital–Fresno
- St. Agnes Medical Center–Fresno*

*Acute care hospitals.

APPENDIX B

Case Mix Data for Selected Fresno Area Hospitals

Hospital	2015	2014	2013	2012	2011	2010	2009	2008
Clovis Community Medical Center (CMC)	1.02	0.98	0.99	0.97	0.94	0.91	0.88	0.88
Coalinga Regional Medical Center	0.94	0.95	0.92	0.92	0.88	0.85	0.88	0.83
Community Regional Medical Center – Fresno (CMC)	1.39	1.37	1.34	1.35	1.32	1.27	1.23	1.20
St. Agnes Medical Center	1.42	1.36	1.29	1.29	1.27	1.26	1.28	1.24
San Joaquin Valley Rehabilitation Hospital	1.20	1.33	1.31	1.32	1.24	1.20	1.23	1.07
Fresno Surgical Hospital	2.31	2.27	2.22	2.09	2.00	1.92	1.82	1.68
Kaiser Foundation Hospital – Fresno	1.29	1.33	1.26	1.28	1.22	1.24	1.23	1.20
Fresno Heart and Surgical Hospital (CMC)	2.06	2.00	1.97	2.05	2.10	2.01	2.04	2.26

Note: Formula for calculating the case mix index (or average Medicare severity diagnosis-related group [MS-DRG] weight) per hospital: Sum of the MS-DRG weights of all records/ total number of discharges. Numbers greater than 100 indicate a higher level of acuity. Numbers less than 100 are a lower level of acuity.

APPENDIX C

Selected Procedures with Annual Volumes at Selected Fresno County Hospitals (2011)

Hospital name	Esophageal resection	Pancreatic resection	Pancreatic resection (cancer)	Pancreatic resection (other)	Abdominal aortic aneurysm (AAA) repair	CABG	Percutaneous coronary intervention (angioplasty with stent)	Carotid endarterectomy
Clovis Community Medical Center (CMC)	3	8	5	3			87	1
Community Regional Medical Center – Fresno (CMC)	1	35	20	15	18	256	382	21
Fresno Heart and Surgical Hospital (CMC)	4	4	3	1	16	171	86	128
Kaiser Foundation Hospital – Fresno					7		2	22

Note: CABG, coronary artery bypass graft.

APPENDIX D

Selected California Hospital Performance Ratings for Coronary Artery Bypass Graft (CABG) Surgery as Compared to the Statewide Average (2011)

Hospital name	Operative mortality[1]	Postoperative stroke[2]	30-day readmission[3]	Internal mammary artery use[4]
Community Regional Medical Center – Fresno (CMC)	Average	Average	Average	Average
Fresno Heart and Surgical Hospital	Average	Average	Average	Average
St. Agnes Medical Center	Average	Average	Average	Average

Source: California Office of Statewide Health Planning and Development (OSHPD), 2011 data.

[1] Operative mortality is defined as patient death occurring in the hospital after CABG surgery, regardless of length of stay, or death occurring anywhere after hospital discharge but within 30 days after the CABG surgery. Hospital ratings are risk adjusted using a statistical technique that allows for fair comparison of hospital outcomes even though some hospitals have sicker patients than average.

[2] Postoperative stroke is defined as a postoperative, central neurologic deficit persisting for more than 24 hours after CABG surgery while in the operating hospital. Hospital ratings are risk adjusted using a statistical technique that allows for fair comparison of hospital outcomes even though some hospitals have sicker patients than average.

[3] Readmission is defined as a CABG surgery patient being readmitted to an acute care hospital within 30 days of being discharged to home or a nonacute care setting with a principal diagnosis indicating a heart-related condition, or an infection or a complication that was likely related to the CABG surgery. Hospital ratings are risk adjusted using a statistical technique that allows for fair comparison of hospital outcomes even though some hospitals have sicker patients than average.

[4] Internal mammary artery (IMA) usage in CABG surgery is an evidence-based indicator of surgery quality. Clinical research shows that IMA grafts used in CABG surgery stay open longer and increase patients' survival. Very low hospital utilization rates may be associated with poorer care. Hospitals are not assessed for very high IMA-usage rates because there is no consensus on what constitutes an optimal rate. Most first-time CABG surgery patients are eligible to receive an IMA bypass.

ENDNOTES

Information about the Fresno, California, healthcare market, including hospital and health system providers, physician and allied health community, and payer and health insurance community was taken from the California Office of Statewide Health Planning and Development (OSHPD) website, and the California HealthCare Foundation, *California Health Care Almanac*. The scenario and persons described in this case are fictitious.

1. The IHI Triple Aim is a framework developed by the Institute for Healthcare Improvement that describes an approach to optimizing health system performance. It is IHI's belief that new designs must be developed to simultaneously pursue three dimensions, called the Triple Aim:
   • Improving the patient experience of care (including quality and satisfaction)
   • Improving the health of populations
   • Reducing the per capita cost of health care

REFERENCES

California HealthCare Foundation. (2009). *California health care almanac*. Fresno: Poor economy, poor health status stress an already fragmented system. Regional markets issue brief, July, 2009. Retrieved May 1, 2012, from http://www.chcf.org/~/media/MEDIA%20LIBRARY%20Files/PDF/A/PDF%20AlmanacRegMktBriefFresno09.pdf

Institute for Healthcare Improvement. (2016). The triple aim. Retrieved June 28, 2016, from http://www.ihi.org/resources/Pages/Publications/TripleAimCareHealthandCost.aspx

Masters, G., & Valentine, S. (2015). Ten trends that will shape healthcare strategic priorities in 2015. The Governance Institute's E-Briefings, *12*(1). Retrieved June 13, 2016, from http://www.thecamdengroup.com/wp-content/uploads/Ten_Trends_That_Will_Shape_Healthcare_Priorities_in_2015.pdf

Office of Statewide Health Planning and Development (OSHPD), Healthcare Information Division. (2016). Retrieved July 5, 2016, from http://www.oshpd.ca.gov/

11

Western Healthcare Systems

A Healthcare Delivery Continuum

Robert C. Myrtle
University of Southern California, Los Angeles, CA

CASE HISTORY/BACKGROUND

The history of Western Healthcare Systems can be characterized as one of progressively responding to current and emerging community healthcare needs. In the mid-1940s civic and community leaders identified the need for a new community hospital. Under the leadership of Davis Mitac, a prominent businessman, a citizen's committee was formed and plans were drawn for building a new community hospital. When Astrid Bennett made a $500,000 contribution for the new hospital in memory of her husband, Freemont, these plans were put into motion. A fund-raising campaign was launched, and Western County citizens responded generously by providing hundreds of thousands of dollars for the hospital.

Western Community Hospital opened in April 1962. As the first hospital built in Western County in 32 years, the new facility relieved a critical bed shortage by adding 169 medical and surgical beds and 32 maternity beds to the community's healthcare resources. Through the years, the community leaders who formed Western Community Hospital stayed involved and provided the progressive thinking and direction that enabled the hospital to assume a leadership position in the healthcare community. This support led to an expansion of beds in 1975 and the addition of a medical office building on hospital property across the street. While modest renovations have taken place since 1975, the size of the hospital has not changed. Of the hospital's 267 beds, 240 are licensed for medical/surgical patients, 12 are intensive care unit–cardiac care unit beds, and 25 are licensed for maternity services. Last year the hospital maintained a 70.1 percent occupancy level.

WESTERN HEALTHCARE SYSTEMS

In June 1993, Western's board of directors asked Health Planning Associates to study the healthcare needs of the community and the changing environmental and economic conditions of Western County and the surrounding metropolitan area. The report noted that the healthcare environment is rapidly changing. While Western Community Hospital has an excellent reputation and attracts many clients from outside its service area, the consultants note that the area surrounding the hospital was growing more slowly than other areas in the county. Although many of Western Community Hospital's patients are wealthy or covered by third-party health plans, the report notes that residents in areas immediately surrounding the hospital are poorer, less well educated, and more likely to be elderly or a member of a minority group. The consultants note that the areas northwest and south of Western Community Hospital are growing more rapidly, with higher proportions of affluent and better-educated residents. While consultants point out that there is no critical need for new hospital beds, they note that a "lack of coordination" in healthcare delivery and the poor operating performance of several hospitals in the area create a strategic opportunity for Western.

Acting on the recommendations of the consultants, Western Community Hospital made a series of decisions to improve its competitive position in its environment while continuing to pursue its mission of providing quality healthcare to the residents of Western's service area. In September 1998, Western signed an agreement to manage Kettering Memorial, a 181-bed, general acute care hospital located in the northeast portion of the county. Six months later Western was asked if it might be interested in purchasing Kettering. The board agreed to purchase Kettering, and Western Healthcare Systems was formed.

Over the years Western responded to economic and environmental changes. In January 2001, Western Healthcare Systems acquired William

Frances Stair Community Hospital. Located in the southern part of the county, this 250-bed hospital provided Western Healthcare with a horizontally integrated delivery system. A few years later they added a full-service inpatient and outpatient rehabilitation center to the William Frances Stair facility. Shortly thereafter they acquired Pleasant Valley Hospital, a 120-bed acute care psychiatric hospital providing a full range of inpatient and outpatient psychiatric services, completing what some had described as a geographically and strategically diversified delivery system.

DEVELOPING A HEALTHCARE DELIVERY CONTINUUM

In 2010, with the passage of the Patient Protection and Affordable Care Act, Western Healthcare Systems' board asked Hospital Planning Associates to provide a comprehensive review of the health, economic, and service delivery conditions of Western County and the surrounding metropolitan areas. Their report indicated that Western Healthcare had been very strategic in its acquisitions. This strategy helped maintain market share in an increasingly competitive environment. The consultants noted that operating margins were better than most facilities in the area, but were declining, primarily because of changes in reimbursement policies and service delivery activities. The consultants stated, "While Western Healthcare Systems has extended its presence in key geographic sectors of the area, it must move beyond its present inpatient focus to encompass an expanded service continuum." The consultant report notes four areas that Western Healthcare Systems should focus on:

1. Acute care: strengthen its position in this area of patient care by establishing centers of excellence and adopting a product-line management strategy

2. Behavioral health: expand the role and function of Pleasant Valley Hospital to create a major behavior health center providing comprehensive treatment, including preventive, therapeutic, and rehabilitative services

3. After care: develop specific services for the care of patients with chronic disease, as well as for those who need outpatient services, day care, home health, hospice, subacute, nursing home and long-term convalescent, or rehabilitative care

4. Ambulatory care: shift its focus from facility-based outpatient clinic care to include freestanding ambulatory and urgent care service centers, clinics, and alternative delivery systems and mechanisms

COMMUNITY HEALTHCARE NETWORK

Shortly after accepting the consultant's report, the Western Healthcare Systems' board was asked by A. P. Wilinski, President of First Western National Bank, if it might be interested in an equity position in Community Healthcare Network, one of the region's rapidly growing multispecialty medical groups. George Harrison and his two sons formed Community Healthcare Network in 1929 shortly after graduating from University Medical School. Harrison Clinic, as it was known at that time, experienced steady growth through the 1930s. In 1946, Dr. Harrison retired. With their father's retirement, the Harrison brothers asked a former university classmate to join their practice on a salaried basis. Over the next five years Harrison Clinic grew and additional physicians were hired. In 1951 the medical group began to experience growing pains. A clinic administrator was recruited, and the five salaried physicians were given full partnership status in the medical group.

The ensuing years saw rapid growth and development in Western County. This growth created an increased demand for medical care, which was met by an increase in the number of physicians affiliated with the medical group. By 1965, the medical staff had grown to 30, housed in two office buildings located in the north-central and western areas of the county.

During the planning for the second clinic, the general partners formed a new corporate entity named the Community Healthcare Network. While Harrison Clinic is a named unit in the new organization, the Community Healthcare Network soon established its own identity as an important healthcare provider in the community. At present, the Community Healthcare Network operates five clinics in Western County, with a sixth under construction. It has 68 physician partners, employs a support staff that numbers over 270 full-time equivalent positions, operates its own clinical laboratory, and has an annual operating budget of $27,094,003.51. It has contracts with four of the six health maintenance organizations operating in the county. All physicians are partners in the corporation and are compensated under a base draw, personal productivity formula system. Other employees are compensated on a salary or contractual basis.

While Community Healthcare Network provides a stable and viable practice environment for its physicians, the group has experienced cash flow and organizational difficulties associated with the recent expansion activities and partnership share refunds to retiring members. Although the group is otherwise financially solvent, it has been exploring several organizational and financial options to reverse its current difficulties. It was this search that brought the group's plight to Wilinski's attention.

THE COMMUNITY HEALTHCARE NETWORK DECISION

With the board's approval, the leadership of Western Healthcare asked Anderson & Anderson, a prominent consulting firm, to study the financial, legal and organizational options that might be worth pursuing. Anderson & Anderson reported that the network's physicians were positive about many aspects of their practice. Turnover within the group was quite low, and because of its reputation and location, it experienced little difficulty in recruiting new members. The consultants pointed out that the group's physicians expressed concern about the competitive changes taking place in the healthcare industry, reporting that some physicians were very unhappy with the continued influx of new doctors to the region and the aggressive moves of several area hospitals to develop satellite clinics and acquire group practices. The report also indicated that several partners felt there was a need for the network to expand into several rapidly growing areas of the county. Funding this expansion, particularly in light of the practice-building activities of different hospitals and partnership fee refunds to a growing number of retiring associates, does not seem possible under the current capitalization plan.

The consultants noted that the network's senior management was capable, although they focused more on operational than strategic issues. Each clinic operated in a quasi-autonomous fashion, with little integration of medical, financial, and administrative systems. Although the network's executive officer had attempted to develop an integrated management and patient care information system, progress was very slow due to the nature of the decision-making processes within the medical group and the concerns of many physicians over how these changes would affect day-to-day operations of the clinics. Any attempt to develop organizational structures and management processes that appeared to reduce the autonomy or control in the clinics was likely to be resisted.

The consultants also pointed out that different members of the medical staffs at Western Community, Kettering, and Stair had stated their concerns about the possibility that Western Healthcare Systems would also acquire group practices to be operated by member hospitals. One of the most vocal physicians in opposition was responsible for nearly 20 percent of admissions to Kettering. Nonetheless the consultants felt that because most of the network's medical staff had privileges at the hospitals operated by Western Healthcare, they felt this concern could be managed or diffused.

These issues notwithstanding, the consultants felt that some form of collaborative or interorganizational arrangement offered considerable strategic opportunities for Western Healthcare. While financing different alliances would create cash flow difficulties in the short run, the longer-term projection was positive. And, since opportunities such as this occur infrequently, it is a course that they recommended Western Healthcare explore.

ASSIGNMENT

You are part of a senior-level planning group that Western Healthcare has formed in response to the consultant's report to review the recommendations of both Hospital Planning Associates and Anderson & Anderson. Using the information in Tables 11.1–11.11, and Figure 11.1, complete the following exercises:

1. Indicate what strategies and actions Western Healthcare should undertake in response to changing conditions and emerging opportunities identified.

2. Prepare an outline describing the risks your strategy entails and the steps Western should take to overcome them.

3. Develop an implementation plan and timetable that identify the level, nature, and means for integrating the strategy you are recommending with the functions and activities of Western's hospitals and other patient care delivery units.

4. Address any other issues critical to the successful implementation of your suggested strategy.

Table 11.1. Western Healthcare Systems facilities

	Western Community Hospital	Kettering Memorial Hospital	William Francis Stair Community Hospital	Clearview Rehabilitation Center	Pleasant Valley Hospital
Beds	367	181	250	NA	120
Personnel full-time equivalent	735	462	691	183	279
Outpatient emergency room visits	93,317	30,577	48,727	106,635	25,419
Gross revenue (thousands)	$75,123	$61,311	$77,985	$9,337	$52,486
Medical staff	375	214	345	37	81
Total Patient days	68,316	45,122	65,426	NA	40,165

Source: Last year's annual report of Western Healthcare Systems.

Table 11.2. Community Healthcare Systems network facilities

	Broadway Clinic	Hillside Clinic	Tivoli Clinic	Harrison Clinic	34th Street Clinic
Medical staff	18	14	12	10	14
Personnel (full-time equivalent)	83	52	38	39	58
Clinic visits	86,112	68,432	53,358	44,986	63,409
Gross revenue (thousands)	$5,652	$4,516	$4,784	$4,104	$4,262

Source: Last year's annual report of Community Healthcare Systems.

Table 11.3. Western County population statistics by health facility planning areas (HFPAs), and major population centers

Geographic area	1960 Census	1970 Census	1980 Census	1990 Census	2000 Census	2010 Census
HFPA 1	58,395	70,075	80,584	97,507	116,444	136,484
Cypress Valley	33,869	41,421	48,677	59,576	71,021	84,585
HFPA 2	50,803	63,768	67,584	86,781	103,964	125,796
Belmont Heights	28,450	36,794	40,903	54,854	62,704	79,069
HFPA 3	76,497	93,199	109,683	134,087	160,650	180,909
Desmond	44,146	53,878	65,492	81,245	95,138	112,358
HFPA 4	123,213	138,817	143,521	150,268	153,424	156,661
Arlington	74,051	82,926	83,257	85,668	88,986	90,096
Western County totals	308,908	365,859	401,372	468,643	534,482	599,850

Source: Western State Department of Health and Human Services, 2012.

Table 11.4. Demographic characteristics of Western County

	1960 Census (%)	1970 Census (%)	1980 Census (%)	1990 Census (%)	2000 Census (%)	2010 Census (%)
Age group						
0–14	40.4	38.7	35.4	26.3	24.9	22.6
15–44	43.1	43.3	45.2	49.6	46.4	43.2
45–64	11.7	13.1	14.2	16.3	18.6	22.6
65+	4.8	4.9	5.2	7.8	10.1	11.6
Ethnicity						
Black	9.6	10.4	10.6	10.9	11.3	11.5
Hispanic	NA	NA	5.9	7.1	7.4	7.9
Other nonwhite	NA	NA	3.6	4.2	4.5	4.7

Note: NA, not available.
Source: Western County Agency for Economic Development, 2010.

Table 11.5. Demographic characteristics of Western County by health facility planning area (HFPA)

	1960 Census (%)	1970 Census (%)	1980 Census (%)	1990 Census (%)	2000 Census (%)	2010 Census (%)
HFPA 1						
Age group						
0–14	41.2	39.5	36.2	31.8	27.7	25.1
15–44	43.5	43.8	45.7	47.9	48.0	48.6
45–64	11.5	12.8	14.0	14.6	16.3	17.1
65+	3.7	3.9	4.1	4.1	7.9	9.1
Ethnicity						
Black	8.5	9.3	9.4	9.7	10.0	10.2
Hispanic	NA	NA	5.2	6.3	6.6	7.0
Other nonwhite	NA	NA	3.7	4.2	4.5	4.8
HFPA 2						
Age group						
0–14	41.9	40.2	38.1	35.1	30.3	26.1
15–44	43.2	44.7	45.3	46.7	47.7	48.6
45–64	11.2	11.3	12.1	12.3	14.1	16.1
65+	3.7	3.8	4.4	5.9	7.8	9.3
Ethnicity						
Black	8.3	8.9	9.1	9.3	9.6	9.8
Hispanic	NA	NA	4.7	5.8	6.1	6.4
Other nonwhite	NA	NA	3.7	4.3	4.6	4.9

HFPA 3

Age Group

0–14	43.0	42.1	41.2	38.4	34.6	33.3
15–44	42.1	42.1	42.2	43.1	43.8	41.4
45–64	11.3	11.8	12.2	13.7	14.9	16.1
65+	3.6	4.0	4.3	4.8	6.8	9.2

Ethnicity

Black	8.5	9.2	9.4	9.7	10.0	10.2
Hispanic	NA	NA	4.7	5.7	6.0	6.4
Other nonwhite	NA	NA	3.8	4.3	4.9	4.9

HFPA 4

Age group

0–14	39.4	38.2	36.0	34.1	32.3	29.6
15–44	43.3	40.6	39.5	37.7	36.5	34.4
45–64	12.2	15.7	17.9	19.5	21.0	23.1
65+	5.2	5.5	6.6	8.7	10.2	12.9

Ethnicity

Black	19.1	10.8	11.1	11.4	11.8	12.0
Hispanic	NA	NA	6.9	7.3	7.7	8.2
Other nonwhite	NA	NA	3.7	4.2	4.5	4.8

Note: NA, not available.
Source: Western State Department of Health and Human Services, 2012.

Table 11.6. Western County acute care facilities by health facility planning area (HFPA)

Facility and location	Sponsorship	Total beds	Medical	ICU/CCU	OB/GYN	Pediatric	Psychiatric	Occupancy (%)
HFPA 1								
Oakwood Community	Nonprofit	125	99	4	16	6		67.7
Valley District	Public	50	38	4	6	4		83.9
Cypress Valley								
Carson Memorial	Nonprofit	85	60	5	19	10		57.3
St. Luke	Nonprofit	150	70	10	30	30	10	67.7
Valley Doctors	For profit	76	62	4	10			54.4
HFPA 2								
University Hospital and Medical Center	Public	250	145	15	50	30	10	80.1
Belmont Heights								
Western County	Public	180	110	15	30	15	10	80.8
HFPA 3								
Overlook Community	Nonprofit	80	62	4	10	4		64.7
Ward Howard District	Public	50	50					57.4
Desmond								
Cedars of Lebanon	Nonprofit	133	94	7	20	12		68.6
Kettering Memorial	Nonprofit	181	123	8	30	20		68.3
HFPA 4								
IHS Doctors	For profit	80	76	4				72.3
William Frances Stair	Nonprofit	250	190	10	30	20		71.7
Arlington								
St. Bernadine	Nonprofit	153	95	8	30	20		67.3
Western Community	Nonprofit	267	195	12	25	25	10	70.1

Note: CCU, critical care unit; IHS, IHS Doctors Hospital; ICU, intensive care unit; OB/GYN, obstetrics/gynecology.

Table 11.7. Western County physician workforce distribution by specialty

Specialty	1960 Census	1970 Census	1980 Census	1990 Census	2000 Census	2010 Census
Primary care specialties	202	223	245	259	365	440
Other medical non-surgical specialties	24	30	34	48	60	70
Surgical specialties	127	159	178	182	210	235
All other physician specialties	138	159	172	197	250	290
Total physicians	491	571	629	686	885	1,035

Source: Western State Department of Health and Human Services, 2012.

Table 11.8. Western County physician workforce distribution by specialty and health facility planning area (HFPA)

Specialty	1960 Census	1970 Census	1980 Census	1990 Census	2000 Census	2010 Census
HFPA 1						
Primary care	24	32	42	48	90	120
Other medical nonsurgical specialties	3	4	6	11	15	20
Surgical	15	22	31	41	50	65
All other physician specialties	16	22	30	44	60	80
Total physicians	58	80	109	144	215	285
HFPA 2						
Primary care	23	30	36	50	70	95
Other medical nonsurgical specialties	3	4	5	9	10	15
Surgical	14	21	26	35	40	50
All other physician specialties	15	21	25	38	50	65
Total physicians	55	76	92	132	170	225
HFPA 3						
Primary care	32	42	57	58	120	160
Other medical nonsurgical specialties	4	6	8	11	20	25
Surgical	19	29	41	41	70	85
All other physician specialties	21	29	40	44	80	105
Total physicians	76	106	146	154	290	375
HFPA 4						
Primary care	123	119	110	93	85	65
Other medical nonsurgical specialties	14	16	15	17	15	10
Surgical	79	87	80	65	50	35
All other physician specialties	86	87	77	71	60	40
Total physicians	302	309	282	246	210	150

Source: Western State Department of Health and Human Services, 2012.

Table 11.9. Type of physician practice arrangement

Health facility planning area	Solo	Partnership	Group	Other	Total
1	62	94	109	20	285
2	53	68	77	27	225
3	52	92	175	56	375
4	29	37	63	21	150
Total	196	291	424	124	1,035

Source: Anderson & Anderson analysis, current year.

Table 11.10. Community Health Network statement of income and expenses for fiscal year just ended

Patient Service Revenue		
Private insurance	$16,430,181.33	
Self-pay	$6,790,325.92	
Medicare	$2,154,622.80	
Medicaid	$1,150,997.46	
Other	$567,876.00	
Gross patent revenue		$27,094,003.51
Less		
Contractual allowances and adjustments	($1,214,422.52)	
Bad debt	($3,206,282.50)	
Total adjustments		($4,420,705.02)
Net patient revenue	$22,673,298.49	
Other operating revenue	$2,392,657.00	
Total operating revenue		$25,065,955.49
Operating expenses		
Physician services	($8,999,673.20)	
Nursing services	($4,005,519.91)	
Other professional services	($804,650.00)	
Administrative services	($399,000.00)	
General services	($536,432.93)	
Office and clerical services	($637,292.05)	
Supplies and expenses	($1,523,960.00)	
Pension and insurance	($4,360,341.16)	
Depreciation	($1,241,334.08)	
Interest	($2,482,668.16)	
Total operating expenses		($24,990,871.49)
Nonoperating revenue		
Rental income	$30,390.00	
Investment income	$243,124.00	
Total nonoperating revenue		$273,514.00
Excess of revenue over expenses		$348,598.00

Source: Community Health Network annual report.

Table 11.11. Western Healthcare Systems statement of operating income and expense for last two years

	Second most recent statement	Previous year's statement
Patient service revenue	$389,499,246.00	$327,584,262.00
Less		
Allowances and bad debt	($87,714,255.20)	($63,605,256.00)
Net patient service revenue	$301,784,990.80	$263,979,006.00
Plus		
Other operating revenue	$10,157,460.00	$5,955,947.20
Total operating revenue	$311,942,450.80	$269,934,953.20
Operating expenses		
Nursing services	($83,256,424.90)	($74,247,098.10)
Other professional services	($134,554,946.40)	($118,028,653.00)
General services	($33,874,111.00)	($33,479,628.00)
Fiscal services	($17,079,984.90)	($14,783,283.90)
Administrative services	($29,332,977.10)	($18,549,054.00)
Depreciation	($12,956,063.40)	($10,753,700.58)
Total operating expenses	($311,054,507.70)	($269,841,417.58)
Operating gain(loss)	$887,943.10	$93,535.62
Nonoperating revenue and expense		
Unrestricted gifts and bequests	$467,310.00	$564,540.00
Income from investments	$6,614,784.00	$5,853,650.00
Gain on sale of investments	$2,550,000.00	$613,000.00
Net nonoperating revenue	$9,632,094.00	$7,031,190.00
Total gain (loss)	$10,520,037.10	$7,124,725.62

Source: Western Healthcare Systems annual report.

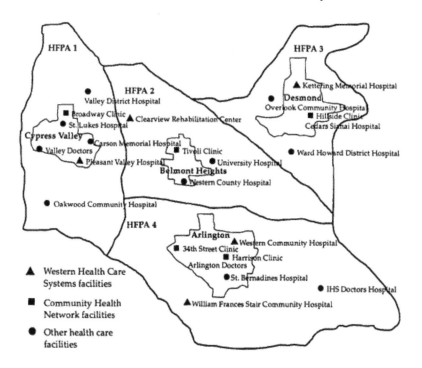

Figure 11.1. Western County Health Facility planning areas. (*Source*: Western Healthcare Systems strategic plan)

ENDNOTE

This case adapted from "Western Health Care Systems," published in *Strategic Alignment: Managing Integrated Health Systems*, Douglas A. Conrad and Jeffrey Hoare, eds., Ann Arbor, MI: AUPHA Press/Health Administration Press, 1994.

PART III

Organizational Management

12

Hartland Memorial Hospital

Part 1: In-Box and Prioritization Exercise

Kent V. Rondeau
University of Alberta, Edmonton, Alberta, Canada

John E. Paul
University of North Carolina at Chapel Hill

Jonathon S. Rakich
Indiana University Southeast, New Albany, IN

CASE HISTORY/BACKGROUND

Hartland Memorial Hospital, established 85 years ago when wealthy benefactor Sir Reginald Hartland left an estate valued at more than $2 million, is a 285-bed, freestanding community general hospital located in Westfield, a ski resort community of 85,000 people. Ridgeview Hospital is the only other hospital in the area, situated some 18 miles away in the village of Easton. Hartland Memorial is a fully accredited institution that provides a full range of medical and surgical services. It has an excellent reputation for delivering high-quality medical care for the citizens of Westfield and the surrounding area.

YOU AND THE HOSPITAL

You are Elizabeth Parsons, BSN, MSN, PhD, Vice President for Nursing Services, at Hartland Memorial. You accepted this position 17 months ago and have been instrumental in introducing a number of innovations in nursing practice and management. In particular, these innovations have included the establishment of job sharing, self-scheduling, and a compressed work week for all general-duty nurses. In addition, you have also developed a new performance appraisal system and are contemplating using it to create a merit pay system for the nursing staff.

Your administrative assistant, Wilma Smith, handles your correspondence, as well as scheduling meetings and conferences. Each morning she opens hard-copy mail and memos and puts them on your desk. She also places hard-copy phone messages on your desk, for those people who did not want to be routed to your voice mail. Although she has access to your e-mail, voice mail, and electronic calendar, she does not routinely monitor them. Wilma is only moderately comfortable with the new modes of communicating, generally preferring the ways of the "pre-electronic" era.

Your second-in-command is Anne Armstrong, who is assistant director for nursing services. Anne has worked at Hartland Memorial for seven years and is very competent. She has only recently returned to work, however, after spending some time in the hospital recovering from the suicide of her husband. A list of the key personnel at Hartland Memorial is presented in Figure 12.1, and selected biographical sketches can be found in Figure 12.2.

THE SITUATION

You have just returned from a needed long weekend off. At your husband's insistence, the two of you left Thursday evening for a mountain resort, and you just got back last night. Long hours, high stress, and constantly being accessible by cell phone, voice mail, and e-mail have been taking their toll—you seem to have been "on-call" continuously for months now. Compounding these "curses-of-the-modern-job" have been meeting the needs ("being there") for your school-age kids, and, a recent development, the demands of addressing your parents' needs as they age. In particular, your mom seems increasingly incapable of taking care of your dad, for whom some other living arrangements may have to be found. Caught between responsibilities with kids and parents (to say nothing about spouse) you are truly in the "sandwich" generation.

The weekend away, however, was wonderful. You were out of cell phone coverage, and the inn did not make their computer generally available

Name	Position
Allan Reid	President and CEO
Scott Little	Assistant to the president
Elizabeth Parsons	Vice president–Nursing Service
Anne Armstrong	Assistant director–Nursing Service
Cynthia Nichols	Vice president–Human Resources
Clement Westaway, MD	President–medical staff
Janet Trist	Nursing supervisor–3 East
Sylvia Godfrey	Weekend supervisor
Jane Sawchuck	Clinical nurse specialist
Norm Sutter	Vice president–Finance
Marion Simpson	Auditing clerk
Fran Nixon	Staff relations officer
George Cross	Nurse's Union representative
Bernard Stevens	Chairman of the board
Wilma Smith	Administrative assistant

Figure 12.1. List of key personnel at Hartland Memorial Hospital.

Elizabeth Parsons	A professionally trained and degreed registered nurse (BSN, MEd). Age 45, with 20 years of progressive management and nursing experience. Married to Neal Parsons, two children, age 10 and 12.
Allan Reid	CEO at Hartland Hospital for 2 years. Age 36, with 5 years of experience as an assistant administrator at a 100-bed rural hospital. MHA degree. Married, two children.
Bernard Stevens	Colonel, US Army Infantry (retired). Chairman of the board for Hartland Hospital for the past 12 years. Age 70. Widower, four grown children.
Clement Westaway, MD	Medical degree from the University of Pennsylvania. Internist. Member of the Hartland medical staff for 30 years and president of medical staff for the past 10 years. Age 64. Divorced, two grown children. Son is resident physician at Hartland.
Anne Armstrong	Assistant director of nursing service at Hartland for the past five years. MSN degree. Age 35. Recently widowed, two children.
Janet Trist	Nursing supervisor. Interrupted career at age 26 to raise her children. Resumed working two years ago. RN (diploma program). Age 41. Married.
Wilma Smith	Administrative assistant in her present position for the past 15 years. Has worked at Hartland for 28 years. Age 50. Single, no children.

Figure 12.2. Brief biographical sketches of key players at Hartland Memorial Hospital.

to guests. In any case, your husband would have probably left you if you'd logged on or called in.

Sunday night after getting home you had planned on logging on and assessing the situation facing you at work, after four blessed days out of touch. The kids, however, needed attention, the dog needed walking, and your mom called and talked for over an hour about what to do about your dad. You never got to your voice mail, either.

It is now 7:45 a.m. on Monday morning, and you have just a little over one hour until your first meeting of the day with Norm Sutter, vice president for finance. You really have to get through your e-mail, voice mail, and the hard-copy items Wilma left on your desk—letters, phone messages, etc.— and take some action before meeting with Norm. You know the rest of the day will be a blur, and you'll have no further opportunities to get caught up. Moreover, new stuff will be constantly coming in and piling up. The refreshed feeling you had after the weekend out of town is rapidly slipping away.

A hard copy schedule of your appointments for the day left on Friday by Wilma is shown in Figure 12.3. You know that it will likely be changing.

(as of 7:45 a.m.; left on your desk by Wilma, Friday afternoon at 5:00 p.m.).	
8:00 a.m.	
8:30	
9:00	Meeting with Norm Sutter
9:30	
10:00	Regular Monday morning meeting with nursing supervisors
10:30	
11:00	Meeting with Clement Westaway
11:30	
12:00 Noon	Lunch with Anne Armstrong
12:30	"
1:00	Orientation talk to new nursing recruits
1:30	"
2:00	
2:30	Meeting of infection control committee
3:00	"
3:30	
4:00	Meeting with Allan Reid
4:30	"
5:00	
5:30	

Figure 12.3. Schedule of appointments, Monday, October 7.

WHAT NEEDS TO BE DONE

The pages that follow show the various e-mails, voice mails, memos, letters, and hand-written messages that Elizabeth finds awaiting her (Figure 12.4). Since Wilma doesn't arrive until 8:30 a.m. Elizabeth has the office to herself. Note that the Hartland Hospital information technology system does a fairly good job of filtering out spam and junk mail. The occasional item does make it through, which Elizabeth immediately deletes. Additionally, however, there are the e-newsletters from The Kaiser Family Foundation, the Commonwealth Fund, American College of Healthcare Executives, etc., to which Elizabeth subscribes, but which she rarely has time to read. She tends to let these pile up in her in-box, sometimes making it hard to find the critical material there. The newsletters that came in over her mini-holiday are not included below.

For each item, indicate on the worksheet (Figure 12.4, Hartland Memorial Hospital, in-box exercise) the course of action you think Parsons should take. Be prepared to defend your underlying rationale. If delegating, identify who should be responsible for each item. *Work sequentially through each item. Do not jump ahead.*

Although you may not have all the information needed to make an informed decision (as in the real world), go ahead and make assumptions that you believe are needed to justify your actions. Make notes of those assumptions on the worksheet.

Item No.	Action Alternatives (check one)	Item Action Content (quick notes/ bullet points)
1. Scott Little (e-mail)	☐ Call Immediately	
	☐ Note to call w/in 2–3 days	
	☐ Email immediately	
	☐ Email w/in day	
	☐ Meet with ASAP	
	☐ Forward to: _____	
	☐ Note to meet w/in 2–3 days	
	☐ Other (specify: _____)	
	☐ No response needed	
2. Mabel Westfield (letter)	☐ Call Immediately	
	☐ Note to call w/in 2–3 days	
	☐ Email immediately	
	☐ Email w/in day	
	☐ Meet with ASAP	
	☐ Forward to: _____	
	☐ Note to meet w/in 2–3 days	
	☐ Other (specify: _____)	
	☐ No response needed	
3. Mom (voice mail)	☐ Call Immediately	
	☐ Note to call w/in 2–3 days	
	☐ Email immediately	
	☐ Email w/in day	
	☐ Meet with ASAP	
	☐ Forward to: _____	
	☐ Note to meet w/in 2–3 days	
	☐ Other (specify: _____)	
	☐ No response needed	

Figure 12.4. Hartland Memorial Hospital, in-box exercise (worksheet). *(continued)*

4. Allan Reid
   (e-mail)

☐ Call Immediately

☐ Note to call w/in 2–3 days

☐ Email immediately

☐ Email w/in day

☐ Meet with ASAP

☐ Forward to: _____

☐ Note to meet w/in 2–3 days

☐ Other (specify: _____)

☐ No response needed

5. Sylvia Godfrey
   (e-mail)

☐ Call Immediately

☐ Note to call w/in 2–3 days

☐ Email immediately

☐ Email w/in day

☐ Meet with ASAP

☐ Forward to: _____

☐ Note to meet w/in 2–3 days

☐ Other (specify: _____)

☐ No response needed

6. Janet Trist
   (e-mail)

☐ Call Immediately

☐ Note to call w/in 2–3 days

☐ Email immediately

☐ Email w/in day

☐ Meet with ASAP

☐ Forward to: _____

☐ Note to meet w/in 2–3 days

☐ Other (specify: _____)

☐ No response needed

7. Westfield High
   School (letter)

☐ Call Immediately

☐ Note to call w/in 2–3 days

☐ Email immediately

☐ Email w/in day

☐ Meet with ASAP

☐ Forward to: _____

☐ Note to meet w/in 2–3 days

☐ Other (specify: _____)

☐ No response needed

Figure 12.4. Hartland Memorial Hospital, in-box exercise (worksheet). *(continued)*

Item No.	Action Alternatives (check one)	Item Action Content (quick notes/bullet points)
8. Marion Simpson (e-mail)	☐ Call Immediately ☐ Note to call w/in 2–3 days ☐ Email immediately ☐ Email w/in day ☐ Meet with ASAP ☐ Forward to: _____ ☐ Note to meet w/in 2–3 days ☐ Other (specify: _____) ☐ No response needed	
9. Wilma (written note)	☐ Call Immediately ☐ Note to call w/in 2–3 days ☐ Email immediately ☐ Email w/in day ☐ Meet with ASAP ☐ Forward to: _____ ☐ Note to meet w/in 2–3 days ☐ Other (specify: _____) ☐ No response needed	
10. Neal (text message)	☐ Call Immediately ☐ Note to call w/in 2–3 days ☐ Email immediately ☐ Email w/in day ☐ Meet with ASAP ☐ Forward to:_____ ☐ Note to meet w/in 2–3 days ☐ Other (specify:_____) ☐ No response needed	

Figure 12.4. Hartland Memorial Hospital, in-box exercise (worksheet). *(continued)*

11. Cynthia Nichols
(e-mail)

☐ Call Immediately

☐ Note to call w/in 2–3 days

☐ Email immediately

☐ Email w/in day

☐ Meet with ASAP

☐ Forward to: _____

☐ Note to meet w/in 2–3 days

☐ Other (specify: _____)

☐ No response needed

12. Marion Simpson
(memo)

☐ Call Immediately

☐ Note to call w/in 2–3 days

☐ Email immediately

☐ Email w/in day

☐ Meet with ASAP

☐ Forward to: _____

☐ Note to meet w/in 2–3 days

☐ Other (specify: _____)

☐ No response needed

13. Wilma
(written note)

☐ Call Immediately

☐ Note to call w/in 2–3 days

☐ Email immediately

☐ Email w/in day

☐ Meet with ASAP

☐ Forward to: _____

☐ Note to meet w/in 2–3 days

☐ Other (specify: _____)

☐ No response needed

14. Cynthia Nichols
(e-mail)

☐ Call Immediately

☐ Note to call w/in 2–3 days

☐ Email immediately

☐ Email w/in day

☐ Meet with ASAP

☐ Forward to: _____

☐ Note to meet w/in 2–3 days

☐ Other (specify: _____)

☐ No response needed

Figure 12.4. Hartland Memorial Hospital, in-box exercise (worksheet). *(continued)*

Item No.	Action Alternatives (check one)	Item Action Content (quick notes/bullet points)
15. Scott Little (memo)	☐ Call Immediately ☐ Note to call w/in 2–3 days ☐ Email immediately ☐ Email w/in day ☐ Meet with ASAP ☐ Forward to: _____ ☐ Note to meet w/in 2–3 days ☐ Other (specify: _____) ☐ No response needed	
16. Wilma (written note)	☐ Call Immediately ☐ Note to call w/in 2–3 days ☐ Email immediately ☐ Email w/in day ☐ Meet with ASAP ☐ Forward to: _____ ☐ Note to meet w/in 2–3 days ☐ Other (specify: _____) ☐ No response needed	
17. Coach Bailey (e-mail)	☐ Call Immediately ☐ Note to call w/in 2–3 days ☐ Email immediately ☐ Email w/in day ☐ Meet with ASAP ☐ Forward to: _____ ☐ Note to meet w/in 2–3 days ☐ Other (specify: _____) ☐ No response needed	

Figure 12.4. Hartland Memorial Hospital, in-box exercise (worksheet). *(continued)*

18. Jane Sawchuck
    (e-mail)

☐ Call Immediately

☐ Note to call w/in 2–3 days

☐ Email immediately

☐ Email w/in day

☐ Meet with ASAP

☐ Forward to: _____

☐ Note to meet w/in 2–3 days

☐ Other (specify: _____)

☐ No response needed

19. Allan Reid
    (e-mail)

☐ Call Immediately

☐ Note to call w/in 2–3 days

☐ Email immediately

☐ Email w/in day

☐ Meet with ASAP

☐ Forward to: _____

☐ Note to meet w/in 2–3 days

☐ Other (specify: _____)

☐ No response needed

20. Scott Little
    (e-mail)

☐ Call Immediately

☐ Note to call w/in 2–3 days

☐ Email immediately

☐ Email w/in day

☐ Meet with ASAP

☐ Forward to: _____

☐ Note to meet w/in 2–3 days

☐ Other (specify: _____)

☐ No response needed

21. Bernard Stevens
    (phone message)

☐ Call Immediately

☐ Note to call w/in 2–3 days

☐ Email immediately

☐ Email w/in day

☐ Meet with ASAP

☐ Forward to: _____

☐ Note to meet w/in 2–3 days

☐ Other (specify: _____)

☐ No response needed

Figure 12.4. Hartland Memorial Hospital, in-box exercise (worksheet). *(continued)*

Item No.	Action Alternatives (check one)	Item Action Content (quick notes/bullet points)
22. Dr. Clement Westaway (e-mail)	☐ Call Immediately	
	☐ Note to call w/in 2–3 days	
	☐ Email immediately	
	☐ Email w/in day	
	☐ Meet with ASAP	
	☐ Forward to: _____	
	☐ Note to meet w/in 2–3 days	
	☐ Other (specify: _____)	
	☐ No response needed	
23. Cynthia Nichols (e-mail)	☐ Call Immediately	
	☐ Note to call w/in 2–3 days	
	☐ Email immediately	
	☐ Email w/in day	
	☐ Meet with ASAP	
	☐ Forward to: _____	
	☐ Note to meet w/in 2–3 days	
	☐ Other (specify: _____)	
	☐ No response needed	
24. Allan Reid (on the phone)	What do you do now?	

Figure 12.4.   Hartland Memorial Hospital, in-box exercise (worksheet). *(continued)*

Team Summary/Consensus:

1. Aside from the last item (#22), which are the four most critical items to address? (Indicate item numbers below.)

   _____

2. Think of reasons why these four items are the most critical. *What professional/personal values and priorities do they reflect?*

Total number of items marked:

_____ Call immediately   _____ Note to call w/in 2–3 days

_____ Email immediately   _____ Email w/in day

_____ Meet with ASAP   _____ Forward to

_____ Note to meet w/in 2–3 days   _____ Other: _____

_____ No response needed

3. Looking back on the work you have just laid out, is it feasible to accomplish in the time constraints faced by this administrator? What happens next? What techniques would your group suggest for Elizabeth to make it successfully through this day?

Notes/Comments:

_____
_____
_____

Figure 12.4.   Hartland Memorial Hospital, in-box exercise (worksheet). *(continued)*

ITEM 1:   E-MAIL

To: Elizabeth Parsons, VP–Nursing Service

From: Scott Little, Assistant to the President

Date: October 4

Time: 8:00 a.m.

Subject: Wandering patients–IMPORTANT!

On Thursday evening, Mrs. Grace O'Brien, a patient with diabetes and Alzheimer's disease, was missing from her room when her daughter came to visit her. It took the staff more than 3 hours to finally locate her. She was found naked and unconscious in the basement washroom of the Stuart Annex. Her daughter is extremely upset and is threatening to sue the hospital.

We don't need another lawsuit!!!

—Scott

ITEM 2:   **LETTER**

September 26

President, Hartland Hospital

Eliz: Please note. What actions are needed?
—A.

Dear Sir,
I have been a patient in your hospital on three different occasions over the last 4 years. In the past I have been very satisfied with the nursing care that I have received; however, my last stay there has left much to be desired. For the most part I have found that many of your nurses are very rude and arrogant. On a number of times when I asked these people for assistance, they would either refuse to help me, tell me they were too busy, or ignore me altogether.

I have great respect for Hartland Hospital and I trust that you would want to correct this problem. My late husband, Horace, was once a trustee at your hospital and would never have allowed this to happen.

Sincerely,
Mable Coleman Westfield

Figure 12.5. Elizabeth Parson's in-box Monday, October 7, 7:30 a.m. *(continued)*

ITEM 3:   VOICE MESSAGE

To: Elizabeth Parsons

From: Your mother

Date: Monday

Time: 7:30 a.m.

(Voice message left at 7:30 a.m. on office phone—you forgot to turn on your cell phone driving to work.)

"Elizabeth, this is Mom. I tried to get you before you left home this morning, but just missed you—Dad got up today upset and saying that he was a burden. He's gone back to sleep now. What should I do? Please call as soon as you get a chance!"

ITEM 4:   E-MAIL

To: Elizabeth Parsons, VP–Nursing Service

From: Allan Reid, President/CEO

Date: October 4

Time: 2:10 p.m.

Subject: EOM

I have heard that a number of other hospitals have been very successful at motivating their staff by implementing employee recognition programs. These programs can go a long way toward increasing employee commitment and morale. I would like to institute an "Employee-of-the-Month" award here at Hartland. I have a few ideas and would like to discuss them with you.

—A

Figure 12.5.   Elizabeth Parson's in-box Monday, October 7, 7:30 a.m. *(continued)*

ITEM 5:   E-MAIL

To: Elizabeth Parsons, VP–Nursing Service

From: Sylvia Godfrey, RN, Weekend Supervisor

Date: October 6

Time: 9:07 p.m.

Subject: Insufficient staffing

Again this weekend we had a number of nurses call in sick and we were subsequently short staffed. I had to call in nurses from the "availability list" that was provided by the Temp Placement Agency. I don't really think these nurses are any good because they are poorly trained and make too many errors. I am sick and tired of having to go through this hassle every single week!

—Sylvia

ITEM 6:   E-MAIL

To: Elizabeth Parsons, VP–Nursing Service

From: Janet Trist, RN, Supervisor–3 East

Date: October 4

Time: 1:23 p.m.

Subject: Scheduling problems

I am really having a problem with this new self-scheduling system that we adopted last month. A number of my junior nurses are refusing to go along with it and are threatening to quit because they always get stuck with the worst shifts. It's affecting the morale on my unit and making my life miserable. We need to discuss this right away.

—Janet

Figure 12.5. Elizabeth Parson's in-box Monday, October 7, 7:30 a.m. *(continued)*

ITEM 7:   LETTER

WESTFIELD HIGH SCHOOL

September 28

Elizabeth Parsons

Vice President–Nursing Service

Hartland Hospital Westfield

Dear Mrs. Parsons:

The Future Careers Club of Westfield High School would like to invite you to be the guest speaker at our November meeting. The meeting will be held on November 14 at 8:00 p.m. in the school auditorium. We would like you to discuss "The Changing Role of the Professional Nurse."

We believe that your presentation will be quite informative for us because several of our students are interested in pursuing a nursing career.

We hope that you will be able to accept this invitation. Please call our sponsor, Mrs. Bonnie Tartabull, to confirm at your earliest convenience. Thank you.

Sincerely,

Kathy Muller
President, Westfield High Future Careers Club

ITEM 8:   E-MAIL

To: Elizabeth Parsons, VP–Nursing Service

From: Marion Simpson, Auditing

Date: October 4

Time: 9:45 a.m.

Subject: Hours of work for part-time nurses

Once again, many part-time nurses are working between 25 and 30 hours per week. If we permit this to continue, under the terms of the collective agreement, we must give full-time benefits to those involved.

The agreement states that full-time benefits must be given to those working in excess of 25 hours per week.

The actual number of hours worked per week for part-timers averaged 24.5 hours for the month of September.

We want to avoid going over!

—Marion Simpson

Figure 12.5.   Elizabeth Parson's in-box Monday, October 7, 7:30 a.m. *(continued)*

ITEM 9:   WRITTEN NOTE FROM WILMA

To: Elizabeth Parsons

From: Dr. Clement Westaway, President of the Medical Staff

Date: October 2

Time: 10:20 a.m.

Subject: Dr. Westaway called, said it was urgent, but did not leave a message.

ITEM 10:   TEXT MESSAGE

Liz, message on answering machine before I left. Something about snacks for Jimmy's softball game on Monday? I'm on the course now. —Love, Neal

---

ITEM 11:   E-MAIL

To: Elizabeth Parsons, Vice President–Nursing Service

From: Cynthia Nichols, Vice President–Human Resources

Date: October 2

Time: 4:45 p.m.

Subject: Sexual harassment charges

STRICTLY CONFIDENTIAL

We have just received a notification from a nurse employed here at Hartland alleging sexual harassment by one of our physicians on staff. The charges, if verified, are extremely serious. The physician involved is Jared Westaway, senior resident, and son of Dr. Clement Westaway.

I would like to appoint you, along with Fran Nixon, from our staff relations department, and George Cross, union representative for the nurses' association, to form a committee to investigate these charges. I have been told that the nurse claiming harassment has already begun legal action, so we need to proceed quickly.

—Cynthia Nichols, Vice President

Figure 12.5. Elizabeth Parson's in-box Monday, October 7, 7:30 a.m. *(continued)*

ITEM 12:   MEMO

To: Elizabeth Parsons, Vice President–Nursing Service

From: Marion Simpson, Auditing

Date: October 3

Subject: Reimbursement for travel

Further to your request for travel reimbursement for your upcoming conference, I regret to inform you that you have already used up this year's travel
budget allocation and therefore will not be reimbursed from this account.

Marion Simpson

ITEM 13:   TELEPHONE MESSAGE

To: Elizabeth Parsons

From: Norm Sutter

Date: October 4

Time: 3:05 p.m.

Mr. Sutter called and asked if the next year's budget projections for nursing
have been finished. He needs these figures by Monday.

—Wilma

ITEM 14:   E-MAIL

To: Elizabeth Parsons, Vice President–Nursing Service

From: Cynthia Nichols, VP–Human Resources

Date: October 4

Time: 11:35 a.m.

Subject: Social media

Elizabeth—Social media, in particular Twitter (which I don't do!) seems to be
becoming more prevalent, particularly among Hartland nursing staff. Potential
problems relate to both patient confidentiality and hospital gossip. We can get
in trouble here! I've heard some of our current "hot button" issues are crop-
ping up! Ideas on how to "nip it in the bud"? Please contact me ASAP.

—Cynthia

Figure 12.5.   Elizabeth Parson's in-box Monday, October 7, 7:30 a.m. *(continued)*

ITEM 15:   MEMO

To: Elizabeth Parsons, VP–Nursing service

From: Scott Little, Assistant to the President

Date: October 3

Subject: United Way Campaign

This is a follow-up to our discussion of last week concerning the appointment of someone from your department to serve as a representative for our hospital's annual United Way Campaign. I need to have the name of your representative by tomorrow, Friday, October 4th.

—Scott

ITEM 16:   WRITTEN NOTE FROM WILMA

Date: October 4

Subject: 2:12 p.m.

Ms. Parsons—Mr. Stevens dropped in and was looking for you. He seemed quite upset and was muttering something about a lawsuit. He wants you to call him as soon as you get back from your trip.

—Wilma

ITEM 17:   E-MAIL

To: Elizabeth Parsons, Vice President–Nursing Service

From: Coach Bailey

Date: October 7

Time: 2:45 p.m.

Subject: Snacks needed!

Ms. Parsons—Left you a voice mail at home this morning. Can you **please** bring the snacks for the team for Jimmy's tee-ball game Monday night? Several other moms have already said they couldn't! Please confirm if this is OK. Thanks so much!! You're the true "Super-Mom"!!

Regards,
Coach Bailey

Figure 12.5. Elizabeth Parson's in-box Monday, October 7, 7:30 a.m. *(continued)*

ITEM 18:   E-MAIL

To: Elizabeth Parsons, VP–Nursing Services

From: Jane Sawchuck, Clinical Nurse Specialist

Date: October 3

Time: 8:34 a.m.

Subject: Nosocomial infections

It has come to my attention that, again last month, we have recorded high levels of *Staphylococcus* and *Pseudomonas* in operating rooms B and C. It is becoming apparent that we need to review our standard procedures in this area before an epidemic breaks out.

—Jane

ITEM 19:   E-MAIL

To: Betty Parsons

From: Allan Reid

Date: October 3

Time: 7:00 p.m.

Subject: Need a favor!

My niece, Jennifer, just graduated from nursing school and will be in town just one day—Monday, October 7. She is looking for a job in her field and I have asked her to talk to you. She is a delightful girl. Would you please see her?

—Allan

Figure 12.5.   Elizabeth Parson's in-box Monday, October 7, 7:30 a.m. *(continued)*

ITEM 20:   E-MAIL

To: Elizabeth Parsons, VP–Nursing Service

From: Scott Little, Assistant to the President

Date: October 4

Time: 7:34 a.m.

Subject: Nurse working illegally

Carmen Espinoza, the woman I talked to you about, was working illegally for us. She was using a stolen Social Security number. The Immigration and Naturalization Services (INS) contacted me yesterday and a representative will be coming Monday afternoon to inquire about the matter.
    Please give me a call right away.

—Scott

ITEM 21:   TELEPHONE MESSAGE

(Wilma intercepted the call and took a message; put note in front of you.)

To: Elizabeth Parsons, Vice President–Nursing Service

From: Bernard Stevens, Chairman of the Board

Date: October 7

Time: 8:55 a.m.

Mr. Stevens just called and says that he needs to meet with you and Allan Reid this morning at 10:00 a.m.

Figure 12.5.   Elizabeth Parson's in-box Monday, October 7, 7:30 a.m. *(continued)*

ITEM 22:   E-MAIL

To: Elizabeth Parsons, Vice President–Nursing Service

From: Dr. Clement Westaway, President–Medical Staff

Date: October 2

Time: 12:34 p.m.

Subject: Nurse–physician relations

Further to our discussion last week concerning the pressing need to improve communication between physicians and nurses at Hartland Memorial, I am hoping that the suggestions that I gave you will be successfully implemented by your staff. Remember, we are all trying to provide the best possible medical care for our patients.

—C.W., MD

ITEM 23:   E-MAIL

To: Elizabeth Parsons, Vice President–Nursing Service

From: Cynthia Nichols, VP–Human Resources

Date: October 3

Time: 2:15 p.m.

Subject: Firing Ms. Jean White, RN

As we discussed yesterday, it is important to conduct the termination interview of nurse Jean White as soon as possible. Her last day of work at Hartland will be October 18 and, according to our collective agreement, she requires 2 weeks' notice. Please call me when the deed is done.

—Cynthia Nichols, VP–HR

Figure 12.5. Elizabeth Parson's in-box Monday, October 7, 7:30 a.m. *(continued)*

STOP!

Do not proceed to ITEM 24 until you have responded
to all previous items.

ITEM 24:   TELEPHONE CALL (**LIVE**)

Time: 9:45 a.m., Monday, October

Allan Reid just calls, and tells you that Mrs. Grace O'Brien, the patient with diabetes and Alzheimer's disease, is again missing from her room, apparently since late last night. He advises you that he was just informed of this by a local newspaper reporter who had gotten wind of the story. He instructs you to call Mrs. O'Brien's daughter to tell her of this recent development before she hears, or reads it in the media. Reid gives you no opportunity to respond, saying, "I have the reporter on the other line and have to go." He then hangs up the telephone.

Figure 12.6. Elizabeth Parson's in-box Monday, October 7, 7:30 a.m. *(continued)*

13

Bad Image Radiology Department

Kurt Darr
The George Washington University, Washington, D.C.

HISTORY AND SETTING

MacMillan Hospital was established in a metropolitan area of the south-eastern United States in the decade following the Civil War. It was named for Abner MacMillan, a successful lumber and hardware merchant whose business had prospered at war's end when there was a great need for rebuilding in his war-ravaged region. The hospital was originally located in a large, colonnaded antebellum home that was MacMillan's residence before his death. In addition to the house, MacMillan had donated the 40 acres on which it stood and $50,000—a large sum in the 1870s—for the charitable purposes to which the hospital was to be dedicated. Originally named for the city in which it was located, the board voted to change the name after MacMillan's death.

In the almost 150 years since MacMillan Hospital was established, it has undergone numerous building projects and renovations. By the early 21st Century it was licensed for 350 beds, but operated only 250, which have an average occupancy rate of 75%. The parcel of land was large enough that construction and renovation could occur without the need to acquire more land. The original house had been restored and is occupied by the hospital's administrative offices.

MacMillan Hospital offers all primary and secondary acute care inpatient services. A few tertiary services are available: autologous bone marrow transplant services, neonatal intensive care, cardiac catheterization, and radiation oncology. Annual outpatient admissions exceed 80,000. Its busy emergency department has more than 45,000 admissions annually. The hospital has just over 1,000 full-time equivalent (FTE) employees. MacMillan has no bargaining units, but there are occasional rumors that union organizers have talked to employees.

MacMillan's service area has two hospitals of similar size that offer similar services. Many area physicians have privileges at all three hospitals. MacMillan has several advantages, however. It has enjoyed a good reputation in its service area and its competitors face natural barriers that include two rivers and a range of foothills. MacMillan's competitors are not served by public transportation; the road system favors it, as well. The service area has several physician-owned, freestanding centers that offer urgent care, imaging, and ambulatory surgical services. A small psychiatric care facility offers inpatient alcohol and drug detoxification services and rehabilitation. MacMillan and its competitors refer complex cases to the university hospital, which is 75 miles distant.

In terms of hospital-based physicians MacMillan has contracts with six different physician groups that independently provide anesthesiology, cardiology, emergency medicine, clinical and anatomical laboratory, hospitalist, and medical imaging (radiology) services. These concessionaires use equity-owner physicians as well as physician employees to provide services. As is true in most hospitals, these clinical departments at MacMillan are closed, meaning that only physicians in the group or employed by the group may have clinical privileges in them. Nonetheless, physicians must go through the usual credentialing process as set out in the professional staff bylaws. Nonphysician staff in these six clinical areas are employed by the hospital, but their work is directly supervised and evaluated clinically by physicians in the specific group. This split between supervision and employment is common in acute-care hospitals. The resulting matrix-type organization facilitates delivery of services by improving coordination and communication, but divides employee loyalty, blurs lines of authority and reporting, and violates Henri Fayol's principle of unity of command. MacMillan has been continuously accredited by The Joint Commission on Accreditation of Healthcare Organizations. The "deemed" status provided by Joint Commission accreditation is important for reimbursement of Medicare and Medicaid patients, which represent 35% of admissions.

BOARD OF TRUSTEES

MacMillan Hospital is governed by a 21-member board of trustees, who are true trustees because they are responsible for the trust originally established by Abner MacMillan. The board is self-perpetuating, which means that it nominates and selects replacement trustees. Trustees serve 3-year terms, and they may be renominated for two additional 3-year terms. One third of terms expire each year. The hospital CEO is an *ex officio* member of the board, but has no vote. Board committees include executive, professional staff organization (PSO), human resources, strategic planning, budget and fiscal, quality evaluation and improvement, and nominating. The executive committee meets monthly and is composed of the chair of the board and the chairs of the seven committees. The board bylaws require that committees meet at least quarterly, but they are subject to call of the chairs.

The board chair is Harriet Buchanan, a retired schoolteacher and community leader. She recently started her second 3-year term as chair and is seen by other board members and management as dedicated, well intentioned, and reasonably effective. The board is composed of interface stakeholders who are social and economic leaders in the community and who are of varying ages and ethnic backgrounds. Three are physicians who are members of the active professional staff at MacMillan and not part of a contract group. The board has been active and successful in strategic planning and fundraising. It emphasizes the hospital's financial performance and uses that as a major basis for judging management's success. Implementation of board policy decisions (resolutions) is left to senior management, and the board does not review day-to-day performance. The PSO committee makes recommendations through the executive committee after it reviews credentialing recommendations of the PSO, which have come to it through the PSO credentialing and executive committees.

THE PROFESSIONAL STAFF ORGANIZATION

The professional staff at MacMillan Hospital is organized, self-governing, and quasi autonomous; like almost all hospital professional staffs, it has chosen not to be a separate corporation. Although legally subordinate to the board of trustees because its bylaws (and revisions), as well as PSO appointments and clinical privileges, must be approved by the board, the PSO sees itself as a partner in the full range of hospital activities. As is typical in private (nongovernmental) hospitals the PSO has bylaws that describe its organizational structure, including officers, committees, and policies. There are also PSO "Rules and Regulations" that include specific procedures and rules. In addition to the vice president for professional affairs (VP/PA) who is appointed by the CEO (with approval of the board) and is part of administration, the PSO elects a president who represents the PSO to administration and the board. PSO standing committees include executive, credentials, bylaws, technology, nominating, quality assurance and improvement, and medical records. The chairs of standing committees serve on the executive committee, whose presiding officer is the president of the PSO.

There are 920 physicians on MacMillan's PSO, of whom 200 are active. In addition to physicians, the PSO bylaws allow doctors of podiatric medicine (DPM), certified registered nurse anesthetists (CRNAs), and certified nurse midwives (CNMs) to be members of the PSO. Podiatrists' privileges are determined individually. Privileges for the CRNAs and CNMs are determined as a group; they have a vote on the PSO, but may not hold office. The PSO bylaws define "active" as physicians who admit five or more inpatients per year. For purposes of defining active, three outpatient admissions are considered equal to one inpatient admission. Only active members of the PSO are allowed to hold office or chair committees. All members of the PSO may vote on general matters such as elections; the vote on matters such as amending the bylaws, however, is limited to active staff.

It is common that hospitals use *locum tenens* physicians to staff hospital-based physician clinical departments temporarily. The PSO bylaws at MacMillan allow appointment of *locum tenens* physicians and state in part:

> All appointments to the PSO shall be reviewed by the PSO department, which is to be the applicant physician's primary department. . . . The department chair shall make a recommendation to the credentials committee as to the appropriateness of the appointment and the suitability of the clinical privileges requested by the applicant, in consultation with such members of the department as are deemed appropriate. All appointments shall be subject to approval by the board of trustees.

Historically, this provision has been interpreted to include *locum tenens* appointments and temporary physicians have been processed consistent with this provision. Ultimately, as is universal practice for hospitals, the board at MacMillan approves all appointments to the PSO and the specific privileges of each individually credentialed member of the PSO, or the credentials held by groups such as the CRNAs.

ADMINISTRATION

MacMillan's chief executive is Jack Gargon, who was appointed 15 years ago. Gargon is 60 years old and holds a master's degree from an accredited health services administration program. He is a Fellow of the American College of Healthcare Executives and has more than 25 years of senior-level experience. A first task on assuming his duties at MacMillan was to reorganize the management hierarchy. One goal was to reduce the number of middle managers in anticipation of reduced federal reimbursement because of implementation of the federal diagnosis-related groups (DRGs) payment system. The resulting structure was much flatter and had fewer middle managers. The board was pleased with the reorganization and other efficiencies Gargon implemented and concluded he was a capable and technically proficient manager. Mr. Gargon's elimination of middle management, however, caused significant grumbling among surviving middle managers who had seen friends and colleagues fired. Satisfied that internal operations were under control, the board increasingly turned its attention to external responsibilities. Gargon's reputation in the hospital is that he is a capable and technically proficient manager who gives his management team wide latitude in decision making. He expects them to solve problems on their own and not to bother him unless his specific assistance or intervention are needed.

Gregory Halton is Gargon's vice president for clinical services (VP/CS). Halton is 27 years old and has been at MacMillan since he completed a postgraduate internship there 5 years ago. Prior to being promoted to VP/CS 2 years ago, he was responsible for strategic planning and marketing. He holds a bachelor of science in health services management and is working part-time on his master's degree; his areas of responsibility include medical imaging. Halton is seen by his hospital colleagues as enthusiastic, hardworking, and job-focused. He can be stubborn, however, and occasionally peers have questioned his judgment.

The guidelines for managers responsible for clinical departments are general and unwritten, but reflect long-standing custom at MacMillan. Managers are expected to focus on the nonphysician staff and to leave the review of physicians' activities to the VP/PA and the PSO. The chief technologist in medical imaging, for example, reports to the clinical department head for clinical matters and to the VP/CS for administrative matters, which results in a matrix-type arrangement. The clinical chief and the responsible manager evaluate performance of support staff in clinical departments jointly. Halton is administratively responsible for the department of medical imaging, which was known as the department of radiology previously.

The VP/PA position has been vacant for 6 months, despite efforts to recruit a replacement for the previous incumbent who retired.

MEDICAL IMAGING

The chief of medical imaging is Harold Goodview, M.D., a board-certified radiologist. Goodview is the majority stockholder in Good Views

Medical Imaging, LLC, the professional corporation that has had an exclusive contract to provide radiographic services at MacMillan for the past 15 years. Goodview's wife and her family are minority stockholders. Two years ago, MacMillan and Good Views signed a 5-year extension of the basic contract. Good Views employs all the radiologists, including Goodview, who is both employee and owner.

The department of medical imaging is extraordinarily busy and has a volume of more than 100,000 cases per year. There are 40 FTE radiologic technologists and 27 FTE file room clerks, secretaries, receptionists, and transporters. The technologists include radiographers, cardiovascular-interventional technologists, sonographers, radiation therapists, and magnetic resonance imaging technologists. Each area of activity has a lead technologist. There is a chief technologist for the entire department who functions as the department administrator. The department performs a wide range of radiographic studies including plain film studies, contrast studies, intravenous pyelograms, magnetic resonance imaging (MRI), computed tomography (CT), needle biopsies, drainages, nuclear medicine, ultrasound, and interventional procedures such as angiograms and stent placements.

The terms of the contract between MacMillan and Good Views are typical for the field. MacMillan Hospital provides and maintains all capital and noncapital equipment. It provides and maintains the space and all supplies and consumables, including disposables. MacMillan employs nonphysician staff. The hospital is paid for its work by budgetarily apportioning part of the DRGs for Medicare and Medicaid patients and by billing other third-party payers and the small number of self-pay directly. Good Views has a contract billing service that bills for the professional fee charged by the radiologists. Part B pays for Medicare beneficiaries; Medicaid, other third-party payers, and self-pay patients are billed directly. Primarily because of the high volume, this basic arrangement has been financially rewarding for both parties.

Relationships with administration have generally been business-like, if distant. Goodview prefers "dealing with the top" and calls Gargon whenever there is a problem that needs attention. Even when there was a VP/ PA, Gargon rarely involved her in any departmental problems. Being bypassed in this manner annoys Halton greatly, but the pattern was established before Halton came to MacMillan. Halton has mentioned the problem to Gargon several times, but Gargon has taken no action. Believing this reflects a lack of support of his role in medical imaging, Halton has been reluctant to challenge Goodview's actions directly. Consequently, Halton has been embarrassed numerous times when he learned about decisions affecting his responsibilities in medical imaging from the chief technologist. Halton's efforts to develop a more effective working relationship have been rebuffed by Goodview.

Historically, Goodview has had difficulty keeping radiologists employed in his company and, thus, in staffing the department. When Good Views Medical Imaging first obtained the exclusive concession to provide radiology services, the group had four equal partners. Over the years, Goodview bought them out when they wanted to leave. His long-term-employed radiologists have become fewer and fewer; currently there are only two, Drs. Banda and Leipzig. In addition, there are several *locum tenens* radiologists.

The chief radiographic technologist is Sally Lebeau, who has been employed in the department for 18 years, during half of which she has been the chief technologist. Lebeau is well regarded by her staff and is seen as fair and reasonable, especially given the fast-paced and intense working environment. Lebeau has tried to implement Deming's quality principles and the methods of continuous quality improvement, but neither Goodview nor the hospital's administration supported her efforts, and they have come to naught. Lebeau is concerned with what she perceives to be a decline in the quality of work in medical imaging. She has tried, unsuccessfully, to discuss her concerns with Goodview on numerous occasions. In the past several years she has seen other developments that raised concerns. First, despite increased volume, the department has fewer radiologists in total. Second, the constant turnover of radiologists and the resulting heavy use of *locum tenens* is very disruptive to the department's work. Third, Goodview does more and more of the work himself—both because of the radiologist staffing problems and because of what Lebeau thinks is an increasing obsession with money. Fourth, without the knowledge of senior administration, Goodview ordered a cable connection so he could follow the stock market and trade technology stocks on line. He is often distracted from reading radiographs and other imaging by stock market developments, especially in the volatile technology stocks, in which he invests heavily.

Lebeau's concerns were such that she went to see Halton. When Lebeau described how she saw the four problems, Halton told her he could do little about the first three, nor did he think they were his responsibility. The number of *locum tenens* physicians and the quality issues had to be addressed by someone else—probably the PSO. Halton seemed incensed, however, that Goodview had been so bold as to order installation of Internet access without clearing it with administration. While Lebeau was in his office Halton called maintenance, which reports to the vice president for support services (VP/SS). The head of maintenance confirmed there was a cable hook-up and the hospital was paying the fee. While Lebeau waited, Halton called the VP/SS, Susan Williams. After a lengthy discussion in which Halton became quite agitated and began to shout, Williams finally agreed to have the cable disconnected the next day. This greatly pleased Halton, who said to Lebeau, "I've been trying to get Goodview's attention; I bet this'll do it. He'll have to come to me to resolve this problem—I'm sure that, over the long term, it will help us develop a better working relationship."

Lebeau was disappointed by Halton's response, especially his feeling that he had no role in quality of services. She thought the cable issue was the least of the problems, even though it was clearly a distraction and Goodview was using hospital resources for his private purposes. When Lebeau returned to medical imaging, she saw several of the staff standing as though transfixed outside the room where radiologists read films. They were listening intently to a heated conversation Goodview was having with an online broker who Goodview alleged had failed to make a trade in time to avoid a significant loss. The language was foul and was becoming so loud patients waiting for procedures could hear it. Lebeau quietly shut the door to the reading room and told the staff to go back to work.

The next day Goodview's Internet connection suddenly went dead, just as he was trying to execute a sell order on a rapidly falling technology stock. He reacted violently and threw the monitor on the floor breaking the screen and chipping the flooring. When he called the cable company Goodview was told the hospital had ordered the Internet service disconnected. Goodview stormed over to "management house" to see Gargon, who was only somewhat successful in calming him before Goodview left his office. After talking to Halton, Gargon basically agreed with his action, but chided him for how he had done it. In the weeks that followed, Goodview brooded about the loss of his cable connection; he frequently cursed out administration. Several times he stated that if he had a bomb he'd blow up "management house."

Goodview's agitation was increasingly reflected in his work. For example, he read mammograms as quickly as he could bring them up on the monitor and dictated reports in groups. He found virtually none that required more than a few seconds of study. When Dr. Leipzig raised a question about the speed of his readings, Goodview said, "Reading mammograms is so simple a one-eyed first-year medical student could do it." To check Goodview's readings, Leipzig reread 100 randomly selected mammograms and found several that warranted follow-up studies, including repeat mammograms and fine needle aspirations. He ordered them without telling Goodview.

Concerned about the mammograms and similar problems, Leipzig followed Goodview's custom and went "to the top" to see Gargon. Gargon was initially noncommittal and told Leipzig that he would have to undertake his own investigation. Gargon called Halton and asked him to speak to Lebeau. When their meeting began Halton asked Lebeau for her comments on the information relayed from Leipzig. Her response was a torrent: poor staff morale, low patient satisfaction, high turnover of radiologists, and Goodview's continuing bad behavior were causing a great deal of stress.

Alarmed, Halton met with Gargon, but they were unsure how to proceed and the meeting produced no plan of action. The following week, Dr. Leipzig resigned, citing in his letter the continuing and significant quality problems in medical imaging. This meant that Drs. Banda and Goodview were the only nontemporary radiologists in the department. The other radiologists in the department were *locum tenens*, who usually stayed only 1–3 months.

The controversy between administration and Goodview and questions about the quality of work in medical imaging were common knowledge in the hospital. Their extent and duration were such, however, that admitting and referring physicians in the community were increasingly concerned about the quality of imaging services their patients would get at MacMillan. Gargon and several board members, including Ms. Buchanan, had received calls from prominent active staff physicians who said they had become uncomfortable referring patients to MacMillan for imaging and that they would use a competing hospital or a freestanding imaging center. In the short term fewer referrals would reduce hospital revenue from medical imaging; in the longer term inpatient admissions would be affected, thus potentially affecting quality of care received by persons in the hospital's service area, but certainly causing a decline in hospital revenue.

Greatly concerned and prompted by a call from the board chair, Harriet Buchanan, Gargon scheduled a meeting with Goodview and Halton. As usual, Goodview arrived late. Looking at Halton he blurted out, "What are you doing here?" With little conviction, Halton replied that as the VP/CS he was administratively accountable for medical imaging and it was his responsibility to be present. Goodview proceeded to harangue Gargon about the poor support he was getting from administration, how the technologists were badly trained and disloyal to him, and the equipment was inadequate for a 21st-century imaging department. All the while he ignored Halton. Gargon began by expressing his concern that there were too few radiologists for the volume of procedures. Goodview said that radiologists were in great demand and he was doing the best he could to recruit additional staff. In the meantime, he, Banda, and the *locum tenens* radiologists could handle the workload. After 30 minutes of heated discussion, the meeting ended with no resolution.

After Goodview left, Gargon told Halton to contact physician search firms and determine whether Goodview was correct about the shortage of radiologists. A week later, in early July, Halton reported the search firms had sent information that radiologists were available in adequate numbers, but they were being attracted to groups that paid better than Good Views. Goodview's salary offers were well known to the search firms—one even called Goodview "a cheapskate." The search firms sent 10 résumés of radiologists who could be employed on a long-term basis by Good Views or who could be hired as *locum tenens*, if the salaries were competitive.

Armed with this information, another meeting was held with Gargon, Halton, and Goodview. Goodview was adamant that he would not bring any more "traitors" such as Leipzig or other full-time radiologists into his company. He felt all of his former full-time radiologists had betrayed his trust and friendship over the years. He said, however, he would consider more *locum tenens* appointments, but only if he really needed them. A week later, in mid-July, Goodview had done nothing about hiring more *locum tenens* radiologists. This prompted Halton to contact the search firms. He asked them to send applications from the 10 radiologists whose résumés they had sent previously. Halton was sure this would force Goodview to take action. Applications received in administration were forwarded to Goodview, who stubbornly ignored them.

CONTRACT TERMINATION

When Gargon arrived at work on August 1 his secretary told him there was a voice mail from the chair of the hospital board that had been received at 5:30 a.m. Buchanan stated she had slept little the night before because the problems in medical imaging were weighing on her mind. She ended her recording by stating something had to be done. She wanted Gargon to review the contract with Good Views to determine how to terminate it. By noon she had called twice to follow up on her request. Gargon put her off until early afternoon; by then he had checked with legal counsel and was able to give Buchanan an informed response. The relevant contract provision stated:

> Either party may, upon demonstration of adequate cause, terminate the contract with a 30-day notice. Cause is defined as either party's: inability to meet the clinical needs of the other; nonperformance of a significant provision of this contract; or actions that interfere with the ability of the other party to perform this contract.

After talking to Halton, who said, "It's about time!" Gargon called Buchanan and told her legal counsel had informed him there appeared to be adequate cause to terminate the contract. Buchanan instructed him to draft a letter advising Good Views Medical Imaging that its contract with MacMillan would be terminated as of September 1. Consistent with board bylaws, Buchanan polled the executive committee, which approved the action. The letter was signed by Gargon and hand delivered to Goodview the same day. Goodview was performing a fine needle biopsy and he asked a technologist to read the letter to him. On hearing the content, he became enraged. He shouted for Banda, who was on a coffee break, to "get in here and finish up this patient." The patient became very agitated and had to be reassured by the technologist before Banda could complete the procedure. Goodview stormed over to "management house" and burst into Gargon's office without being announced. Gargon's executive assistant was so concerned about Goodview's rage and the potential for violence that she called security and asked them to send two officers to the administrative suite immediately. Goodview left shortly thereafter, vowing to get the "meanest, nastiest lawyer in town."

Goodview's attorney petitioned the court for a temporary restraining order (TRO), arguing that contract termination would cause irreparable economic harm to Good View's Medical Imaging and would also irreparably harm Goodview's professional reputation. The TRO was granted despite arguments by MacMillan's lawyers that focused on the need to provide quality imaging services and maintain the quality of patient care. The TRO prohibited MacMillan and its management from interfering in the role of Good Views Medical Imaging and its agents and employees in the medical imaging department of MacMillan. Less than a week after the TRO was granted, Goodview filed suit against MacMillan for breach of contract and defamation. Gargon and Halton were named personally as having "conspired to deprive Goodview of his business and professional livelihood and of causing irreparable harm to his professional reputation." In addition to economic damages for breach of contract, the lawsuit asked that the court award punitive damages based on the alleged conspiracy and bad faith on the parts of Gargon and Halton, as agents of the hospital. Given the urgency of the situation, MacMillan was successful in gaining an early trial date on the breach of contract and defamation lawsuit. Trial was scheduled for December 1st, even as the TRO remained in effect.

BREAST CANCER AWARENESS MONTH

As it had done for the past 8 years, MacMillan Hospital's "Health-Promotion Promotion" program designated October as breast cancer awareness month. Local radio and television stations aired public service announcements that urged women older than age 45 to go to MacMillan for a free screening mammogram. Special efforts were directed at MacMillan Hospital staff. The "Health-Promotion Promotion" used flyers, bulletin board notices, social media, and public address announcements in the cafeteria to encourage women older than 45 to be screened. The continuing shortage of radiologists and pending legal proceeding made the extra workload seem especially burdensome this year.

Cowed by the TRO and the pending lawsuit for breach of contract and defamation and concerned there might be charges of harassment, which could result in being held in contempt of court or prompt another lawsuit, Gargon and Halton stayed away from medical imaging and Goodview. Emboldened by the initial success of obtaining the TRO, Goodview was even more critical of administration and his behavior became increasingly bizarre. Lebeau's stress level was so high she sought medical attention and was prescribed a mild tranquilizer. To the technologists and other staff, the situation was overwhelming; morale sank even lower and there was talk of a mass resignation. Only the perseverance of Lebeau gave the staff some encouragement.

A MacMillan Hospital housekeeper, Amelia Tendo, presented herself at medical imaging early one morning in October for a screening mammogram. She said she had felt a small lump in her right breast and was concerned about it. Goodview read the mammogram in his usual fashion and diagnosed the lump as benign and "nothing more than a calcium deposit in an overly anxious female." Reassured, Tendo asked that a copy of the report be sent to her primary care physician.

THE FIRST TRIAL

In preparing for trial, attorneys for MacMillan and Goodview/Good Views took depositions (questions answered under oath) of the major parties in the case. Without exception, persons employed by the hospital, including radiologic technologists, stated in their depositions that Goodview's work in managing and providing radiologic services was well below acceptable levels and his actions that effectively resulted in inadequate radiologist staffing had put and were putting patients at risk. Testimony such as this was necessary because the hospital had the burden of proving that the grounds for termination specified in the contract had been met. In addition, the hospital had retained two medical experts who stated, after reviewing Goodview's readings, diagnoses, and the depositions of the other deponents, that Goodview's work fell below the standard of care.

Except for tepid support from Banda and the *locum tenens* radiologists, Goodview had few allies in the hospital. He did have an expert witness who stated his work and Good Views' performance of the contract were acceptable and within the range of performance for departments of radiology nationwide.

The trial commenced December 1st and lasted 5 days. The witnesses who appeared were those who had given depositions. Goodview could not restrain himself when he testified, and he proved to be his own worst enemy, even as he tried to present himself as a poor physician who was being bullied by an overwhelming bureaucracy. The jury found in favor of the hospital and against Goodview and Good Views Medical Imaging on both the breach of contract and the defamation claims. The verdict caused the judge to vacate the TRO.

Hospital administration was jubilant and, with Good Views' contract terminating in 30 days, it immediately began to recruit a new radiology group. Radiologists who had been part of Good Views were contacted. Dr. Leipzig said he was interested and he set about organizing a radiology group.

SECOND LAWSUIT

Ms. Tendo, who had had the screening mammogram in October during breast cancer awareness month, continued to be concerned by the lump in her right breast. When she performed her intermittent breast self-examinations over the next several months it seemed to be growing. Whenever her anxiety rose, she recalled Dr. Goodview's reading and diagnosis that it was only a calcium deposit and was reassured. Six months later, in April she had become convinced the lump was substantially larger and she scheduled an examination with her gynecologist. He immediately ordered a mammogram at a freestanding imaging center, which led to a fine needle aspiration. After other tests, the final diagnosis was cancer of the right breast with metastases to one lung, nearby lymph nodes, and liver. She died 3 months later. Within a year, Ms. Tendo's estate sued Dr. Goodview, Good Views Medical Imaging, and MacMillan Hospital for medical negligence.

DISCUSSION QUESTIONS

1. Identify the issues in the case.

2. Prepare a time line of major events in the case. Determine the points at which intervention by hospital administration or the board might have prevented the problems in medical imaging from developing as they did. For each intervention point, outline the intervention that should have been taken.

3. What is the role of hospital executives in monitoring quality and intervening, as needed, in the delivery and/or quality of clinical services?

4. Identify points at which hospital administration should have intervened to lessen the probability of Dr. Goodview's failure to diagnose Ms. Tendo's breast cancer.

5. What steps should be taken by MacMillan Hospital to resolve the lawsuit brought by Ms. Tendo's estate? Is an apology part of an appropriate response?

6. What actions, if any, should be taken against Messrs. Gargon and Halton? Who should take them?

ENDNOTE

This case used by permission of the author. Copyright © 2017 Kurt Darr.

14

Westmount Nursing Homes

Implementing a Continuous Quality Improvement Initiative

Kent V. Rondeau
University of Alberta, Edmonton, Alberta, Canada

Shirley Carpenter took a deep breath and looked at her watch. It was 3:40 p.m. and just 20 minutes were left to get ready for her meeting with the board. She knew there was going to be a difficult confrontation and believed that many board members would call into question her leadership skills and administrative judgment. She felt that her well-earned reputation as a brilliant strategist and dynamic change agent would be put to a severe test. She needed to find a way to calm the widespread fear that the total quality management (TQM) initiative she had worked so hard to implement at Westmount Nursing Homes was badly off the rails. She wondered what had gone wrong and how it could be saved.

BACKGROUND

Carpenter came to Westmount 22 months ago to assume the role of president and chief executive officer. Westmount Nursing Homes, Incorporated is a for-profit chain of seven nursing homes located in a northeastern state. Since 1953, it had grown from a single 42-bed residential facility for affluent seniors, to a dynamic company composed of four divisions: 1) the Facilities Division, managing skilled nursing homes; 2) the Home Care Division, operating homemaker and nursing services for seniors in their own homes; 3) the Commissary Services Division, operating a central kitchen preparing and distributing meals to four of its nursing homes, two small local hospitals, and elderly people in their own homes; and 4) the Consulting Division, marketing management consulting and accounting services to a variety of clients in the long-term care industry. Westmount's statement of profit and loss for the past 3 years can be found in Table 14.1.

Westmount continues to search vigorously for opportunities to expand its core business. Last year, it began a comprehensive day care program for seniors at five of its nursing homes. Recently, discussions have been undertaken with Breton Funeral Homes to purchase its assets, including four family-owned funeral establishments. Westmount has also commenced negotiations with a regional chain of drug stores to lease them commercial space in its three largest nursing homes. It also is exploring the establishment of a home care alliance with two other hospital-based home care programs in order to attract new managed care contracts and to improve referrals from existing contracts involving their parent hospitals.

Over the past 2 years, under the leadership of Carpenter, Westmount purchased two additional nursing homes, increasing its total skilled

Table 14.1. Westmount Nursing Homes, Incorporated statement of revenue and expense (years 201x–201z) (figures in thousands of dollars)

Year	201x	201y	201z
Facilities Division			
Revenue	15,640	18,622	26,453
Expenses	12,458	15,140	22,512
Profit margin (%)	20.3	18.7	14.9
Home Care Division			
Revenue	1,741	2,254	3,060
Expenses	1,360	1,752	2,493
Profit margin (%)	21.9	22.3	18.5
Commissary Services Division			
Revenue	1,382	1,940	2,188
Expenses	1,162	1,614	1,870
Profit margin (%)	15.9	16.8	14.5
Consulting Division			
Revenue	—	42	426
Expenses	—	16	230
Profit margin (%)	—	61.9	46.0

nursing bed complement by almost 43%. A strategic planning process began last year. Out of this initiative came Westmount's formal declaration to pursue the goal of becoming the "home of choice" for the elderly in the tristate area. Its primary target market was identified as affluent seniors who desire a broad range of single access, high-quality health and social services. This strategy was based on the belief that to survive in a rapidly changing healthcare environment, customers require "one-stop shopping" for a wide variety of services outside of the acute care setting. Westmount firmly believes that future success will go to those proactive organizations that achieve a vertically and horizontally integrated delivery system.

SHIRLEY CARPENTER

Shirley Carpenter, R.N., M.B.A., came to Westmount Nursing Homes two years ago from Grasslands Community General Hospital, where she had been the vice president of nursing. Grasslands is a 325-bed acute care hospital located in a rapidly growing community in the Midwest. At Grasslands, Carpenter was widely received as a dynamic and resourceful leader who was not afraid of making the difficult decisions that went with her job description. She was primarily responsible for Grasslands' radical redesign of its patient care delivery system toward a highly integrated patient-focused approach. The changes she had initiated saved the hospital more than $1.7 million per year on direct patient care services, while at the same time lowering hospital length-of-stay and improving patient outcomes. When the press got wind of Grasslands' successful reorganization, the hospital and Carpenter received a great deal of local and national media attention. Grasslands became recognized as an innovative organization at the cutting edge of excellence in patient care delivery. It wasn't long before Carpenter was being asked to speak at forums about a wide variety of healthcare issues. She also received additional recognition when she was selected as "one of the most outstanding young healthcare executives in the nation."

Although the changes Carpenter had instituted were widely acclaimed as successful, she did have her detractors. Her direct, no-nonsense style was often seen as confrontational, and many found her to be intellectually intimidating. On several occasions she had openly chastised staff members with whom she took issue. Although she was greatly respected and even admired by her staff, people tended to give her a wide berth on most issues. Carpenter demanded perfection from her staff, but also held herself up to the very highest level of performance expectation. She once stated, "You've got to be visible and out front if you're going to navigate an organization toward progressive change. This requires that you stand behind your words and accept the consequences of your convictions. Complacency never got the job done. Too many people are attached to the status quo. You can't make an omelet without breaking a few eggs."

George Pearson had been the chief executive officer at Grasslands during Carpenter's tenure. Pearson once stated that Carpenter was "the daughter I never had." He had given her wide latitude and regularly deferred to her judgment in most areas related to running the hospital. Everyone had assumed that Pearson had been grooming Carpenter to take over the hospital upon his pending retirement. When he retired, the selection committee did the unexpected and chose another candidate. Carpenter was devastated. Six weeks later she left Grasslands for Westmount Nursing Homes.

A NEW DIRECTION FOR WESTMOUNT

Carpenter's arrival at Westmount created a great deal of anticipation and excitement. Her reputation as a healthcare innovator and progressive change agent was now well-established. Over the years, Westmount had languished through a series of rather bland administrators who lacked the vision that could move the organization forcefully into the future.

The first year of Carpenter's tenure at Westmount was marked by a number of bold initiatives on her part. Soon after arriving, she was able to resolve the threat of loss of licensure and potential funding on two of its nursing homes that had been cited for a number of violations. Carpenter also instituted a broad and sweeping reorganization at Westmount in creating the four operating divisions. In addition, after securing support from her board, Carpenter began a very aggressive program of asset diversification because the firm had relied for too long on revenues from its affiliate nursing homes. Declining reimbursement rates, coupled with full occupancy, meant that Westmount had to broaden its base of revenue. This was partially achieved by expansion of its home care and food commissary services, and by establishing a consulting division to market management services to a variety of clients in the long-term care industry. In particular, the consulting division was thought to have significant growth potential due to a perceived lack of expertise by most local consultants on long-term care management issues. During this period, Westmount also purchased two additional homes with the option of acquiring three more. The firm spent more than $1.5 million on renovations to these facilities.

Within 18 months, Carpenter had implemented a number of innovative programs at Westmount focused on providing augmented services to its seniors and, in addition, expanded employee services. Carpenter formed and chaired a quality-of-work-life committee aimed at improving conditions for Westmount's employees and staff. Morale in all of the homes had suffered after years of neglect. At the time of Carpenter's arrival, the turnover rate of staff nurses and nursing assistants at Westmount was among the highest in the state. To reverse this, a recognition program and performance-based pay system were implemented to identify and reward outstanding individual and group achievement. A career planning and inventory program was developed to assist employees in identifying their career goals and charting a path toward those goals. In addition, the staff education and development program was greatly expanded. All employees were openly encouraged and received financial support to acquire their high school equivalency, or to seek further education and skills enhancement. Westmount also established a progressive literacy program to address literacy issues in the workplace. The quality-of-worklife committee estimated that about 35% of the workforce at Westmount had deficiencies in reading and writing. Carpenter once stated, "Organizational excellence comes about only when people are sufficiently motivated and empowered to make a difference. The bedrock of staff empowerment is knowledge and education. This requires a significant investment in the intellectual potential of each employee. Our people are our most important asset."

THE TOTAL QUALITY MANAGEMENT INITIATIVE

Three months after arriving at Westmount, Carpenter initiated a strategic planning retreat to identify Westmount's preferred future. One conclusion emerging from the retreat was that there was a need to find a way to better address quality-of-care issues in delivering services to seniors. Carpenter latched onto the notion that total quality management (TQM) would be the vehicle through which Westmount could achieve the cultural transformation articulated in its vision statement, which included a statement that "Westmount Nursing Homes, Incorporated believes in striving for excellence in everything we do."

Carpenter quickly became immersed in the burgeoning literature on TQM. Her interest in, and passion for, its possibilities grew when she learned about quality management as a part-time doctoral student at the local university. In fact, she was so determined to become an expert in its theory and application that she began to explore the possibility of focusing her doctoral dissertation on the subject.

Her faculty advisor and mentor was Dr. Daylon Quinby, a sage yet crusty academic, now nearing retirement. Carpenter asked the venerable professor if he would "mentor the quality improvement journey at Westmount." Quinby readily agreed, and was soon found wandering around the grounds at all hours observing people at work or showing up quite unannounced at management committee meetings. Several staff members found Quinby to be "an odd old duck" whose presence was widely seen as annoying, if not unnerving. Most people did not know why he was there; some speculated that it was management's way of spying on them.

One of Quinby's first actions was to evaluate the organizational culture in the seven nursing homes. Findings from the cultural audit used to assess readiness to pursue organizational change indicated that much work would be required to transform Westmount. In particular, the professor found that prevailing work practices at Westmount were, in many respects, antithetical to the philosophy of TQM. Quinby announced the findings of the cultural audit at the annual general meeting of the board, management, and staff. He stated in his address that "if Westmount is to successfully implement total quality management, no less than a complete and unequivocal repudiation of current workplace values and norms needs to be achieved." Quinby concluded that "the management in the nursing homes consistently demonstrates patterns of practice that are overly autocratic, rigid, and dysfunctional. All too often, management treats its employees like children. Staff widely believes that management does not value them. An overly confrontational atmosphere, based on a deeply rooted disrespect for management, has created an atmosphere of skepticism and cynicism pervading work in many of the homes." Quinby cited several examples from incidents he had observed. Needless to say, the conclusions he stated were not well-received by a number of staff and managers.

Soon after the cultural audit feedback session, Carpenter and 12 senior managers embarked on a 10-day educational retreat to learn about TQM and the leadership skills needed to successfully navigate the workplace cultural transformation it required. Although the retreat was located on a resort island in the Caribbean, Carpenter impressed on her managers that the time spent was not a paid holiday, but an opportunity to acquire new leadership and management skills. When the news broke that management had gone to a resort for a "working retreat," many employees openly questioned why they needed to "go so far away to learn how to manage better at home." When the senior managers returned from the retreat, most could scarcely contain their enthusiasm and set about immediately to apply the principles they had learned. A quality council was quickly formed, chaired jointly by Carpenter and Quinby. The quality council was charged with leading and directing the TQM transformation at Westmount. Its membership consisted of the directors of the seven homes and the divisional directors of home care, commissary services, and consulting services, along with senior representatives from human resources and strategic planning. Within two weeks, executives in each of the homes and divisions were busy holding educational seminars for their middle managers and supervisors on the philosophy, tools, and techniques of TQM.

Not long afterward, under the supervision of the quality council, the first quality improvement (QI) team was formed. Led by Carpenter and facilitated by Quinby, a seven-member multifunctional team of service providers suggested innovative ways to dramatically reduce the waiting time for nursing response to requests from bedridden residents. Within two months, 23 QI project teams were established, addressing quality-related problems ranging from improving resident food to designing a new commercial exercise video program for seniors. Table 14.2 is a list of early quality improvement projects at Westmount. Initial interest and excitement generated by many employees for the TQM initiative at Westmount convinced Carpenter that she was onto something big.

Table 14.2. Westmount Nursing Homes, Incorporated, quality improvement projects

QI Program	Responsibility
1. Client satisfaction survey	Headquarters
2. Family satisfaction survey	Headquarters
3. Nursing response times	Facilities
4. Seniors' exercise video	Headquarters
5. Staff retention study	Facilities
6. Family relations study	Headquarters
7. Medication errors	Facilities
8. Suggestion system design	Headquarters
9. Resident fall study	Facilities
10. Wandering patients study	Facilities
11. Employee recognition program	Headquarters
12. Patient accounts	Headquarters
13. Food quality	Facilities
14. Food preparation	Headquarters
15. Pet therapy	Headquarters
16. Job redesign	Headquarters
17. Physician reimbursement	Headquarters
18. Physician satisfaction	Headquarters
19. Ethical review	Facilities
20. Grounds beautification	Facilities
21. Resident transportation	Facilities
22. Self-scheduling	Facilities
23. New ventures	Headquarters

Yet, many of her junior managers were privately expressing fear that the changes, which were now transforming Westmount's once placid culture, were happening all too fast. Vice President of Finance Norm Taylor's opinion was shared by many other managers at Westmount: "It's a proven fact that people in the long-term care industry really can't absorb organizational change as easily as those working in acute care settings. People here just have too much respect for tradition and past practice."

For her part, Carpenter was strongly convinced that these changes could not occur fast enough. Carpenter stated, "I don't believe in waiting around and hoping that quality comes your way. That just never happens. I like to create it through a planned, deliberate approach. One small improvement leads to another, and soon you've got tangible results. The fact is, people like to associate with excellence."

THE WESTMOUNT BOARD RESPONDS

The board of Westmount was never really very enthusiastic about Carpenter's TQM makeover. Explained to them as a tool to enhance productivity and to create a long-term competitive advantage in Westmount's chosen markets, the board reluctantly gave its approval "to implement a TQM program, as long as it wasn't too costly." The chairperson of the board was Dr. Ann Howard, age 57, a highly respected family physician with a specialty in geriatric medicine and long-time board member. Howard was not convinced that TQM could work at Westmount, and stated, "Total quality management might be all right for building cars, but I just can't understand how it can work in a nursing home. Anyway, I read somewhere that this TQM stuff is just an expensive fad, and that over 80% of healthcare organizations who have tried to implement it have failed. Can we really afford to waste our time on something with such a spotty track record? Perhaps Carpenter should be focusing her efforts and the organization's money on proven management methods."

Shirley knew that the turnaround at Westmount would not happen overnight. She attributed the board's indifference to ignorance and fear, and resolved that she would not be deterred from her quest to transform Westmount. "Give me a couple of years and you won't recognize this place," she was heard to have said.

LABOR CONTRACT NEGOTIATIONS

Several months after the TQM initiative had begun, Westmount began contract negotiations with the local chapter of the United Federation of Nurses, which represented Westmount's 214 registered nurses and nursing auxiliaries. Carpenter believed in taking a hands-on approach to dealing with the unions, and insisted on conducting all negotiations personally. In the beginning, management at Westmount felt that contract discussions would be straightforward and would proceed with little of the rancor that had characterized much of their collective bargaining in the past. In the earliest months of the TQM initiative, Westmount had witnessed a remarkable improvement in workplace morale. It was hoped that improved morale would pay an important "peace dividend" in the organization and win important concessions from the union.

In fact, all three of the unions representing non-management employees at Westmount believed that the active participation of their membership in TQM demonstrated their steadfast commitment to finding new ways of working responsibly with management. For many years, the fractious nature of their contract negotiations had left both sides bitter after they had concluded.

From the union's vantage point, negotiations were aimed at improving the collective bargaining agreement by obtaining significant wage gains and achieving formal union representation on the Westmount board. Two issues were of particular significance during contract talks. First, the union sought to replace the merit pay plan for registered nurses with an across-the-board pay increase for all nurses. Most people felt the merit pay plan conceived to reward top performers was not working very well. Many viewed it as a complicated and subjective protocol that caused a great deal of confusion and bitterness in its application. Second, the union sought protection against what it felt was management's abhorrent practice of substituting RNs with nursing assistants and other personal care workers. The union claimed that management was using lower-paid nursing auxiliaries for tasks that are outside their scope-of-practice and should be done by RNs.

Early in the contract negotiations it became apparent that they would be very difficult. In its opening address at the negotiation table, the union stated that its "price of compliance" with Westmount's total quality program was significant wage increases for its membership. Carpenter countered by offering to provide job security and suggesting the formation of a committee to study questions of nurse staffing mix. She also stated that she was in favor of allowing limited union representation on the board. This was consistent with her idea of incorporating more vibrant forms of shared governance in the workplace. Carpenter insisted, however, that the merit pay plan must remain in place. As its primary architect, she felt a deep personal commitment to its continuation. Carpenter stated, "You've got to have a way of rewarding those people who consistently perform above the call of duty. That's what quality service is all about. Money is a great way to motivate people. To ignore the impact that it has on the performance of employees is to remove a very powerful weapon from your arsenal." After several heated meetings, the negotiations seemed to be at an impasse.

THE BOARD STEPS IN

It was soon apparent to the Westmount board that contract negotiations with the nurses' union were not going well. The executive committee of the board met with Carpenter to determine an appropriate strategy to help reach an agreement. After much heated discussion, they decided that management should take a more direct approach in dealing with the union. The board chair, Ann Howard, summed up the attitude of the board in saying, "You can't allow a union to ruin the financial viability of your enterprise. The truth is 80% of our costs are direct expenditures for labor. If we are ever to reverse our fiscal problems around here, we need to lower our labor costs. These people have to realize we're all in this thing together." The board also gave a thumb's down to the idea of allowing union representation on the board. Howard remarked, "You know, this move to democratize the work place by giving the union a seat on our board is just rampant socialism. You give these people an inch and they take a mile."

When Carpenter returned to the bargaining table, she brought along Quinby to assist in discussions. Unfortunately, he was not able to break the impasse. His abrasive and authoritarian manner further alienated the union and created additional tensions at the table. With no new offer made by either side, no resolution on any of the major outstanding issues could be achieved. Carpenter suspended negotiations by claiming that the union was being inflexible while "holding the residents of the homes ransom for spite."

THE FLASH POINT

At this point the executive committee of the board began to make direct overtures to union representatives requesting an informal meeting to "determine if there were not avenues of mutual interest that could be explored." Howard and two other board members met in private with the union negotiators and suggested the possibility of major staff cuts if the union did not agree to make significant wage concessions. The union representatives countered by insinuating that the Westmount management was bargaining in bad faith. Robert Sawyer, the union's chief negotiator, said, "We will not be bullied into signing a collective bargaining agreement that does not have the best interests of our membership at heart. We have showed our willingness to bargain in good faith by engaging in activities aimed at improving productivity. The participation of our members in these efforts is often unpaid and obviously unappreciated." The meeting ended with the union threatening to boycott further participation by its membership in future quality improvement activities. According to Sawyer, "If we are going to be treated with such contempt, I can only recommend to my membership that we suspend our active participation in the program immediately."

As Carpenter prepared for the 4 P.M. board meeting she was frustrated and angry that persons and events had conspired against her. She had always felt pride in her ability to control any agenda. Her record of achievement was one of soaring accomplishments. She wondered how she could regain control of her board and move ahead with the important reforms she had initiated.

ENDNOTE

This case used by permission. From *Cases in Long-Term Care Management* by Donna Lind Infeld and John R. Kress. (Chicago: Health Administration Press, 1995, pp. 85–95.)

15

District Hospital

A Lesson in Governance

Cynthia Mahood Levin
Healthcare Consultant, Palo Alto, CA

Kurt Darr
The George Washington University, Washington, D.C.

HISTORY

Barclay Memorial Hospital (BMH) has enjoyed a reputation for excellent medical care in an affluent community for over 70 years. In the mid-1940s, its community was mainly agricultural, but urbanization was beginning. Hospitals in the region were operating at capacity. Community members and physicians proposed a solution to the problem of overcrowding at local hospitals: form a hospital district supported by the community through a tax. Voters approved the hospital district in 1945 by a 5 to 1 margin. The first decision was to select a 15-acre campus. In 1947, voters approved an $8 million bond issue to finance construction and operation of a 275-bed hospital. The tax district spans seven townships that elect five district community members to a governing board for the district hospital's four entities, which include the hospital, joint ventures that operate an urgent care center and a hospice, and the hospital foundation.

THE PHYSICIAN-HOSPITAL ORGANIZATION

About 15 years ago, the district hospital board and the CEO devised a strategic plan to form a physician-hospital organization (PHO) with Valley Physician Group (VPG). VPG was formed in 1951 when a number of physicians agreed they could provide better care to their patients by sharing resources and ideas. Over the years, VPG expanded as more physicians and physician groups joined. Currently, VPG has more than 315 full-time physicians in 28 specialties and subspecialties.

Joining with VPG to form a PHO required that BMH change its legal status from a public (governmental) hospital to a private, not-for-profit hospital. The new hospital governing board was responsible for the PHO. Within two years, the PHO was going bankrupt because of poor management and a lack of focused leadership. Infighting among VPG and non-VPG physicians began as the hospital deteriorated financially and employee morale plummeted. With the help of consultant Gregory Schilling, the district board, which had not disbanded, fought the not-for-profit governing board and successfully returned BMH to hospital district control. Being a tax district (governmental [public]) hospital confers several benefits on BMH: public hospitals are a political subdivision of the state with certain legal advantages; board members are elected by voters in the tax district; financial surpluses are reinvested in the hospital; and it has authority to levy a tax on homeowners in the district. Schilling was asked to become the new CEO immediately following dissolution of the PHO. See the timeline in Figure 15.1.

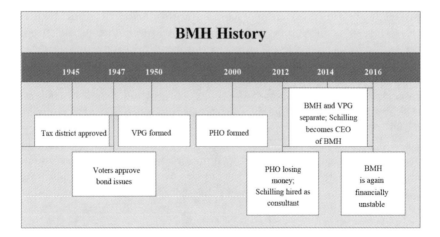

Figure 15.1. Timeline of major events in history of Barclay Memorial Hospital. BMH, Barclay Memorial Hospital; PHO, physician–hospital organization; VPG, Valley Physician Group.

MARKET POSITION

The healthcare market in the area included five hospitals in close proximity. One was a major teaching hospital; another was a county hospital that provided services to the indigent. In addition, there were numerous physician groups. Originally, BMH provided only outpatient surgery, a birthing center, psychiatric unit, and a senior center. Today, the hospital offers a comprehensive range of services: cancer, urologic, cardiac, and vascular surgery; neurology; orthopedic and spinal surgery; men's and women's health services; mental health services; geriatric, palliative, and hospice care; diagnostic services; digestive health; emergency services; primary care, including mother-baby health and pediatrics; rehabilitation medicine; pulmonary services; and a sleep lab.

Currently, BMH is licensed for 390 beds. Last year it operated 378 beds, with an average daily census of 249. Annually, BMH provides services of all types to the 118,177 persons living in the service area. BMH has 17,731 inpatient discharges, 6,224 inpatient surgeries, 4,347 outpatient surgeries, and 51,989 ER visits. The numbers reflect decreased volumes in most service lines. The average length of stay (ALOS) is 4.2 days. ALOS has increased somewhat because a change in state law now allows new mothers to be hospitalized longer than 24 hours after a normal delivery. The 4,912 newborn deliveries last year were a record; it is likely the number will increase because BMH is the desirable maternity hospital in the area. Nurses are attentive and maternity units have only private, newly renovated patient rooms. Outpatient visits totaled more than 113,265 last year and should continue to increase as technology allows less invasive treatment. Projections show a potential to increase occupancy if more surgeons admit at BMH *and* the processes for delivery of services become more efficient. This will make the hospital more profitable. Transplant surgery should generate more revenue, however. Orthopedics is another service line that could be expanded; it has only 40% of the estimated market. BMH is, however, competing with the neighboring teaching hospital for this patient population. Total full-time employees (FTEs) is 3,205. This is a higher-than-average FTE ratio compared to area hospitals. More FTEs result in higher salary and benefit costs. There are 455 physicians on the active medical staff, which reflects a decade-long decline. The number of hospital volunteers decreased from 890 last year, as well. BMH had gross revenue of $610 million in the last fiscal year, with an operating budget of $570 million. Managing to budget has been difficult. A hiring freeze mid-year showed positive results initially, but after three months some nursing units had nurse–patient ratios that were too low. Figure 15.2 shows the current organization of BMH.

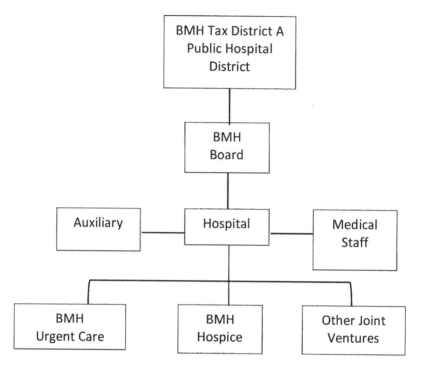

Figure 15.2. Organization of the Barclay Memorial Hospital District.

THE DISTRICT BOARD

The BMH board has five members elected by voters in the tax district to serve three-year terms (see Figure 15.3). The CEO is hired by the board. The chairman of the board, Dr. Larry Harvey, is an orthopedic surgeon with privileges at BMH. His position and authority in the hospital have raised questions of conflicts of interest. He has used his authority to disregard requests from the operating room supervisor to arrive on time for his cases. Harvey's tardiness means his patients must wait for their procedures to begin and highly paid hospital staff are idle. Harvey threatened to have the orthopedic surgery department manager fired because she tried to control excessive use of supplies and pressed him to keep to his schedule.

According to estimates of demand included in marketing analyses, the orthopedic surgery service line should produce a profit; instead, its small market share results in a loss. Furthermore, the payer mix for orthopedics was 50% government insurance coverage for the indigent, which pays only 30% of charges. When the subject was broached by Schilling,

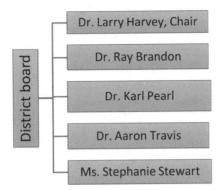

Figure 15.3. District board members.

Harvey threatened to admit his patients at a competing hospital. Harvey often became emotional in meetings and accused Schilling of yelling at him. Eventually, Harvey stopped returning Schilling's phone calls. Compounding these problems was Harvey's difficulty in separating his anger about reductions in healthcare reimbursement and the hospital's rocky relationship with the VPG physicians from his clinical work in the hospital.

Dr. Ray Brandon is also an orthopedic surgeon. Brandon was on the district board when there was a PHO, but he took a more passive role. During a closed-door meeting of the board he did not hide his animosity toward the VPG physicians who formed the PHO with the hospital. He, too, was frustrated by declining reimbursement. In addition, he was frustrated by the breakdown in the relationship between physicians and hospital governance. Occasionally, Brandon appeared to disregard state law applying to governance of tax district hospitals. The "open meetings" law requires that board members only discuss district hospital matters in meetings open to the public. Meetings in which proprietary information is discussed are exempt from the open meetings requirement. During a "closed" board meeting at which proprietary matters were being discussed, Brandon stated he wanted to discipline physicians who refused ER call. After the "open" board meeting that followed, Brandon took the hospital attorney aside and asked her to research legal action against physicians who refused ER call. Schilling had advised board members to approach the ER call issue more diplomatically and not attract media attention. Schilling used a politically acceptable solution by analyzing benchmarking data from area hospitals and offering to pay on-call physicians at market rates. Physician groups were asked to bid to take ER call.

The third member on the district board during the years of the PHO was Dr. Karl Pearl, a neurologist with privileges at BMH. He is the most bitter of the board members about how VPG "ruined" the PHO, and he is publicly critical of VPG. Pearl resented the decreases in healthcare reimbursement and he often pontificated about it at board meetings. As with the other physician board members, Pearl's clinical privileges at BMH are perceived as a potential conflict of interest. He has publicly criticized the large size of the management staff. The CEO took this as a personal affront and believed it adversely affected the morale of his staff.

The fourth member of the board is also a clinician. Aaron Travis, DO, is an osteopath with privileges at a competing community hospital. He respects Schilling and accepts his advice. Travis boasts of "saving" the hospital during the PHO by asking "a few simple questions" about the hospital's performance that, at the time, no one could answer. This led to other questions. The result was greater transparency and, eventually, a financial turnaround for the hospital. Unfortunately, Travis has limitations that affect his ability to be an effective board member. He is openly angry about his experiences during the PHO, such as when his car was vandalized and he received threatening phone calls. Since Travis has privileges at a competing hospital, some question his loyalty to BMH and commitment to it.

The fifth board member, Stephanie Stewart, is a community business woman. She respects Schilling and is willing to work with him. Stewart had difficulty grasping the complexity of hospital operations and its finances when she was first a board member. To her, it made no sense that the hospital is not paid its charges for services. She wants to be a team player and becomes frustrated at times with the physician members' negativity. Often, she and Travis have asked physician board members to "move on from the past." The breakdown in communications with the CEO was apparent to Stewart.

THE NEW CEO

Three of the five district board seats stood for election in 2012. Two of the three current members remained on the board because there were no other candidates. Before the November elections, the board asked Schilling to become the new CEO. Schilling was the former CEO of a not-for-profit hospital and had spent his entire 40-year professional career as a hospital administrator. Schilling has a history of back problems. When he arrived on the job he appeared to be in good health. As noted, he was originally hired by the district board as a consultant to help the hospital dissolve its relationship with VPG in the PHO. He successfully returned the hospital to district control and eliminated the hospital's $3 million per month deficit within his first year as CEO. The number of FTE hospital employees had decreased significantly during the affiliation with the PHO. This kept expenses for salaries and benefits at a lower percentage of hospital revenue, but Schilling wanted to increase employee morale by hiring more staff, reinstating salary increases, and improving benefits. He also began to put resources back into the hospital by making desperately needed upgrades to the facility. These changes increased employee trust and respect for Schilling, while his warmth and caring attitude helped him gain employees' loyalty. However, these changes also caused the hospital to start losing money again.

LEADERSHIP STYLE

Board members, physicians, and employees gave Schilling accolades for returning the hospital to profitability. Schilling's leadership style, however, was criticized when later financial projections showed a $30 million loss for the following year. Physicians described his leadership style as patriarchal and paternalistic. Physicians, nurses, and managers were accustomed to a culture of teamwork that had been supported and fostered by the former CEO. Schilling became frustrated when his authority was questioned, not only by the medical staff and nurses, but by his executive team. Schilling felt that members of his team did not have the experience to support his turn-around efforts. Most were good at taking direction from him and his COO, but they felt the absence of a strategic plan impeded their ability to focus on a common goal. Schilling delegated the authority to conduct executive team meetings to his COO, Daniel Porter. Porter was not well respected by the management team because of his authoritarian leadership style and his lack of listening skills. The dynamic in executive meetings was such that participants would either begin arguing with each other or nobody would contribute ideas. A lack of leadership was becoming apparent throughout the organization.

LOSING SUPPORT

By improving morale, renovating the facility, and recruiting former members of his executive team, Schilling stabilized BMH. A strategic plan was developed and presented to the board. Schilling's decision to keep the strategic plan confidential until it was ready to be launched, however, made some managers, physicians, and hospital staff uneasy. Because of the politics involved when physicians think their prerogatives are threatened, it was proving impossible to increase market share of revenue-generating services. When pressed to expand the orthopedic and transplant surgery service lines by recruiting new surgeons, the physicians affected threatened to admit to competing hospitals. The orthopedic and transplant surgeons had been at BMH for years and were comfortable with their departments' status. Added to the equation was the physician board members' reluctance to make enemies. The PHO experience had left a bitter taste in the mouths of these board members; they seemed paralyzed by past events. Schilling began to lose support.

The board even criticized successful decisions made by Schilling. The last major decision the board made at his recommendation was to end risk pool agreements with insurance companies. Schilling had presented two options to the board: increase revenue or decrease expenses. The board agreed to decrease expenses by renegotiating the hospital's risk pool contracts, but later claimed Schilling waited too long to present this information to them. In fact, Schilling had tried to persuade the board to exit risk pool agreements for more than 2 years.

A TROUBLED PHYSICIAN

The vice chief of staff, Clara Mavory, M.D., is an anesthesiologist who practices at BMH. She was praised for her commitment to the hospital's survival as a freestanding facility. Mavory had helped lure Schilling from a neighboring hospital to return BMH to district ownership in 2014. Mavory had a troubled history with VPG; she was asked to leave after being disciplined for disruptive behavior seven years prior to establishing her own medical practice. Mavory had a troubled history at BMH, too. A peer review file on Mavory's clinical performance prepared by the BMH quality department showed several instances of questionable clinical judgment prior to 2015. Also, the file included complaints about Mavory's inappropriate behavior toward patients and hospital staff. As Mavory's friend, Schilling felt protective of her. And, he had a sense of obligation toward her for his position at BMH. Although her peer review file had gone to a peer review committee of BMH physicians, no disciplinary action resulted. Schilling kept Mavory's file locked in a cabinet in the clinical quality department office. According to the hospital attorney, the only way to remove a physician's clinical privileges is to substantiate evidence of poor-quality medical practice using procedures required by the medical staff bylaws.

One year after Schilling became CEO in 2014, Mavory began to demand confidential records, including legal and peer review files. Mavory disagreed with many sections of the medical staff bylaws and recommended revisions. This slowed preparation for The Joint Commission on Accreditation of Healthcare Organizations (The Joint Commission) survey because the quality department had to focus on the hospital's legal counsel's review of proposed revisions to the medical staff bylaws. The Joint Commission requires bylaws changes to be in effect a year before a survey. When Mavory did not receive the confidential files she demanded, she criticized Schilling publicly and began to persuade other physicians to distrust his leadership. She had done the same thing to the prior administrator. Also in 2015, board members began to feel bullied by Mavory. The three physician board members with clinical privileges at BMH disagreed with Mavory's demands, but found it easier to acquiesce than challenge her.

Later, in 2016, Schilling realized how useful the information in her peer review file could have been in stopping Mavory from causing a rift between the medical staff and administration. The file existed and still could be used. Because Schilling and Mavory had become adversaries and because a long time had elapsed since the events as now it was over a year, reporting Mavory would seem vindictive, however. Schilling's only recourse was to persuade the board to support him in blocking her demands for confidential information. Over the last year, however, Schilling received no support from the board in disciplining Mavory for her disruptive behavior toward hospital staff. Schilling's numerous attempts to contact the board chair, Dr. Harvey, had been futile. Harvey would not return his calls.

Schilling wrote memoranda to board members when Mavory demanded information. The memoranda included responses to Mavory and explanations to the board as to why certain information was confidential or not appropriate for her to have. No board members answered Schilling's memoranda. Verbal communications had become infrequent and were limited to board meetings. Harvey, along with other board members, felt Schilling was not healthy enough to continue as CEO. Their concerns about Schilling's health diminished their trust of his decision making. They preferred to ignore Mavory rather than deal with her. As fellow clinicians, the physicians on the board were reluctant to criticize Mavory.

REORGANIZING THE BOARD

Schilling trusted his intuition and 40 years of experience as he tried to make better use of the two board members who supported his ideas and remained loyal to him. He developed a plan to organize the board into subcommittees to maximize the influence these two board members had on the other three. Subcommittees included strategic planning, finance, emergency room on-call coverage (ad hoc subcommittee), and governance. Each subcommittee had two board members, the CEO, and designated administrative staff. The proposal for the new subcommittees was presented at an evening public (open) board meeting and was passed unanimously by the board. This restructuring was the first step toward solving the communication problems and increasing the level of trust the other three board members had in Schilling.

SUCCESSION PLANNING

Schilling's contract would end in the fall. Should he retire or should he seek to renew his contract? As much as he did not want to admit it, his health was deteriorating, and maintaining tumultuous relationships was becoming too demanding. Surgery relieved a back condition, but his general health improved only minimally. Schilling had succeeded in what he had been hired to do—get BMH back into district control and stabilize it. Continued success depended on regaining support of his board and the trust of the medical staff. After adding staff and upgrading the hospital, however, expenses substantially exceeded revenues. Projections showed BMH would soon repeat history by losing $3 million a month. Patient volumes in most services were very low. Nursing ratios were high, but the culture of the organization demanded lower nurse–patient ratios in return for not increasing salaries, a compromise that a strong in-house nursing union supported.

Unfortunately, most board members were not interested in following the CEO's advice to improve the numbers because they had lost confidence in his judgment. As the date for his contract renewal neared, employees, too, began to question Schilling's continuation as their leader. Morale declined further as employees began to fear the instability of a possible change in leadership. Employees feared a for-profit hospital system would buy the hospital. This would change the culture of BMH, and likely lead to lay-offs. During the PHO period, employees had been laid off, salaries frozen, and benefits cut. The employees did not want that to happen, again. After receiving a phone call from a BMH employee, a statewide union used local leadership to try to organize non-nursing employees. Nurses and facility engineers were already unionized. Schilling did not have the energy to stop expansion of the unions, which could ultimately organize all nonsupervisory employees.

A NEW CHIEF OF STAFF

Dr. Mavory was elected vice chief of staff after successfully running against several opponents. The medical staff bylaws provided that the vice chief

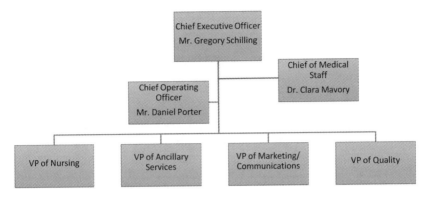

Figure 15.4. BMH organization chart.

of staff automatically becomes chief of staff if the election is uncontested. Mavory had stated she would refuse to take the salary usually paid to the chief of staff because she considered it a conflict of interest. As the election neared, her only opponent withdrew after Mavory confronted him by telling him his candidacy was causing a rift in the medical staff. His withdrawal made an election unnecessary and Mavory became chief of the medical staff (see Figure 15.4). A chief of the medical staff is an adviser to the CEO and a buffer between the CEO and the chiefs of the clinical departments and specialties. Typically, the chief of the medical staff is a confidante to the CEO and a sounding board for clinical matters. This senior member of the executive leadership solves clinical problems and manages medical issues before they become matters that adversely affect a hospital. Dr. Mavory, however, acted out of self-interest and did not perform these duties.

In response to Mavory's criticism of his power over the board, Schilling recommended a change to the hospital bylaws to make the CEO a nonvoting member of the board. As Schilling's energy and involvement waned due to his health problems, Mavory requested that the hospital board make her a voting member because she was chief of staff. These actions required changes to both the hospital bylaws and the medical staff bylaws. The board did not act on either request.

CAUSING TURMOIL

After Mavory became chief of the medical staff, she continued to make enemies of the VPG physicians by attacking them in the medical staff newsletter and at medical staff executive committee meetings. Seven years earlier, Mavory had been forced out of VPG because of disruptive behavior. Schilling was sure this caused her animosity toward the VPG. Since VPG physicians are 50% of BMH physicians, admitting their patients to BMH is essential to its financial health. Schilling thought Mavory's disruptive behavior would eventually subside if she were not confronted. He hoped that by ignoring Mavory she would lose her audience. This was not the case, however. On a weekly—and sometimes daily—basis, she demanded access to computer files, legal correspondence between medical staff office employees and the hospital attorney, and files on medical malpractice cases. Mavory demanded the right to attend confidential department meetings and verbally abused physicians who disagreed with her. She constantly tried to pit the medical staff against administration and appeared to want the physicians to become a union bargaining unit.

OBSTRUCTING PREPARATION FOR THE JOINT COMMISSION

At a meeting that focused on preparing for The Joint Commission survey, Mavory demanded a change in a diagram that showed the flow of communications in the hospital. During the last Joint Commission visit surveyors praised BMH for its excellent communication process, which they said was a model for how other hospitals could expedite communications through layers of bureaucracy. However, Mavory argued the chart showed the medical staff reporting to the CEO.

As soon as she became chief of medical staff, Mavory tried to dissolve the medical executive committee and change the membership of most physician committees. She wanted representatives of administration removed even if they were support staff to the committees. These changes would violate the medical staff bylaws and could compromise The Joint Commission accreditation survey, which was only six months away. The only Type 1 violation (the most serious kind) the hospital received in the previous survey was the medical staff's failure to comply with its own bylaws. Mavory wanted the vice president of quality, Harold Fredrick, excluded from all meetings and eventually fired. Mavory said she did not like Fredrick because they had a personality conflict. Mavory interfered in various ways with implementation of policies and procedures that she disliked. She added and removed appointments to joint medical staff and administrative committees and stalled medical staff bylaws revisions for months and even as long as a year (see Figure 15.5). According to the vice president of quality, this jeopardized Joint Commission accreditation because all recommendations by the medical staff chiefs' committee (MSCC) that require board approval must be in place for at least a year before a Joint Commission survey.

REMOVAL OF COMMITTEE MEMBERS
. . . A committee member appointed by the chief of staff may be removed by a two-thirds vote of the Medical Staff Chiefs' Committee. A committee member appointed by the department chief may be removed by a two-thirds vote of the department medical staff membership or the Medical Staff Chiefs' Committee . . .

Figure 15.5. Proposed medical staff bylaws provision thwarted by Dr. Mavory.

The manager of the medical staff office resigned, citing high levels of stress over the last year. Mavory told hospital employees and physicians that she considered herself everyone's boss. When copy room staff told her she could no longer make personal photocopies at hospital expense, she told the supervisor, "Do you know who I am? I am the most powerful physician in the hospital. I am your boss. You will do as I say!"

COMPENSATION FOR ER ON-CALL PANEL

Mavory seemed to search for issues or problems to pit BMG's physicians against administration. Knowing physicians wanted to be paid to take ER call, she coached one plastic surgeon to take this issue to the MSCC. When some members of the MSCC asked the plastic surgeon for benchmark data on what other hospitals paid ER on-call physicians, the plastic surgeon said he was "too busy" to do the research. The plastic surgery group was the most frustrated with not being paid for ER on-call. They gave administration a deadline to begin on-call payments that the hospital could not meet. No physician would agree to research or benchmark how much other hospitals were paying physicians for on-call. A few board members wanted to report physicians to the state for refusing to take call. Patients not treated in the ER because there were too few physicians, or if the ER had no specialists to meet their medical needs had to be transported to other hospitals. Some board members were concerned this was a violation of the Emergency Medical Treatment and Active Labor Act, which could lead to large fines for the hospital and bad public relations. Administration thought this was unlikely, however. The two board members on the on-call subcommittee came to the MSCC meeting to show their willingness to resolve the issue and to get feedback from the physicians as to what they believed the solution to be. They were well received by the physicians attending the meeting after board members encouraged the physicians to help solve the problem. Ultimately, the CEO proposed an acceptable solution: physicians would be paid $500 to carry an ER pager; physicians asked to come to the ER would be paid $1,500 per 8-hour shift.

NO STRATEGIC PLAN IMPLEMENTED

The board refused to sell or close the money-losing cancer unit because its oncologists would admit patients to a competing hospital. They also worried that VPG doctors would be overcompensated because of the financial arrangement. Schilling believed the board was uneasy about a change in hospital services. After the PHO problem, they seemed reluctant to cut services that could make even one hospital physician angry, or add services that could "overcompensate" physicians.

Dr. Mavory's replacement as vice chief of medical staff was the secretary/treasurer of the medical staff, Dr. Barry Landon. He was the only cardiovascular surgeon at BMH. This violated state law that required hospitals performing open-heart procedures to have a two-surgeon team. When the director of strategic planning, Kelly Nelson, asked Landon about recruiting another cardiovascular surgeon, Landon wanted to have her fired. Landon felt threatened by Nelson's recommendation. He wanted complete control over open-heart surgery. Mavory supported Landon's efforts to remove Nelson, calling her "no good."

SCHILLING'S RESIGNATION

Schilling decided to resign. He did not want to be blamed for BMG's demise and felt responsible for solving its financial problems. His attempts to rebuild relationships with the board and chief of medical staff had been futile. His poor health meant Schilling had no energy to improve relationships with employees, managers, and physicians. Schilling agreed to stay until the district board hired a consultant as interim CEO.

CONSULTANT HIRED

Jenna Carson agreed to take the position as interim CEO of BMH. Carson's 20 years of experience as a "turnaround" expert made her an obvious choice. She had many decisions to make in her new role. As she thought about the future, several questions came to mind.

DISCUSSION QUESTIONS

1. How could she improve the financial position of BMH?

2. What strategies should be used to increase patient volumes?

3. Should she use the old strategic plan or develop a new one?

4. Would the board support her decisions? Her recommendations to it?

5. Should she try to prevent nonunion employees from unionizing?

6. What steps were necessary to control the chief of medical staff?

7. What is the priority of preparing for The Joint Commission survey?

8. What could she do to assist board members in governing BMH?

9. How could the executive team become more effective in improving BMH's performance and help it become a market leader?

10. How should these questions be prioritized?

ENDNOTE

This case used by permission of the authors. Copyright © 2004–2016 by Cynthia Mahood Levin and Kurt Darr.

16

Restructuring Decision Making at Holy Family Hospital

Overcoming Resistance to a Shared Governance Program

Kent V. Rondeau
University of Alberta, Edmonton, Alberta, Canada

Sally Brooks, RN, MSN, was baffled and just a bit angry. Her great effort to introduce shared governance and distributed leadership for the nursing staff at Holy Family Hospital was being met with indifference by many and with downright hostility by the rest. She could not understand the resistance from nurses and physicians to even consider adopting a new approach that she believed would dramatically revolutionize clinical decision making at the hospital. Shared governance is an important new initiative—the aim of which is to distribute decision-making authority more widely to hospital nursing staff. By creating new organizational structures and by implementing a directed professional practice model that would more fully engage, enable, and empower her staff, Brooks believes she would be able to more effectively utilize their full scope of talents and experiences. After all, she thought, "Doesn't everyone want more power and authority at work?"

As the newly hired vice president for Nursing Care at Holy Family Hospital, Brooks was eager to make her mark in the 440-bed community general hospital by promoting and adopting what she considered "progressive management practices." As a nursing leader in her previous job, she had seen the power of shared governance in action. Indeed, shared governance works by dispersing decision-making authority to a larger cadre of employees, typically involving nurses, physicians, and administrators who hold membership in a governing council, or on its various committees. The rationale for distributing leadership more widely in the hospital is that, by empowering employees to engage in activities outside traditional job descriptions, artificially imposed organizational silos and rigid occupational hierarchies that affect quality of care can be eliminated. Through staff engagement and commitment programs such as shared governance, people begin to take more responsibility for the things they do and develop an appreciation for the larger picture that is often seen as external to their traditional fields of responsibility.

In her previous employment at a large and prestigious teaching hospital, shared governance and other forms of distributed leadership were well-regarded practices with a proven track record of success. Accordingly, she believed the practice of shared governance would be easily accepted at Holy Family. When Brooks thought about the power of this progressive innovation to change the organization and its people in a positive and dramatic way, she reflected on her own personal leadership journey. "It was really through shared governance that I began to see its promise for tapping the full potential of nursing staff, as well as enhancing my own role in the process," she thought. "It was my involvement with this program that exposed me to my own leadership abilities and talents. Without this exposure, I would not be where I am today."

While Brooks was fully committed to introducing shared governance to all nursing staff, she was also keen to extend it further by involving the medical staff and administration. The hospital executive director, Roger Steele, was generally supportive of the idea of distributed leadership at Holy Family if it would improve patient care quality and reduce operating costs. However, he was concerned that shared governance might slow decision making by creating additional bureaucratic hurdles. Indeed, the last accreditation review noted that Holy Family "suffers from slow and convoluted decision making as a consequence of having too many administrative committees with little coordination among them."

The physicians were highly supportive of efforts to improve patient care quality at Holy Family, but worried that the potential of programs like shared governance would not improve communication between doctors and nurses. Dr. Stan Jonas, the chief of staff, was on record as being frustrated by the quality of the relationships between the hospital's physicians and nursing staff, which had become increasingly strained in recent years. Dr. Jonas stated his position on the matter rather succinctly: "Nurses have to remember that they are here to serve patient needs and carry out the commands of the attending physicians by working in ways consistent with their legally mandated scope-of-practice."

INTRODUCING SHARED GOVERNANCE TO THE NURSING STAFF

The meeting with her nursing staff at which Brooks introduced the idea of a shared governance approach to manage clinical decision making at Holy Family Hospital did not go well. As she thought back, she realized the staff concerns were a laundry list of reasons why it shouldn't be done. One nurse manager stated she had read somewhere that the track record on nursing shared governance was decidedly mixed. Another said a local nursing home had tried to introduce it a few years ago and abandoned shared governance after it didn't work. "I don't think we should be pursuing theoretical approaches to management unless there is convincing evidence they work in practice," she declared.

One experienced nurse reminded the group she had "no free time" to participate in the program; patient care responsibilities, administrative duties, and dealing with demanding doctors filled her day. "I can't meet after my shift as I have family responsibilities," she claimed. Another asked if she had to do extra work to serve on a shared governance committee and if she would be paid extra for her participation. "I don't think I'm paid enough as it is, given all that I do around here."

One young nurse hired in the past year stated she was "too new" and didn't have enough experience in managing complex care for very ill patients. "I don't feel competent enough to make decisions that could affect whether someone lives or dies," she stated. A senior nurse with over 30 years of experience at Holy Family commented that doctors have always made the real decisions around here. "They won't cede any clinical decision making power to us. Anyway, I don't see why we have to change how things are done as the system has worked pretty well for us in the past, hasn't it?" Another nurse asked what would happen if the shared governance committee made one decision and it was overruled by the director of nursing or by the hospital administration. "I don't want to serve if I don't have any real power," she asserted.

A nursing aide asked if the members of a shared governance commit-tee could be held accountable and legally liable for decisions that turned out bad. "If that's the case, I don't want any part of this program!" Two nurse ward managers asked about the limits on decision-making authority under a shared governance model. "In what areas will we have a say and will we be restricted from having input on things that are really important to us?" An experienced nurse remarked that she doubted hospital admin-istration and staff physicians would ever participate in structural changes aimed at curtailing their decision-making authority. "I've been around here for over ten years and I know that the 'suits' and especially the 'docs' are never going to give nurses more power!"

One senior nurse manager openly questioned the wisdom of allowing junior staff to make important decisions when they haven't earned their spurs. "I have worked hard to become a nurse manager here, done lots of committee work, gone back to school for my MBA, and stuff like that. I don't think it's fair that others should be given authority when they have not earned it," she declared.

The nurse union representative cautioned everyone that false ideas like distributed leadership programs are really management's way of "extracting more work off the backs of workers. Anyway, it's the responsi-bility of management and the doctors to make decisions, and not us. That's why they make the big bucks, isn't it?" Furthermore, she claimed that pro-grams like shared governance were "illegal" because they operate outside the collective bargaining process, and are really meant to circumvent that process. "If management tries to establish this program here, you can be sure that our union will grieve it," she asserted.

Finally, one elderly nurse nearing retirement stated that, in her day, ideas like distributed leadership and shared governance "would not pass muster." "I think that we too easily get caught up in every little new thing that comes along. This stuff is entirely unproven and is just another stupid management fad that will soon pass. Just ignore it and it will go away!"

As Brooks braced herself against the onslaught of resistance to shared governance, she recalled all the reasons to implement it at Holy Family. Her belief in the benefits of shared governance gained from witness-ing it firsthand at her previous place of employment provided her with confidence that it had the power to transform what she perceived as a rigid, authoritarian, top-down culture at Holy Family. Brooks believes the "physician-centered" ways of doing things at Holy Family silenced, sub-merged, and subordinated nurses under physician control and dominance. "We cannot improve patient care quality here until we have liberated all the human capital of our nursing staff. Shared governance is the means to do just that!"

SHARED GOVERNANCE AS A SOLUTION AT HOLY FAMILY?

Shared governance in management involves an administrative body through which a group of employees exercises its full authority based on their knowledge, skills, and experience. It refers to a group decision-making process that is cast on the bedrock of professional collegiality, egalitarianism, workplace democracy, and shared accountability for the outcomes of those decisions. A broadly shared governance structure describes a partnership between managers and clinical staff, including physicians and other healthcare providers. An underlying premise of shared governance is that staff nurses at every level of the organization should govern their professional practice while being included in all decisions that directly or indirectly affect their patients. Two assumptions are often associated with this form of clinical decision making: first, previous forms of governance will be distributed from traditional managers to clinical staff following the implementation of shared governance, and second, it assumes that nurses, generally, want to be full participants in decisions that affect them.

From a managerial perspective, shared governance is complementary to a number of high-involvement employee work practices, including self-managing work teams, continuous quality improvement teams, nursing cross-training programs, and employee suggestion programs. All these programs require fully engaging providers in the totality of the work enterprise. Nurse empowerment is considered the means by which this engagement occurs because those with the relevant knowledge need to inform decision making since they operate at "the-point-of-care." Shared governance involves a nurse empowerment structure that articulates this requirement because nurses (along with other healthcare providers) operate extensively at this interface.

The literature on shared governance suggests it involves a dynamic structure focused on four critical principles: equity, partnership, ownership, and accountability. *Equity* refers to integration of the nursing duties and roles needed to achieve common goals based on the willingness of each member to contribute to the greater good. *Partnership* requires development of relationships among diverse staff to promote mutual respect, effective communication, and enhanced collaboration to achieve organizational objectives. The principle of *ownership* refers to recognition by the individual of the value of their efforts, knowledge, and aptitudes to organizational performance, while *accountability* involves a willingness to invest in decision making that produces a shared sense of responsibility for individual and collective outcomes. Nursing shared governance is a managerial innovation that legitimizes nurses' control over their practice while extending their influence into administrative areas previously controlled by administrators and clinical areas under the purview of physicians.

Shared governance is not a new idea. Indeed, in the past three decades, forms of it have been implemented with varying degrees of success. Its implementation has been euphemistically described as "very tricky" and akin to "pinning Jell-O to a wall." The shift from traditional models of nursing practice to one of shared governance involves structural change. Indeed, structure is vital to making shared governance work. Healthcare organizations that implement nursing shared governance create organizational structures or permanent committees that address issues such as nursing practice, administration, quality of care, research, and education.

Three primary models of shared governance have emerged in practice. The *councilor model* is the most common. Here, a coordinating council integrates clinical and administrative decisions made by managers, physicians, and nursing staff holding membership on various subcommittees. The *administrative model* continues the traditional bureaucratic structure but splits the organizational chart into two tracks with either an administrative or a clinical focus—although membership in both tracks usually includes managers and staff as implementation progresses. Third is the *congressional model*, which maintains the traditional structure but empowers nurses to vote on issues as a group.

Does shared governance work? There is evidence it has the potential to provide significant benefits to the organization and its nurses. Nevertheless, many healthcare organizations have been unable to realize them. Many studies of the effectiveness of shared governance lack conceptual and methodological rigor that makes it difficult to draw definitive conclusions. Their conclusions draw on anecdotal evidence of success with subjective appraisals of outcomes that include better relationships and team harmony, fewer job-related conflicts, greater job and career satisfaction, improved communication, collaboration, personal and professional growth, and lower turnover. A major problem in determining the effectiveness of shared governance is the absence of valid and reliable standards assessing the extent to which its principles and practices are embedded in the organization. Multiple definitions and conceptualizations of shared governance make comparing studies difficult. A shared governance program in one healthcare organization may be structurally dissimilar and engage decision-making spheres differently than shared governance in another.

A major benefit touted by proponents of shared governance is its potential to improve the work environment of nurses, as well as their satisfaction and retention. A few case studies of single organizations report benefits to nursing, but definitive empirical information of implementing shared governance is mixed. Although some anecdotal cases report improvement in the nursing work environment when autonomy, communication, and practice are consistent with professional ideals, these results have not been consistent over the range of studies with multiple designs, sampling, and measurement strategies. Evidence that shared governance leads to improved team dynamics, such as team cohesion, commitment, and conflict resolution, is also somewhat mixed. Similar to evaluation of other outcomes of shared governance, consistent relationships between shared governance and nurse satisfaction have not been found. In some instances, nurse satisfaction was found to improve when shared governance was implemented; other studies reported no change, or a decrease in nurse satisfaction.

An important contributing factor in explaining the failure of shared governance to realize many of its performance enhancements may be that, as a care delivery model, it requires a major shift in how organizations are typically managed. Most proponents of shared governance stress the need for a supportive organizational culture in which it can take root. Shared governance is a way of conceptualizing workplace democracy and empowerment and includes new structures that must be created to support and extend it. As such, it usually requires changes involving a significant transition as to how managers, nurses, physicians, and organizational systems interact. Part of the journey in implementing shared governance is the high degree of emergent learning that will take place along the way. Implementing structural, process, and cultural changes in complex dynamic systems cannot be mapped precisely before the process has begun. It has been stated that implementing this kind of change is like "opening a door into the soul of the organization. You really don't know exactly where it is going to take you or what you will encounter along the way!"

ADDRESSING RESISTANCE TO SHARED GOVERNANCE AT HOLY FAMILY HOSPITAL

Comforted by her belief in the totality of benefits that could be derived by implementing shared governance at Holy Family, Brooks was, nonetheless, distressed as she thought about how she might proceed and how to answer the questions from the nurses who were reluctant to embrace it. Brooks knows that shared governance requires a strong, supportive culture and strong leadership that will nourish its implementation. Of the six nurse managers at the meeting, two offered only mild support for the idea, while the others were highly skeptical that it could be implemented successfully. An important factor present at Holy Family is a strong, top-down autocratic culture that seems to stifle management innovation. Historically, most important decisions were made by hospital administrators and physicians. Nurses were expected to perform their clinical duties and had narrow, clearly defined, predetermined circumstances in which they could exercise discretion. Nurses had never questioned the existing power structure. Indeed, most nurses had grown comfortable with the status quo in which they worked under rigid scope-of-practice limits.

Brooks knew nurses at Holy Family were deeply suspicious of her motivation for introducing shared governance. The previous director of nursing had tried unsuccessfully to implement a number of management reforms, including nurse self-scheduling, job-sharing, self-managing nursing teams, and a cross-training initiative. All the initiatives were introduced with great fanfare but were abandoned soon after their introduction because they were not working. Often these innovations were abandoned after criticism by a few vocal nurses or by the nurses' union and never had a chance to take root. The hospital had used significant resources to train staff for their new roles and had even purchased a new software program to help nurses job-share and self-schedule their work shifts. Quietly, however, administration made known its skepticism that these "innovations" would significantly reduce nursing costs and improve patient care quality. In retrospect, the impetus for implementing these initiatives followed soon after a consultant's management study showing nurses suffered from problems of morale, stress, burnout, and absenteeism, all of which led to costly turnover. The hospital board was alarmed by the findings and mandated that the executive director do something to address the issues. However, hospital management never seemed fully committed to addressing the problems with the nursing staff.

As Brooks thought about her next meeting with the nursing staff she contemplated how she might reduce the reticence and resistance to the shared governance initiative. She remembered a quote from a paper she had read about employee involvement programs: "We presume that nurses want to participate in decision making, but this assumption is not valid . . . if nurses have authority for decision making, that does not mean they will choose to exercise it." She wondered if empowerment was one of those ideas that is "good in theory" but "unworkable in practice." She wondered if she were trying to introduce the program too quickly, or without sufficiently preparing her staff for change. "Maybe I can make the program voluntary and only involve those who want to participate," she thought. "Would that even be workable because it is contrary to the central tenets of shared governance?"

She knew that shared governance required a compatible organizational culture and that the top-down culture at Holy Family was incompatible. She wondered if she should first change the culture to make it more compatible with shared governance before introducing it, or should she introduce shared governance to leverage the needed cultural change? She understood she would be able to choose the shape and model of shared governance that fits the needs at Holy Family. "Perhaps we can start the process by involving the nursing staff, or perhaps just the nursing staff on a single unit. Then, if it works, add the hospital administration and physicians," she thought. Yet she wondered if there is enough benefit to be gained if the hospital administration and physicians are not involved from the beginning.

She wondered about the prospect of winning the support for the program from nurses, only later to have it rejected by the physicians and senior management. While the hospital executive director and chief of medical staff remain skeptical with respect to the benefits of distributed leadership, she knew her strongest resistance came from her nursing staff, most notably the nurse managers and supervisory staff, who feared that shared governance might make their jobs redundant. As she contemplated a new strategy to win nursing's approval and support and find a way to make it happen, she was bolstered by her unshaken belief that shared governance was the best way to transform nursing practice at Holy Family. Given the rough landscape ahead, how should she proceed?

PART IV

Organizational Effectiveness

17

Attica Memorial Hospital

The Ingelson Burn Center

Bonnie Eng-Suess
Dignity Health, Fullerton, CA

Robert C. Myrtle
University of Southern California, Los Angeles, CA

INTRODUCTION

In late 2013, Attica Memorial Hospital purchased and absorbed its nearest competitor, Delphi Hospital, in what was termed an alliance. Attica Memorial's plans were to consolidate duplicate services and to realign remaining units. Services unique to the acquired hospital were evaluated to determine if they could survive the alliance. Services not essential to the community or that added minimum value to Attica Memorial would not be supported. The Ingelson Burn Center was a unique service line that Attica Memorial evaluated as part of this realignment.

BACKGROUND

Attica Memorial and Delphi Hospitals competed for more than 40 years for patients, physicians, and favorable insurance reimbursement. They were nonprofit, acute care facilities in Norton County. They were less than a half mile apart and offered similar services, which created a fiercely competitive environment. Many Attica Memorial physicians had privileges at Delphi Hospital and could admit patients to either. Physicians admit to a hospital based on their judgment about the hospital's ability to meet patient needs, the physicians' previous experiences with the hospital, and, to some extent, patient preference. The hospitals competed for resources such as staff and health plan and medical group contracts. Before Attica Memorial acquired Delphi Hospital, health plans and medical groups pitted the hospitals against each other to obtain favorable financial relationships. Attica Memorial CEO Richard Ponti had formed the opinion that "Any contract rate is a good rate," even if the health plan reimbursed the hospital at the state's minimum for an open-heart procedure. When Delphi's parent organization placed the hospital for sale, Attica Memorial saw a strategic opportunity to purchase a long-time competitor and strengthen its position in the marketplace.

The initial plan of the alliance was to have both hospitals as recognizable "Center of Excellence" facilities by completely realigning the services between the two facilities. As a result, Attica Memorial transitioned into an acute care inpatient facility; Delphi became an ambulatory care outpatient pavilion. The original Attica Memorial facility became Attica Memorial East Campus (AMH East Campus) and Delphi was renamed Attica Memorial West Campus (AMH West Campus). By combining resources with Delphi Hospital, the new Attica Memorial became a stronger, more vital community resource. The new entity could expand its spectrum of patient care by offering new services, more outreach, improved access to care, and an increased focus on quality. Achieving the efficiencies promised by consolidating redundant services, however, required careful evaluation of each department and service line, transfers of personnel, and, inevitably, layoffs.

MACRO ENVIRONMENT

Before the 1980s, hospitals were unconcerned about reimbursement. They were paid fee-for-service (i.e., their charges were paid at full-price, or at rates negotiated with a third-party payer). The 1980s, however, brought dramatic changes to the healthcare environment. These changes were driven by the large increases in the cost of healthcare due to increased costs of pharmaceuticals, aging of the population, advancements in medical technology, shortages of nurses, increases in the number of sicker patients, and large amounts of federal and state money pouring into the healthcare system. In California, this led to development of managed care organizations (MCOs). MCOs monitor hospital services closely to control costs. Health maintenance organizations (HMOs) dictated lengths-of-stay and reimbursement rates for hospitals. This made maintaining or expanding market share in Norton County extremely difficult. In response, demand for healthcare services shifted dramatically from inpatient to outpatient settings. This resulted in too many hospital beds for the declining number of inpatients. At the same time, the federal government attempted to contain and reduce costs by reimbursing hospitals under the federal inpatient prospective payment system (IPPS) diagnosis-related groups (DRGs) rates. Reimbursement from health plans and Medicare and Medicaid declined substantially. Hospitals saw revenue shrink on lower reimbursement and discounted fee-for-service rates. This made it difficult to cover costs.

COMPETITIVE ENVIRONMENT

In Norton County, competition was fierce for market share because there were too many hospitals within a small geographic area. There are 7 hospitals in a 5-mile radius of Attica Memorial. All of them competed for patients, physicians, and health plan contracts. In a 10-mile radius, Attica Memorial's competition increased to 16 hospitals. The managed care penetration in Norton County was approximately 52%—almost double the national average of 28%—thereby creating concerns about managing risk and contract liability (Kaiser Family Foundation, 2015).

There were too many hospital beds in 2015, and the number was increasing. The hospital average daily census in the state was 59%; Norton County's hospitals' average daily census was slightly lower at 53% (California Health Care Foundation, 2015). Another external threat to hospitals was California Senate bill 1953 (SB 1953). This legislation mandated retrofitting existing hospitals to current building seismic safety codes by the year 2020 and would require significant capital expenditures and interruption of services at many hospitals. In addition, the healthcare market was experiencing a nursing shortage, thereby increasing costs and competition for nursing staff.

ANALYSIS OF THE INGELSON BURN CENTER

Nature of Burn Injuries

Burn injuries are unique. Burn is a service line unlike obstetrics, for instance. Obstetricians can estimate how many deliveries they will perform in a given time based on patient base. Burns are caused by fire, sun, chemicals, heated objects, heated fluids, and electricity. Burns are diagnosed as minor (needing non-emergent care) or major (needing life-saving emergency care). Burns are staged depending on damage to body tissue as first, second, or third degree.

Burn Statistics

In the United States, approximately 2.4 million burn injuries are reported per year. Medical professionals treat approximately 486,000 of these injuries; 40,000 are hospitalized. Of those hospitalized, 20,000 have major burns involving at least 25% of their body surface. Approximately 4.500 burn patients die, and approximately 1 million sustain substantial or permanent disabilities (CDC, 2015).

Children age newborn to 2 years are the most frequently admitted patients for emergency treatment of burns. Most burns for these children occur in the kitchen. The next most common area is the bathroom, where they are scalded by hot water. Scalds are the leading cause of accidental death in the home for children from birth to age 4 and are 40% of the burn injuries for children to age 14 (CDC, 2015).

Burn Center Background

In 2003, Dr. Craig Ingelson felt there was a need to provide his unique standard and continuum of care to burn victims in three large counties by establishing a burn center in Norton County. It would serve as a regional center of excellence by using the same coordinated approach to the acute, surgical, and rehabilitative continuum of burn services he provided at Ingelson Burn Center, 50 miles from Delphi Hospital. In 2007, Ingelson and Delphi Hospital established the Ingelson Burn Center as a state-of-the-art, licensed 6-bed inpatient unit coupled with a dedicated outpatient burn center adjacent to the hospital. Dr. Ingelson was named medical director. The Ingelson Burn Center of Norton County earned a reputation for excellent care and superior outcomes achieved by a highly motivated and trained team. The burn center received referrals from other hospitals, employers, insurance companies, and fire departments for both acute inpatient care and continuing outpatient reconstructive surgery and therapy.

Patient Care

Patients arriving at the emergency department of Ingelson Burn Center are met by a team of emergency medicine physicians, nurses, and emergency medical technicians, all of whom are trained in burn care. They conduct a preliminary assessment and perform emergency treatment. The emergency team is in contact with the burn surgeons headed by Ingelson, and they relay information regarding the patient's injuries. The patient is admitted to the inpatient burn unit in which the patient's injuries are monitored for 48–72 hours post admission. Burn care specialists coordinate care.

Staff

The burn team includes plastic surgeons; neurologists; psychologists; infectious disease physicians; neonatologists; pulmonologists; ophthalmologists; nurses; occupational, physical, recreational, respiratory, and speech therapists; and case managers.

Staff are trained in current treatment protocols for burn care and receive continuing education. In addition, all staff is ACLS (advanced cardiac life support) certified and ABLS (advanced burn life support) trained.

Nurse staffing in the inpatient burn center is based on the ratio recommended for a critical or intensive care patient. All specialists are trained in emergent, acute, immediate, and progressive treatment of burn injuries and are assigned as-needed after an evaluation of patient needs. The burn center has four full-time scheduled RN staff, one part-time, and one *per diem* nurse. Normally, the patient–staff ratio is 1:1, 2:1, and 3:1, respectively, based on patient classification and patient care needs.

Staffing is continuously assessed and adjusted based on patient census and condition, staff experience and training, technology used, and supervision needed. Policy requires not fewer than two nursing personnel physically present in the unit when a patient is present, and at least one of the nursing staff members is an RN.

On average, 20% of Ingelson's patients are children. To serve this special population, the burn center has a bilingual licensed clinical social worker on staff who is approved by state children's services. The social worker provides recreational therapy and works with the children and their families to address concerns and fears in dealing with their burn injuries.

Communication among the burn team and a patient's employer, insurer, and medical management representative is critical to delivering quality care. To maintain continuous flow of communication among members of the team, the burn center coordinated weekly patient care conferences moderated by the case manager. The purpose of the conferences is to discuss and evaluate inpatient and outpatient cases to ensure a full continuum of patient care.

Quality/Image

Ingelson is a nationally recognized plastic surgeon, who graduated from Emory University and the University of Tennessee Medical School. He is board certified in general surgery and plastic surgery. Ingelson has a unique method of treating burns, based on extensive use of surgery when he debrides and grafts burn patients. His method is less painful than traditional debridement and grafting. He combines a large burn and reconstruction surgical practice with an aesthetic (cosmetic) surgical practice. The Ingelson Burn Center of Norton County has earned a reputation for excellent care and superior outcomes from a highly skilled and patient-focused team.

License Requirements

A hospital burn unit must comply with the California State Code of Regulations for both state operations codes and state building codes.

State Operations Codes California State Department of Licensing, regulations require that a burn center is a dedicated, closed unit. To treat severe burns, beds must be licensed to treat only burn patients. In addition, the diminished immune response of burn patients requires that the unit be isolated. A burn unit

- is defined as an intensive care unit (ICU) with services and staff specializing in burn treatment, used solely to treat burns or similar/related conditions.

- must be configured to prevent through traffic.

- must have a minimum of 4 beds and no more than 12.

- must treat at least 50 burn patients per year.

State Building Codes According to the architecture firm with which Attica Memorial has a contract, a burn center is defined in the state building code as a unit that meets requirements for operation of an intensive care unit, and has space for rehabilitation and respiratory care services.

The code does not state that any referenced areas may be shared, but only that the design guidelines for a burn center must comply with requirements needed for an intensive care unit, rehabilitation unit, and respiratory care service. Given the unique nature of the treatment and potential for airborne contamination in a burn center, the architects believe it is the intention of the code to designate this department to function as a stand-alone department or unit. In the past, the state health and licensing office categorized the Ingelson Burn Center as a separate unit for treatment of burn patients.

Burn center regulations parallel state building codes for operation of an intensive care unit. The following summarize key requirements pursuant to the state building code:

- At least one negative pressure isolation room provided for patients with an airborne communicable disease

- A nursing station with a control desk, charting space, lockable medicine cabinet, refrigerator, and hand washing fixture

- At least 132 square feet of floor space per bed with no dimension less than 11 feet, at least 4 feet of clearance around the bed, and at least 8 feet between beds

- Twenty-four-hour coordination and physical space requirements for respiratory and rehabilitation care

Physician and Nursing Supervision

There are specific California state operation codes and regulations for supervision of a burn center. The state code requires that Attica Memorial provide medical and nursing staff with significant burn care experience and training as follows:

- Two board certified or eligible surgeons experienced in burn treatment shall be responsible for supervising and performing burn care.

- Continuous in-house physician coverage is required.

- A registered nurse with at least 6 months' experience in treating burn patients and with evidence of burn care continuing education shall be responsible for nursing care and management in the burn center.

- A registered nurse with at least 3 months' experience in treating burn patients shall be on duty each shift.

Members of the medical and nursing staff at Attica Memorial and Delphi Hospitals were interviewed to determine their level of experience and interest in treating burn patients. The interviews found that many RNs trained in burn care had resigned from Delphi Hospital. It was the judgment of the Attica Memorial intensive care unit (ICU) and critical care unit (CCU) leadership that Attica Memorial staff did not have the competencies in burn treatment to provide the level of care.

STATE CHILDREN SERVICES IMPACT

California State Children Services (SCS) regulates treatment of children age birth to 21 years with disabilities resulting from congenital anomalies or severe debilitating injury who are Medicaid beneficiaries. SCS certification is vital to operation of the burn center. According to the director of business development for Ingelson, SCS patients are 74% of pediatric inpatient burn volume and 26% of all pediatric outpatient visits in 2014.

For the first and second quarters of calendar year 2015, 59% of inpatients and 31% of outpatients were SCS.

SCS CERTIFICATION REQUIREMENTS

SCS guidelines provide for specialized care of pediatric patients and for adults with delayed mental development in an acute care environment. These guidelines consist of policies and procedures designed to support the psychosocial and emotional well-being of pediatric patients. SCS certification requirements have very little effect on the normal operations of a burn unit. The following are SCS requirements:

- Pediatric playroom and age-appropriate toys
- Increased security provisions for pediatric patients
- Specialized pediatric burn intake and admission nursing protocols
- Cribs and crib nets functional 24 hours
- Pediatric crash carts, thermometers, scales, BP cuffs, and so forth
- Pediatric physical therapy available 24 hours
- Child life therapist available 24 hours

SCS Current State

The Ingelson Burn Center applied for SCS certification 3 years ago, but was granted only provisional status because the burn center had not fulfilled all requirements of the Department of Health Services. The provisional status expires October 31, 2016. If provisional status expired without immediate written notification to SCS regarding the future of the center, the burn center would no longer be reimbursed for treating the largest percentage of its pediatric patients. Recertification was unlikely if provisional status lapsed.

Even if provisional status were renewed after October 31, 2016, SCS cannot be applied to the burn center at Attica Memorial East Campus since SCS status is not transferable from one facility to another. Applying for SCS accreditation is an extensive process that can take more than 2 years. Without SCS, the burn center could not treat pediatric patients and would have to transfer them to University Hospital, 5 miles to the south. University Hospital treats pediatric burn patients under its SCS medical center umbrella status; however, the medical center is applying for SCS certification specifically to treat pediatric burn patients, which would be a threat to Attica Memorial's ability to capture this important burn population.

FACILITY CONSTRAINTS

Based on findings regarding the licensing and regulatory requirements of operating a burn center, the burn unit must be located near critical or intensive care because of the severity of burn injuries and complications that could arise. Because infection is so threatening to a burn victim, both positive and negative pressure rooms are required for the most critical patients. Children typically comprise 50% of burn patients. To treat pediatric burn inpatients, SCS requires a playroom in the burn unit. The playroom is where parents visit their children, adolescents visit their friends, and staff or social workers perform play and recreational therapy with children. According to the burn center business director, the existing playroom is too small (190 square feet) and must be expanded by 5%.

A hydrotherapy room is a critical element in treatment of severe burns. Hydrotherapy cleanses and disinfects the burn, allows dressings to be removed, and performs gentle skin debridement.

Hyperbaric oxygen therapy (HBO) is the second critical element in treating burns. HBO is a process that places patients in an environment in which they breathe, and their burns are surrounded by, a high concentration of oxygen at two to three times atmospheric pressure. HBO has proven effective in promoting rapid healing.

Equally important is the third element—the outpatient burn clinic, located near Delphi Hospital. At the outpatient burn clinic, patient progress is continually monitored and modified when appropriate, not only by the physicians, psychologist, and nurses, but also by the therapists and the burn case manager.

CAPACITY ANALYSIS

Based on the licensing and regulatory requirements for a burn center, a capacity analysis was conducted to integrate a dedicated burn unit into the Attica Memorial East Campus physical plant. The current East Campus ICU/CCU space is a potential location for the burn center. Two capital build-out scenarios were considered: (1) integration of a burn unit into current ICU/CCU configuration, and (2) expansion of inpatient space through a full unit build-out. Based on ICU/CCU post–campus integration capacity constraints and state operations and building codes, it was found to be infeasible to integrate a burn unit into the ICU/CCU. Therefore, a new unit would have to be built to accommodate. The architecture firm estimated the total cost for a dedicated six-bed burn unit would be approximately $3,386,461; a dedicated four-bed burn unit would cost approximately $3,176,657. It was much less costly to move

Table 17.1:   Ingelson Burn Center summary (without loss of SCS)

	FY 2015	FY 2016	FY 2015	FY 2016
Contribution Margin				
Net Revenues	$4,013,120.83	$4,018,575.18	$4,013,120.83	$4,018,575.18
Less:				
Variable Expenses	$2,040,509.26	$2,210,353.71	$2,040,509.26	$2,210,353.71
Fixed Expenses	$913,773.48	$912,262.72	$913,773.48	$912,262.72
Total	$1,058,838.09	$895,958.75	$1,058,838.09	$895,958.75
Impact to Inpatient Surgery	$404,866.80	$404,866.80	$404,866.80	$404,866.80
Burn Center Net Margin	$653,971.29	$491,091.95	$653,971.29	$491,091.95

	Moved to Present Rehabilitation Space at Attica Memorial East		Moved to Attica Memorial East (full build-out Expansion)	
Capital Expense— 6 Beds	$1,730,510.17	$1,730,510.17	$3,386,461.38	$3,386,461.38
Capital Expense— 4 Beds	$1,552,153.98	$1,552,153.98	$3,176,657.75	$3,176,657.75
Analysis				
Payback (in years)— 6 Beds	2.65	3.52	5.18	6.90
Payback (in years)— 4 Beds	2.37	3.16	4.86	6.47

the burn unit to the Attica Memorial rehabilitation space: approximately $1,552,154 for four beds, or approximately $1,730,510 for six beds (see Table 17.1).

PHYSICIAN RELATIONS

Ingelson is medical director of the Ingelson Burn Center. He does not, however, admit patients at Delphi Hospital. Ingelson and his burn surgeons are only on site for complex and acute burn patients; otherwise, Dr. Fred Peace is the local burn physician who manages burn cases that come through the Ingelson Burn Center. Peace reviews the burn cases with Ingelson to confirm a treatment plan. All phases of inpatient care are coordinated on the same unit and are supervised by Ingelson and his team. Nurses, therapists, and other allied health professionals have been trained

Table 17.2. Ingelson Burn Center summary (with loss of SCC)

	FY 2016	FY 2016
Loss of State Children Services		
Loss of Contribution Margin	$242,407.35	$242,407.35
Lost Savings	$215,642.00	$215,642.00
Burn Center Net Margin	$26,765.35	$26,765.35
	Present Rehabilitation Space at Attica Memorial East	Moved to Attica Memorial East (full-build out expansion)
Capital Expense—6 Beds	$1,730,510.17	$3,386,461.38
Capital Expense—4 Beds	$1,552,153.98	$3,176,657.75
Analysis		
Payback (in years)—6 Beds	64.65	126.52
Payback (in years)—4 Beds	57.99	118.69

to treat burn injuries and related issues. After discharge from inpatient status, care continues at the outpatient burn clinic. There, physicians and staff who know the case work with patients and their families to achieve maximum physical and emotional recovery.

Edward Totino, former CEO of Delphi Hospital, stated that Ingelson is an extraordinary physician entitled to special treatment. Whenever Ingelson was needed at Delphi, the hospital provided limousine service for his trip to the burn center. Totino gave a firm warning that if Attica Memorial did not treat Ingelson well, Ingelson would leave and establish a burn center elsewhere. A burn center without Ingelson would no longer be a center of excellence in Norton County. Therefore, burn patients would use burn centers that were not as effective. In addition, the hospital would lose a vital source of revenue generated by the Ingelson Burn Center (see Table 17.2).

PHYSICIAN POLITICS

When Attica Memorial CEO Rick Ponti surveyed physicians with admitting privileges at both Attica Memorial East and West Campuses, those who knew of Ingelson had negative comments about him. They said Ingelson is a "Diva Physician." They disliked the fact that administration gave Ingelson special treatment and treated him better than other physicians. Attica Memorial East Campus physicians had mixed feelings

Table 17.3. Impact on inpatient surgery contribution margins.

Total inpatient Cases	1420
Average Gross Revenue per Case	$75,791.20
Average Deduction per Case	$51,496.66
Net Revenue per Case	$24,294.54
Average Variable Cost per Case	$14,291.03
Average Direct Fixed Cost per Case	$2,217.61
Average Contribution Margin per Case	$7,785.90
Number of Inpatient Procedures Impacted Each Week by Underutilization of Blocked Operation	
Underutilized Room Time per Week	1
Impact per Week	$7,785.90
Number of Weeks per Year	52
Impact per Year	$404,866.80

Note: According to Jamie Patel in the Surgical Services Department at AHM West Campus, Dr. Ingelson on average underutilizes his operating room time by 3 hours each week. Assuming that the average inpatient surgery takes 3 hours and the operating room time is near or at capacity, the underutilization of operating room will impact 1 surgery per week

about bringing the Ingelson Burn Center to their facility. Some were indifferent to the burn program; however, there was a lack of support from the general and plastic surgeons interviewed. They did not like Ingelson's practice of reserving large blocks of OR time each week because the time was typically underutilized (see Table 17.3).

Ingelson met with Ponti and his executive team to tour the East Campus. It was noted that Ingelson's choice of where to place the burn unit would be extremely expensive to build if regulatory requirements were met. Building a dedicated unit would require removing structures and shifting services. Ingelson's request to convert the RNs' rest area to the burn pediatrics playroom was not well received by Debra Walker, VP of Patient Care. Similarly, converting the physician workout room to hyperbaric use was not well received by physicians.

COMMUNITY IMPACT

Ingelson's dedication to superior patient care, continuing education, and community outreach, has earned the burn center the respect and support of local fire departments. Interviews with local firefighters show support for the Ingelson Burn Center. One firefighter had been treated at Ingelson and was extremely satisfied with the outcome. A local fire department spokesperson stated they preferred treatment at Ingelson to that at University Hospital. The firefighters stated in their memorandum of understanding that if they were ever badly burned, they would prefer to be treated at Ingelson rather than other burn centers.

The progressive group health-care consultants claimed that burn units should admit 100 patients annually for 3 consecutive years to maintain the appropriate level of proficiency. Based on Norton County statistics, University Hospital admitted approximately 384 burn patients from 2008 to 2014 and its burn center was meeting American Burn Association's standards. The Ingelson Burn Center had approximately 279 admissions for the same period. In addition, 85% of the burns treated in Norton County were 0%–20% burns and not considered "severe." Lower severity burns can be treated in nondedicated inpatient units and emergency departments. These statistics suggest there might not be enough projected demand for two burn centers in Norton County.

Dr. Matthew Suess, Medical Director of Norton County's Health Care Department, stated that a preliminary study of burn treatment in Norton County indicated University Hospital provided more than adequate coverage for the county. Suess did not support continuation of the Ingelson Burn Center and did not support Dr. Ingelson's method of treating burns with extensive plastic surgery. Suess stated that low volume of burn cases made it unnecessary for Norton County to have two burn treatment programs. He said the county would not be negatively affected if University Hospital were the sole provider for burn treatment.

OPPORTUNITY FOR MARKET GROWTH

Ingelson Burn Center's status as a center of excellence had the potential to brand Attica Memorial and increase volume. As part of its continuum of care, Ingelson provided outreach and educational services to pre-hospital personnel (e.g., emergency medical technicians), emergency department staff, schools, employers, and insurance carriers. The center hosted educational seminars, participated in community and employer health fairs, and provided in-service training that utilized materials on burn safety, first aid for burn injuries, and breakthrough treatment of burn injuries and similar information. In addition to hosting burn education seminars, Ingelson held an annual burn survivors' reunion for former and current patients and their families and friends.

Opportunities for market growth could be dimmed, however, by competition from University Hospital's burn center. University Hospital had a Level 1 trauma center designation and reported treating 123 inpatient burn cases in 2015. Without Level 1 trauma center designation, Ingelson was limited to receiving only burn patients and was unable to treat patients with combinations of burn and non-burn injuries. According to Norton County Emergency Medical Services, in the past 3 years burn volume had trended down from 23% to 15% of all emergencies.

Treating workers' compensation patients was likely to be limited because patients must either predesignate a program or wait 30 days post-admission to transfer to a different burn center. In an interview, Dr. David Carpenter, owner of a large medical group that had a contract with Attica Memorial, stated his medical group would not use Ingelson for workers' compensation patients because of its high costs. Ingelson's use of plastic surgery to treat burns had impressive outcomes, but costs were high. Carpenter referred his group's workers' compensation patients to University Hospital because it had good outcomes and costs were within the norm.

PROFITABILITY

Based on financial data provided by Delphi Hospital's decision support system and factoring in the impact on inpatient surgery, the Ingelson Burn Center's net margin in FY 2015 was $653,971. Net margin in FY 2016 decreased to $404,867 (see Table 17.1).

If Ingelson were moved to Attica Memorial East Campus, the capital expense for a full build-out expansion of six beds was $3,386,461, based on both FY 2015 or FY 2016 financials. The payback for this capital investment was 5.18 years based on FY 2015 patient volume and revenue, or 6.9 years based on FY 2016.

If the burn program were moved into the current rehabilitation space at Attica Memorial East Campus, the capital expense could be reduced to $1,730,510 for six beds, with payback of the full build-out expansion in 2.65 years based on FY 2015, or 3.52 years based on FY 2016 (see Table 17.1).

Moving the Ingelson Burn Center to the East Campus, whether into a new building or into existing rehabilitation space, however, meant that loss of SCS certification had to be considered. Because SCS status would not transfer to the AMH East Campus, the financial health of the program would quickly worsen. According to the financial analysis for FY 2015, the SCS contribution to margin that would be lost was $242,407. The lost savings for surgery call coverage was $147,869, and the lost savings for a blood bank technician was $67,773; therefore, the total net margin was only $26,765. Without SCS certification, the payback of the capital investment in the burn program for a full build-out expansion for six beds was 126.52 years; if the program moved to the AMH East Campus rehabilitation space, the payback for six beds was 64.65 years. The dramatic financial impact of the loss of SCS status could make it financially untenable for the hospital to support such a unique program (see Table 17.2).

The practice of reserving large blocks of OR time for the Ingelson Burn Center physicians would dramatically affect the Attica Memorial Surgical Services if the burn center moved to AMH East Campus. The Ingelson group currently scheduled two 4½ hour OR time blocks per week at the West Campus in anticipation of as-needed surgery. Attica Memorial's surgical services coordinator stated it was standard practice at East Campus to release OR time 72 hours in advance. The Ingelson group, however, released its block OR time only 14 hours in advance—at 5:00 p.m. the day prior to block time that had no scheduled surgeries. The surgical services coordinator stated late cancellations by the Ingelson group results in idle OR time and affects OR scheduling and, therefore, hospital revenue.

Attica Memorial East Campus OR suites are being utilized at or near capacity and constraints on OR scheduling are anticipated when services from the West Campus are integrated. In addition, interviews with Attica Memorial West Campus Surgical Services staff revealed that the Ingelson group was currently under- utilizing its block schedule by 3 hours each week, which affected inpatient surgery at the Attica Memorial East Campus facility. The practice of reserving large blocks of OR time might reduce Attica Memorial East Campus surgical services revenue by $404,867 (see Table 17.3). When the capital expenditure for a new, six-bed, dedicated burn unit at the East Campus of $1,730,510 (using rehabilitation space), or $3,386,461 for the full build-out, was added to a decrease in the overall inpatient surgery contribution margins (see Table 17.2), the burn program would have a negative impact on the East Campus balance sheet.

EASE TO IMPLEMENT

The proposal to close the Ingelson Burn Center was met with great resentment by the former Delphi Hospital's staff and administration. Delphi's former CEO believed Ingelson's burn treatment methods and outcomes were far superior to competitors that used medical residents to treat burn patients. In addition, with provisional SCS status, Attica Memorial West Campus could increase volume and surpass University Hospital, its nearest competitor. The alliance's plan for an East Campus acute care facility and a West Campus ambulatory care facility would, however, require moving Ingelson to the East Campus and building a new intensive care burn unit and hyperbaric facilities.

Establishing the burn center at the East Campus would require investment to train emergency clinical and critical care staff in emergency burn care. In addition, during the transition, burn staff would train the East Campus clinical staff that will be providing burn treatment. Furthermore, some current Ingelson nurses stated they preferred to not work with Ingelson and burn patients, and wanted to transition out of the burn unit.

Ingelson had a history of high nursing staff turnover because, as one burn nurse stated, working with Ingelson could be challenging. This turnover added to costs because nursing staff had to be recruited and trained.

THE INGELSON BURN CENTER DECISION

After Ponti reviewed the burn center analysis, he knew a decision as to the fate of the program had to be made. In order to clearly delineate the implications of whichever course was taken with the burn center, Ponti had to take a number of issues into consideration. In deciding, Ponti knew that the community impacts and emotional issues could not be overlooked, but that the financials were vital to the decision about whether to continue the burn center. Three alternatives resulted from the analysis: (1) Status quo—the Ingelson Burn Center remains at Attica Memorial West Campus, the former Delphi Hospital; (2) Relocation—the Ingelson Burn Center moves to Attica Memorial East Campus; (3) Termination—Attica Memorial closes the Ingelson Burn Center.

ENDNOTE

This case used by permission of the authors. Copyright © 2016 by Bonnie Eng-Suess and Robert C. Myrtle. *Note:* Names and identifying characteristics have been changed to ensure anonymity.

DISCUSSION QUESTION

1. What should Ponti do?

REFERENCES

California Hospitals: An Evolving Experiment, California Health Care Almanac. (2015). California Health Care Foundation. Retrieved from http://www.chcf .org/publications/2015/08/california-hospitals

Centers for Disease Control and Prevention. (2011). National Hospital Ambulatory Medical Care Survey: 2011 Emergency Department Summary Tables. Retrieved from https://www.cdc.gov/nchs/data/ahcd/nhamcs_emergency/2011_ed_web_ tables.pdf

Centers for Disease Control and Prevention. (2015). Retrieved from https://www .cdc.gov/masstrauma/factsheets/public/burns.pdf

Kaiser Family Foundation. (2015). State Health Facts. Retrieved from http://kff .org/other/state-indicator/hmo-penetration-rate/?currentTimeframe=1&select edRows=%7B%22nested%22:%7B%22california%22:%7B%7D%7D%7D

18

Pediatric Dental Care Center

Eleanor Lin
Children's Dental Health Clinic, Long Beach, CA

CASE HISTORY/BACKGROUND

Dr. Blake Johnson, executive and clinical director of the Pediatric Dental Care Center (PDCC), summarized the situation facing the clinic's leadership and board in 2016.

> In a climate where federal and state reimbursements are insufficient to cover our costs, how is the clinic supposed to survive since the majority of our patients require federal and state aid for payment of services? In only one out of the past 6 years did the PDCC generate surpluses sufficient to cover the full cost of doing business. We are at a crossroads now as to how to change our strategy. How could we uphold our mission to provide oral health services to the underserved children in the greater South Bay Community, when the clinic is already running at a loss, with little prospect for increased reimbursement for treating Medicaid patients, which account for about 80% of our patient population?

Recent trends in healthcare had challenged both PDCC's financial health and its mission. Dr. Johnson is determined to continue providing dental treatment to one of the most vulnerable populations, Denti-Care (dental Medicaid) children. His vision is that all children, especially those who are uninsured and/or indigent, should have access to and receive excellent, comprehensive dental care. The clinic has always had a large patient volume. After the 2007 recession, however, demand for services soared.

Due to reductions in reimbursements—now approximately 35% of the national average—many private pediatric dentists dropped out of the government-insured programs, even as an increasing number of families were qualifying for Medicaid.

Initially, PDCC's main clinic was located inside South Bay Memorial Hospital. About five years ago the hospital renovated clinic offices next to the inpatient tower, and the clinic had to move to the clinic building. Housed in a state-of-the-art building, PDCC was able to implement an electronic dental record system and added new equipment, including digital X-rays. Because the clinic is right next to the hospital PDCC's dentists with surgical privileges use the hospital's operating room to perform oral surgery. This unique arrangement differentiates the clinic from competitors and gives it a marketing advantage.

However, in recent years, the clinic has been unable to cover its expenses. Partly, this is because the rent in the new building is much higher than when it was housed in the hospital. Compounding the problem were reimbursement rates that had not changed since 2000 and a 10% across the board funding decrease in 2013 because of the state's burgeoning budget deficit. While the state rescinded the across the board budget reductions in 2015, reimbursement rates have not changed.

Like PDCC, the hospital is also experiencing decreases in reimbursement for Medicaid and Medicare patients. To respond to changes caused by the Affordable Care Act, as well as offset declines in reimbursement, the hospital is exploring the possibility of having one of its outpatient clinics become designated as a federally qualified health center. Aware of PDCC's financial situation, the hospital encouraged it to become part of the federally qualified health center proposal.

THE ORGANIZATION

History of the Pediatric Dental Care Center

The PDCC was founded in 1932 as a not-for-profit organization. Its mission is "to deliver oral health education and comprehensive treatment for economically disadvantaged children, including complex medical considerations, while providing premier treatment in pediatric and multispecialty dentistry."[1] Helped by its relationship with South Bay Memorial Hospital, the PDCC expanded its services to include dental care for disabled children. In 2016, the clinic provided dental services to 10,000 children who made 33,000 visits to the main clinic, as well as to two satellite clinics located in Center City and Belle Vista Island. A dental education center is located in the main clinic and a mobile clinic travels into the community to treat those who cannot come to it. This commitment to serving the

Table 18.1. Six-year financial results

	6/30/11	6/30/12	6/30/13	6/30/14	6/30/15	6/30/16
Assets						
Current assets						
Cash	$300	$300	$295,726	$351,008	$322,632	$263,521
Savings and temporary cash investments	$758,547	$702,297	$1,396	$180	$180	$0
Pledges and grants receivable—net	$521,220	$433,640	$254,913	$155,962	$103,018	$50,500
Accounts receivable—net	$94,771	$84,289	$116,576	$75,335	$96,541	$358,966
Prepaid expenses and deferred charges	$371	$371	$0	$0	$0	$0
Subtotal	$1,375,209	$1,220,897	$668,611	$582,485	$522,371	$672,987
Noncurrent assets						
Land, buildings, and equipment at cost	$3,116,802	$3,406,504	$4,010,612	$4,085,617	$4,148,237	$4,357,618
Less accumulated depreciation	$985,815	$1,127,464	$1,275,045	$1,420,783	$1,584,944	$1,761,651
Subtotal—land, buildings, and equipment	$2,130,987	$2,279,040	$2,735,567	$2,664,834	$2,563,293	$2,595,967
Investments—publicly traded securities	$5,074,322	$5,646,158	$5,649,023	$5,574,716	$5,536,835	$5,134,810
Other assets	$47,755	$47,755	$104,359	$27,134	$20,990	$12,231
Subtotal	$7,253,064	$7,972,953	$8,488,949	$8,266,684	$8,121,118	$7,743,008
Total assets	$8,628,273	$9,193,850	$9,157,560	$8,849,169	$8,643,489	$8,415,995

(continued)

Table 18.1.   Six-year financial results *(continued)*

	6/30/11	6/30/12	6/30/13	6/30/14	6/30/15	6/30/16
Liabilities						
Current Liabilities						
Accounts Payable and Accrued Expenses	$141,512	$175,860	$169,206	$209,904	$158,157	$191,434
Other Liabilities	$136,900	$0	$0	$224,279	$0	$0
Subtotal	$278,412	$175,860	$169,206	$434,183	$158,157	$191,434
Noncurrent Liabilities						
Long-Term Debt	$632,631	$685,208	$636,264	$577,531	$518,800	$460,068
Subtotal	$632,631	$685,208	$636,264	$577,531	$518,800	$460,068
Total liabilities	$911,043	$861,068	$805,470	$1,011,714	$676,957	$651,502
Unrestricted	$1,463,635	$1,636,683	$2,501,294	$1,947,853	$2,238,731	$2,421,347
Temporary restricted	$1,437,605	$1,227,324	$355,026	$413,454	$279,133	$314,158
Permanently restricted	$4,815,990	$5,417,825	$5,495,770	$5,476,148	$5,448,668	$5,028,988
Subtotal	$7,717,230	$8,281,832	$8,352,090	$7,837,455	$7,966,532	$7,764,493
Statement of activities						
Income						
Contributions and grants	$1,043,053	$1,283,723	$1,052,569	$749,572	$942,997	$1,298,649
Program Services revenue	$1,743,251	$1,786,154	$1,749,625	$1,543,617	$1,824,639	$1,657,221
Investment income	$373,463	$368,119	$402,804	$377,491	$95,383	$21,061
Other revenue	$0	$0	$25,161	$0	$0	$0
Total revenue	$3,159,767	$3,437,996	$3,230,159	$2,670,680	$2,863,019	$2,976,931

Expenses

Grants and assistance to individuals	$12,500	$8,000	$3,500	$4,000	$4,000	$0
Salaries and wages	$1,457,588	$1,556,441	$1,249,791	$1,388,160	$1,390,283	$1,567,406
Employee benefits	$166,633	$326,463	$188,290	$232,427	$213,721	$258,380
Fees, dentists	$1,078,301	$1,017,299	$1,117,103	$931,911	$822,663	$744,648
Office expenses	$258,113	$151,012	$176,424	$164,228	$159,923	$146,692
Rent	$108,534	$145,247	$119,449	$122,347	$123,768	$113,980
Depreciation	$179,006	$150,050	$147,581	$160,299	$164,161	$176,706
Dental supplies	$183,220	$152,657	$170,348	$159,942	$156,231	$165,670
Total expenses	$3,443,895	$3,507,169	$3,172,486	$3,163,314	$3,034,750	$3,173,482
Operating surplus (deficit)	($284,128)	($69,173)	$57,673	($492,634)	($171,731)	($196,551)

underserved is best captured by the phrase in its logo and letterhead "every child deserves to smile."

Dr. Blake Johnson

Dr. Johnson's relationship with the PDCC started in high school when his parents encouraged him to research career choices such as law, medicine, and dentistry. He shadowed a practitioner of each profession and was especially drawn to the staff at the PDCC. He volunteered at PDCC during high school and college while he earned his business degree. Following graduation, he went to the University of the Pacific School of Dentistry.

On graduating from dental school, Johnson worked part time as an associate dentist and continued working at the PDCC. A year later, he and his twin brother opened a private office and practiced there for about 8 years. Then he bought out his brother and became a solo practitioner. After a year in solo practice, and even though his business was booming, Johnson felt some emptiness regarding his profession. He wondered if he could do more.

Through personal contacts, he heard about a dental clinic being established for HIV/AIDS patients at the St. Joseph's Medical Center. He sold his practice and became director of that program, but he continued to work part time at the PDCC. A year later, the PDCC's clinical director wanted to step down and Johnson was recommended for the position. Once he found a qualified replacement for his directorship at the HIV/AIDS clinic, Johnson accepted the position as PDCC's clinical director. Five years later, PDCC's executive director asked Johnson to replace her on her retirement. Even though this added significant administrative responsibilities, Johnson accepted the challenge and became executive director while continuing to serve as clinical director.

As a leader, Johnson had a reputation as a hands-on manager. His director of operations said, "He is everywhere at once, but he always gets things done. Since he has practiced at the clinic himself, he has a rapport with the general and specialty dentists who work here. They know he understands their perspective in providing patient-centered treatment. He has worked with all of the veteran staff here as well, so he is very well liked. Whenever he does a walk-through of the clinic he will offer to jump in and help if the dentists are running behind schedule. This attitude of helping out wherever it's needed is the culture that pervades here. He has established a norm here where there is no such thing as 'my work,' but the 'team's work' instead. The work culture at the clinic is one of family. Everyone helps one another, and everyone is motivated to do the best work possible efficiently."

THE STAFF

Healthcare Providers

The PDCC employs 6 general dentists, 2 orthodontists, 4 pediatric dentists, 1 endodontist, 1 oral surgeon, and 1 dental anesthesiologist (when there are intravenous sedation cases). The PDCC also provides training for the region's school of dentistry's residency programs. There are 2–3 oral surgery residents who come one day per month and 3 full-time pediatric residents who see patients daily at the PDCC. The regional U.S. Veterans Affairs Hospital also sends an endodontic resident for training one day a month.

The PDCC attracts dentists who enjoy working with underprivileged children and giving back to the community. Although the majority of dentists at the clinic have their own successful full-time practices, they see their PDCC practice as rewarding, part-time community work. They like the work, they like the fact that patients are appreciative, and they like the people with whom they work. This commitment is not without some personal sacrifice, however. To meet the needs of children on Belle Vista Island, 25 miles off shore, dentists have to take a ferry several times a month. Other dentists sometimes work in the clinic's mobile dental trailer to examine children at schools they visit.

Dentists work 7:20 a.m. to 3:30 p.m.; other staff work 7:20 a.m. to 4 p.m., Monday through Friday, with a 70-minute lunch break. Each dentist works with a dental assistant. As in private practice, dentists typically treat two patients simultaneously. This method allows the dentist to dedicate one chair to patient treatments that require a longer time and the other chair to examinations lasting 10–15 minutes.

The back-office clinic staff helps with clinical work and sterilization, and a front-office staff handles billing, scheduling, and clerical work. Dental assistants regularly rotate among the clinic's dental specialties to keep their skills sharp and versatile. Some assistants even rotate to work at the front desk with billing and scheduling. This proves helpful because if clarification is needed for coding or eligibility during a procedure, dental assistants with experience working at the front desk can answer these questions without stopping treatment.

The dentists usually work different days, so they don't have much contact with each other. However, the dental assistants and dentists have established good rapport because most have a long-term working relationship with the clinic. Some pediatric dentists were pediatric residents recruited by PDCC for part-time employment. Dental assistants who rotated through PDCC during their training also wanted to work at the clinic, but openings are scarce. As Johnson proudly put it, "We have a lot of life-timers."

Because PDCC is a children's dental clinic, the dentists and their staff have seen many patients grow up. Many patients feel close to the dentists even though a patient might see many different dentists during their treatment at PDCC. Patients are not assigned to a specific dentist. Instead, when appointments are made the patient will see whichever dentist is working that day. Since each general dentist works one or two days a week, it is common that more than one dentist completes a patient's treatment plan. This process increases collaboration and oversight because the treating dentist reviews the work of the previous dentist before proceeding with treatment. The dentists believe this ensures the clinic's standard of care is high because the quality of work one day is visible to a different dentist at the next appointment.

Johnson knew that, although he could not pay competitive salaries to attract high-quality dentists, he could offset this disadvantage by providing a rewarding and enjoyable experience to the dentists who worked there. Since most of the dentists are part time, Johnson felt that the most effective use of their time was treating patients rather than participating in the clinic's staff meetings. While this approach creates an environment in which dentists feel their services are valued and make an impact, most learned little about the financial and operational challenges at the clinic. Without a way for dentists to get information about the issues faced by the clinic they had to rely on their staff to "fill them in." Unfortunately, most staff were not able to provide the detailed information the dentists sought.

The most expensive treatments performed at the clinic are procedures involving a dental surgeon and a dental anesthesiologist. Reimbursement for these services pays some of the additional expense but does not cover the actual cost of providing the care. This is true for nonsurgical dental procedures too. The problem of "less than cost" reimbursement is exacerbated when residents provide care because the reimbursement rate for their services is much lower than that received by a fully licensed dentist.

Even though the dentists are key to providing patient care, Johnson believes it's the clinic staff who make it different from other area dental clinics. This view of the importance of staff to the clinic's operations is reflected in its pay and benefits. Dentists are generally compensated at a rate lower than the market average, but dental assistants and clerical staff are paid at market rates. Since nearly all staff are women, the organization adopted policies that reflect that reality. Among the more significant is the paid maternity leave policy and flexible work schedules that allow staff to deal with the inevitable family or childcare issues.

More than half of employees have benefited from these policies. These "progressive" policies can cause significant problems scheduling employees, which reduces efficiency. Despite the problems, however, most staff enjoy working at the clinic and working as a team. Because of the camaraderie, they know each other well, and some have formed friendships that continue outside work. Even though there isn't much room for advancement, most find the work they do and the team-oriented environment unique to the PDCC.

THE PATIENTS

One factor that makes working and volunteering at the PDCC unique is the patients, who are grateful for getting the care they need in a way that makes them feel special. Most patients are poor, and finding affordable dental health services is difficult. While most patients (about 75%) are covered by Denti-Care (Medicaid), reimbursement for those services fails to cover the cost of care. The next largest group (17%) is covered through a public–private partnership between the county department of health services and private, community-based providers, who try to meet the needs of families who do not qualify for Medicaid or other assistance programs. The remainder (roughly 8%) of patients are billed on a sliding scale according to income. Reimbursements from non-Denti-Care sources are higher than those from Denti-Care, but here, too, costs are not covered.

While 85% of pediatric patients are bilingual, 90% of parents speak only Spanish. This is problematic; the majority of dentists have limited Spanish proficiency. Most office staff are bilingual in Spanish and English, so dentists often have to rely on bilingual assistants to translate treatment information, postoperative instructions, and information for patients and families. Since dental treatment makes many people nervous, talking about the procedure in the patient's native language is important. Staff does an excellent job providing a calming atmosphere for children, but that does not overcome the problem of most dentists being unable to communicate directly with parents about the treatment and associated risks.

The clinic averages 225 new patients monthly. Key factors attracting patients to the clinic are its reputation and the affordability of its services. Unfortunately, what was affordable for patients was not affordable to the clinic. In 2013, the state program, Denti-Care, reduced benefits because of poor economic conditions. This resulted in fewer covered patients, and those who were covered had limits on the number and types of treatment that would be reimbursed. While the state recently rescinded these across-the-board reductions in its Medicaid programs, the clinic still had financial shortfalls. Johnson notes that, although the clinic has been somewhat successful in offsetting deficits with grants and fundraising, it has been increasingly difficult to find enough donor support to cover reimbursement shortfalls.

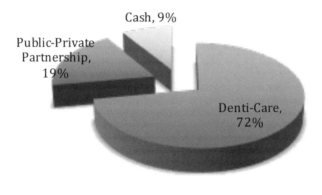

Figure 18.1. Payment mix.

The effects of reimbursement that did not cover the cost of care, increasing dental needs in the community, and the inability of fundraising to provide enough support were a threat to the long-term viability of PDCC. The largest expenditure in clinics like PDCC consists of salaries and wages. Other clinics report that salaries and wages account for 74% of total budget. In contrast, salaries and wages at PDCC are higher. Nonetheless, the PDCC board and senior executives feel that current salary and benefits are appropriate and fair. Unfortunately, continuing reimbursement shortfalls may force management to eliminate one full-time equivalent dentist and reduce the days of coverage by community-based dentists.

RESPONDING TO THE CHANGING ECONOMIC LANDSCAPE

Faced with declining revenue and increasing demand for services, the state made severe cuts to a range of safety net programs. Since healthcare is a major budget item, the state opted to meet increased need by reducing reimbursement for most services, as well as limiting the number of services provided and the frequency with which they are offered. These changes rippled through the provider network, causing some to limit services or reduce access to patients they would otherwise serve.

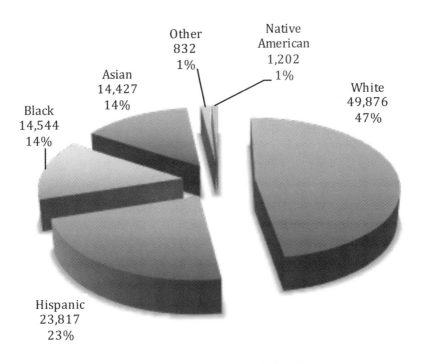

Figure 18.2. Pediatric population in South Bay.

The impact on the PDCC was significant. Consistent with their mission, however, they strove to provide the same quality and amount of care. Simultaneously, the PDCC sought ways to improve efficiency and find other sources of revenue. One way to increase revenue was to join The Children's Clinic (TCC) at the South Bay Memorial Hospital and become a federally qualified health center. Federally qualified health centers must provide primary care for all ages. They are reimbursed with a more generous capitation rate. Required services include preventive health, mental health and substance abuse, transportation, and dental care for adults and children on site or by arrangement with another provider.[2]

In his report to the board, Johnson noted that generous reimbursement as part of a federally qualified health center would improve the PDCC's financial status. As an example, he noted per visit reimbursement ranged from $100 to $400 per patient, depending on the treatment. By comparison, reimbursement for similar treatment under Denti-Care was no more than $80.

One challenge to qualifying as a federally qualified health center is that at least 51% of the clinic's board members must be persons served by the organization. Since a federally qualified health center must serve all of the underserved population, PDCC might be required to treat adults. Such a change would mean a major investment of time and money for training and supplies and development of new treatment protocols. A federally qualified health center designation alone would not provide the funding to meet higher-cost procedures, such as operating room time and intravenous sedation. An additional concern is that the federally qualified health center payment system might incentivize providers to provide less treatment, or to spend less time with each patient. And, as with any government program, what might be economically feasible today may not be in the future.

As Blake Johnson reflected on changes in the healthcare environment, he wondered how the organization should respond. He wondered if there were other collaborative options with the children's clinic or other organizations that might not require changes to PDCC's governing board or its range of services.

DISCUSSION QUESTIONS

1. Is the PDCC at a crossroads?

2. Must the PDCC change its operational strategy?

3. How can the PDCC meet its mission to provide oral healthcare to underserved children in the greater South Bay community?

4. How should PDCC respond to the request to partner with the hospital and the children's clinic and become a federally qualified health center?

5. What other options should be considered?

ENDNOTES

1. From PDCC's website. The mission statement was used for 8 years on PDCC's Internal Revenue Form 990 filing.
2. Information on federally qualified health centers and the dental services required may be found at http://www.ada.org/en/public-programs/action-for-dental-health/access-to-care/federally-qualified-health-centers-faq; http://www.bphc.hrsa.gov/programrequirements/index.html.

19

Radical Innovation on the Idaho Frontier

Bengal Telepharmacy

Julie Frischmann
Idaho State University, Pocatello, ID

Neil Tocher
Idaho State University, Pocatello, ID

Alexander R. Bolinger
Idaho State University, Pocatello, ID

CASE HISTORY/BACKGROUND

As Brad Huerta, CEO of Lost Rivers Medical Center (Lost Rivers Medical), a critical access hospital in rural Arco, Idaho, cut the tape at the ceremonial grand opening of the Bengal Telepharmacy, he almost had to pinch himself. The dream of partnering with Idaho State University's College of Pharmacy to solidify the financial viability of his hospital seemed so out of reach when he and a colleague discussed it over beers those many months ago. Their idea, which once seemed doomed, now had become one of the most innovative health initiatives in the state. Huerta smiled as he reflected on the satisfying end of Bengal Telepharmacy's long journey to become reality.

A RURAL HEALTH CONUNDRUM IN EASTERN IDAHO

The Lost Rivers region of Idaho is the size of Rhode Island, but with a population of only 8,000. The region is anchored by Arco, a quaint community where the local doctor knows your family and the local pharmacist fills your prescriptions without immediate payment. In 2013, the underpopulated, but geographically vast region of Lost Rivers had only one retail pharmacy, one hospital pharmacy, and one pharmacist. A second pharmacist had been employed at Lost Rivers Medical but left in 2012 for a more lucrative job.

Steve Streeper, the local retail pharmacist, was in his 80s and knew that retirement was near. As a lifelong member of the community, he did not want to retire and leave Arco and the Lost Rivers region with an important gap in services. Furthermore, selling his retail pharmacy was his retirement plan; until he sold it, he couldn't afford to retire. Streeper had attempted to sell previously, but the pharmacy had been on the market for years with no prospective buyers.

Streeper was realistic. He knew it would be difficult to sell his pharmacy in a town like Arco, whose future was, at best, uncertain. The primary industries in the region—molybdenum mining and a federal nuclear energy facility—were either downsizing or subject to unpredictable swings in employment. Furthermore, the Affordable Care Act had imposed new requirements for electronic medical records, which required an investment that Streeper was reluctant to make at the end of his career.

Streeper was not the only one with concerns about the future of pharmacy services in Arco. After losing his hospital's pharmacist in 2012, Huerta found temporary replacements to cover the pharmacy part time, including the director of the Idaho State University (ISU) pharmacy program, Kerry Casperson, and Wade Flowers, the chief pharmacist at Bingham Memorial Hospital. Both men lived at least 2 hours by car from Arco; neither was willing or able to work at Lost Rivers Medical full time.

In Huerta's search for a permanent full-time pharmacist at least two forces were working against him. The first was the community itself. Arco was in such a remote, unpopulated corner of Idaho that the federal government designated Lost Rivers Medical not only as a critical access hospital but also as a "frontier" hospital, which is a category based on population density for regions that are not large enough to be classified as rural. The population of Arco is aging and declining in number. It had 896 residents (down 10% from the census of 2010). Primary sources of employment were a federal government–sponsored nuclear research laboratory, mining, farming and ranching, and tourism in the rugged Lost River Mountains and their crystal-clear trout streams. Tourism was seasonal, however, and most federal employees who worked at the laboratory lived in bigger cities on the Snake River plain and took a bus to work each day. The mean annual family income of Arco is only about $35,000.

Second, Huerta was contending with the unfavorable economics of hiring a full-time pharmacist. The former pharmacist at Lost Rivers Medical made $100,000 annually and left for a position paying $115,000. Pharmacists in the state capital, 200 miles distant, had an annual median income of $120,000. Lost Rivers Medical was unable to pay competitive salaries; its offer of $100,000 was ranked in the bottom 5% nationally. Furthermore, when Huerta took over Lost Rivers Medical, the hospital was losing money and verged on insolvency. Even if he could persuade a pharmacist to work full time at the hospital, Lost Rivers Medical could not afford to pay a six-figure salary.

The economics of hiring a full-time pharmacist appeared insurmountable, but Huerta could not eliminate pharmacy services for reasons of patient care and accreditation. The link to patient care and quality is obvious. Lost Rivers Medical must remain accredited by The Joint Commission on Accreditation of Healthcare Organizations, which requires hospitals to have access to pharmacy services.[1] Thus, Huerta had to find a creative solution to provide pharmacy services at a cost Lost Rivers Medical can afford.

A DIFFERENT CHALLENGE AT ISU

While Huerta contemplated how to maintain pharmacy services at Lost Rivers Medical, Kerry Casperson faced a challenge of his own at ISU. The state board of pharmacy required that ISU's College of Pharmacy students complete at least one clinical rotation at a rural location, defined in the 2010 census as a location with 2,500 or fewer people. The rural rotation prepares graduates to serve the nearly 30% of state residents who live in rural locations. It is difficult for ISU to find enough rural clinical sites for these rotations because many small, family-owned pharmacies that used to dot the state have closed.

ISU is about 100 highway miles from Arco on a winding, two-lane road. Lost Rivers Medical's retail pharmacy is in the rural clinic closest to ISU. Casperson watched Huerta's struggle to find a pharmacist for Lost Rivers Medical with concern. He did not want to lose the nearest rural pharmacy. If the Lost Rivers retail pharmacy (Streeper's) closed and Lost Rivers Medical was unable to hire a new pharmacist, ISU would have to send its pharmacy students to rural pharmacies on the west side of the state five to six hours away. Kerry knew that asking students to live across the state would be inconvenient for them and would potentially diminish the attractiveness of ISU's pharmacy program.

ENTER THE 340B DRUG PROGRAM

The 340B drug discount program is part of the Veterans Health Care Act of 1992 (Public Law 102-585). The program requires pharmaceutical companies to provide outpatient drugs to eligible healthcare organizations, such as critical access hospitals, at wholesale prices. The 340B program enables economically vulnerable hospitals (e.g., those in rural areas) to provide lower-cost pharmaceuticals to patients. It was thought the 340B program would permit covered entities "to stretch scarce federal resources as far as possible, reaching more eligible patients and providing more comprehensive services" (U.S. House Committee on Veterans Affairs, 1992).

For healthcare entities with few resources, the 340B program offered an important source of revenue. Specifically, the 340B program allowed covered entity clinics and hospitals, such as Lost Rivers Medical, to pay a reduced price for certain outpatient medications and to retain the difference between the price it paid for the drug and federal government reimbursement (Pollack, 2013). The 340B program had caused controversy and had been contested by lobbyists for the pharmaceutical industry. Among other concerns, the pharmaceutical industry objected in principle to the government dictating what they were allowed to charge for the medications they sold. A Government Accountability Office report acknowledged that the 340B program needed closer oversight to prevent drug manufacturers from overcharging participating hospitals and, in turn, that some participating hospitals had been using the proceeds of the program inappropriately (U.S. Government Accountability Office, 2015). Despite the ongoing controversy, the 340B program remained popular with advocates for rural hospitals and had not been changed as of July 2016.

Eligibility for 340B is defined in the law and includes federal Health Resources and Services Administration–supported health centers, Ryan White clinics, state AIDS drug assistance programs, Medicare/Medicaid disproportionate share hospitals, children's hospitals, critical access hospitals, and other safety net providers. Critical access hospitals such as Lost Rivers Medical are designated by the U.S. Department of Medicare and Medicaid Services. To be certified as a critical access hospital, hospitals or medical centers must meet the following criteria:

- Be in a state with a flex program[2]

- Be in a rural area

- Provide 24-hour emergency services

- Be more than 35 miles from any other hospital

As a critical access hospital, Lost Rivers Medical was eligible for the 340B drug program. Huerta saw that program as a source of revenue enabling both the retail and the hospital pharmacies to survive—at least in the short term. Lost Rivers Medical signed up for the 340B program and sold drugs to Streeper's pharmacy in Arco at wholesale prices. The 340B program led to a net profit on pharmaceutical sales of about $30,000 per month for Streeper's pharmacy and about $10,000 per month for Lost Rivers Medical. This revenue was the same as filling 120 to 130 prescriptions per day. Huerta calculated that filling 100 prescriptions per day was the breakeven point. This revenue brought both Streeper's pharmacy and Lost Rivers Medical back to profitability but did not resolve the issue of Streeper's impending retirement.

THE GRAND IDEA

Back at ISU, Casperson contemplated where to send students for rural rotations if both pharmacies in Arco closed. As fate would have it, Casperson chatted with Huerta at the ISU Division of Health Sciences Christmas party. Casperson mentioned his concern that Streeper's pharmacy would close, which would force ISU to find another rural clinic site. Huerta shared his concerns about the future of Lost Rivers Medical if both pharmacies closed.

As the conversation continued over adult beverages, Huerta and Casperson devised a plan to save Streeper's pharmacy in Arco and provide a rural clinical rotation for ISU pharmacy students. Casperson would convince the ISU Foundation, a fundraising entity managed by prominent university alumni and private donors, to purchase Streeper's pharmacy for the university. The idea was a natural fit with the foundation's mission to raise private funds to support the long-term academic goals of the university.

In the weeks that followed, Casperson approached foundation board members with the plan he and Huerta had discussed. Foundation board members liked it. To purchase the pharmacy, however, the board required a guarantee that it would operate at a profit. Thanks to the 340B program, that condition could be met. Thus, in an unprecedented arrangement for the state of Idaho, ISU bought Streeper's pharmacy in Arco. It appeared the concern that Lost Rivers' pharmacy would close was resolved. However, one last issue remained: although the university owned the pharmacy, the sale did not include hiring a full-time pharmacist.

Neither Casperson nor Flowers wanted to work full-time at Lost Rivers Medical. Huerta had not found a permanent replacement pharmacist and doubted it would be possible if a market-rate salary were not paid. At that point, Casperson suggested establishing a telepharmacy in Arco. Telepharmacy is a concept whereby a pharmacy technician at a remote site prescribes medication under the supervision of a pharmacist. When a customer at the remote site presents a prescription, the pharmacy technician fills it as a pharmacist watches via live video. The pharmacist monitors the transaction, verifies the accuracy of the prescription, and verbally confirms the prescription by video, phone, or fax before it is delivered to the customer. Thus a pharmacy technician (whose salary is less than half that of a pharmacist) becomes the pharmacist's "hands."

The concept of telepharmacy was not new. Western states with large rural populations had experimented with it for a decade. However, telepharmacy had never before been approved in Idaho. Moreover, Idaho does not have a history of innovative healthcare solutions, and Casperson knew that persuading the Idaho State Board of Pharmacy to approve such a venture would require creative advocacy and lots of work. Meanwhile, Huerta worried about resistance to telepharmacy among the residents of Arco. He suspected that its aging population and that of the surrounding area would resist losing the personal touch of a resident pharmacist and would not accept the idea of telepharmacy without a fight. Huerta, then, faced a dilemma. Without community support, the proposed telepharmacy partnership with ISU could be doomed in the long term. Without telepharmacy, however, Lost Rivers Medical would not have access to pharmacy services. Without the ability to provide pharmacy services, Lost Rivers Medical would not be able to use the 340B program and it would likely lose its Joint Commission accreditation, without which it would be hard-pressed to survive. The challenge, then, was clear. Huerta had to convince Arco residents that telepharmacy would save the hospital and the community.

TELEPHARMACY PLATFORM AND THE IDAHO STATE BOARD OF PHARMACY

Casperson and Huerta prepared to be advocates for their cause. There was no need to prove the efficacy of telepharmacy as it had already been proven in rural North Dakota as early as 2001. Similarly, there was local and national evidence that telepharmacies were needed in rural areas. Since 2006, 300 rural pharmacies in the United States had closed, including four in Idaho. Telepharmacy had the potential to greatly expand access to quality healthcare in rural and medically underserved areas, but only if Huerta and Casperson could convince the Idaho State Board of Pharmacy of its benefits.

In March 2014, Huerta and Casperson presented their proposal for the ISU–Lost Rivers Medical Bengal Telepharmacy partnership to the Idaho State Board of Pharmacy. As Casperson had predicted, there was opposition from some members of the board. One member of the board, a practicing pharmacist, was adamant that telepharmacy would "steal" jobs from local pharmacists. Huerta explained how he had worked for years to hire a full-time pharmacist at Lost Rivers Medical and that Streeper had sought to sell his pharmacy for years before the ISU Foundation purchased it. If either Lost Rivers Medical or Streeper had found a pharmacist to work in Arco, the Bengal Telepharmacy proposal would never have come to the board.

Huerta asked if protecting pharmacists' jobs fit with the board's mission. Huerta read aloud from the board's mission statement: "Our mission is to promote, preserve and protect the health, safety, and welfare of the public by and through the effective control and regulation of the practice of pharmacy." "Sure," Huerta said, "protecting jobs is important, but the board's own mission, first and foremost, is to provide services for the public." Furthermore, Huerta stated his willingness to abandon the Bengal Telepharmacy proposal if a pharmacist were willing to move to Arco and accept a salary affordable to Lost Rivers Medical. No one on the state board volunteered. Nonetheless, the Idaho State Board of Pharmacy voted to reject the Bengal Telepharmacy proposal.

IF AT FIRST YOU DON'T SUCCEED . . .

Huerta and Casperson were incredibly frustrated. They had cleared daunting hurdles, including persuading a university foundation to purchase a pharmacy and negotiating a partnership that overcame the regulatory obstacles preventing a university healthcare program and a hospital from working together. Now they had been stymied at the final barrier by members of the Idaho State Board of Pharmacy, who prioritized protecting a few potential pharmacist jobs above healthcare benefits to thousands of Idaho residents. Huerta described his frustrations to ISU pharmacy student Tami Taylor, who had not heard of telepharmacy. Intrigued, Taylor researched telepharmacy in other states and agreed with Huerta and Casperson that ISU's agreement with Lost Rivers Medical was the answer for Arco. Casperson, Huerta, and Taylor brought the issue back to the Idaho State Board of Pharmacy at its next meeting, but with a change in strategy. This time, Taylor would present the proposal.

At the meeting, Huerta, Casperson, and ISU's College of Pharmacy alumni looked on as Taylor made her presentation. She spoke about her research on the success of telepharmacy in other states and how Idaho lagged in addressing rural healthcare needs. Taylor explained that, as a pharmacy student who would soon be graduating, she was also concerned about protecting pharmacists' jobs in the state. However, she stressed that in the midst of the changing economics of healthcare, Arco (and small towns like it) no longer had the population to support pharmacists like herself at market-rate salaries. From her perspective, telepharmacies are a viable way to provide prescription medications to the elderly, a population most in need of pharmaceutical services and for whom driving for hours on icy roads in the winter would be hazardous.

Taylor's argument was persuasive; the Idaho State Board of Pharmacy approved the Bengal Telepharmacy with the following stipulations:

1. The telepharmacy is not allowed to compete with any local pharmacy.

2. Pharmacy students are not allowed to administer medicine. A pharmacist is required to monitor the pharmacy technician from multiple camera angles at all times.

3. The telepharmacy must be co-located (i.e., share a physical site) with a hospital.

SELLING THE IDEA TO THE PUBLIC

Huerta, Casperson, and Taylor were delighted. Huerta began to make plans for the Bengal Pharmacy to move into vacant clinic space in the Lost Rivers Medical. Many things had to be done. For instance, by July 2014, the ISU Foundation agreed to pay $100,000 for renovations. These renovations included installation of new broadband fiberoptic cables and phone lines to improve data transmission and to install cameras to satisfy the mandate of the Idaho State Board of Pharmacy. To enhance the comfort level, a new heating, ventilating, and air conditioning system was added. New flooring, windows, and lighting would improve the work environment. ISU's College of Pharmacy would hire a pharmacist to oversee Streeper's former pharmacy practice full time. The goal was to fill the first prescription in summer 2014.

Even as he began renovating the pharmacy space, Huerta knew that without community acceptance the concept of telepharmacy could not achieve long-term success. Huerta and Casperson brainstormed ideas to make the telepharmacy's services more appealing to a potentially skeptical public. One source of resistance was the slightly higher price of medications at Bengal Telepharmacy than at major retailers, such as Walmart. Huerta feared residents averse to change would drive 60 miles over two-lane roads to the closest Walmart (a round-trip of four hours in the winter) to save $2.00 on a prescription.

To add value to services offered in Arco, Huerta suggested Bengal Telepharmacy and Lost Rivers Medical offer free home delivery. He created a chart (Table 19.1) that compared the cost (including mileage and driving time) of using Bengal Telepharmacy or Walmart.

Table 19.1. Cost and time comparison of Bengal Telepharmacy versus Walmart

Filling location	Average prescription cost (generic)	Average mileage cost (round-trip)	Total
Bengal Telepharmacy	$6	$0	$6
Walmart	$4	$17	$21
Savings per prescription	($2)	$17	$15
Average annual savings by staying in Arco (12 refills)	($24)	$204	$180
Average annual time saved			30 hours

A SUCCESS STORY

In its first few months, Bengal Telepharmacy was accepted by the Arco community. However, Huerta saw more opportunity. Only 10% of the community regularly used the telepharmacy. Nearly 65% of Arco's population was over age 45 and, according to Huerta, the majority of them preferred to interact with a pharmacist face to face—even if that meant making a long and sometimes treacherous drive. Thus, in addition to home delivery, Lost Rivers Medical and Bengal Telepharmacy implemented a private consultation room to personalize the experience whereby the patient and pharmacist converse via video conference. More of the community accepted these enhancements and the increased utilization led to higher profits.

To gain more community support and integration, Bengal Telepharmacy began a pharmacy program partnership with Butte High School, the regional high school in Arco. Junior and senior students interested in attending ISU to study pharmacy were allowed to assist the pharmacy technicians on site and gain valuable experience. Arco parents and students saw this opportunity as a connection with ISU that opened a door to attending college. This was not trivial in a town historically supported by farming, ranching, and mining and whose children would be first-generation college students. Some even wondered if the Bengal Telepharmacy partnership would train a pharmacist who one day would come home to serve the community full time.

THE END—OR, ONLY A BEGINNING?

As Huerta relived the long journey to bring Bengal Telepharmacy to Arco, Gary Michaelson, president of the Lost Rivers Medical Center Foundation and a former patient at Lost Rivers Medical, stopped by for a visit. Michaelson, a long-time resident of Arco, believed that Bengal Telepharmacy was a lifesaver to the extent that the presence of the pharmacy allowed Lost Rivers Medical to continue to exist as a Joint Commission–accredited hospital. In the recent past, Michaelson had suffered a massive heart attack. A cardiologist estimated that Michaelson could not have survived the 60-mile drive across the eastern Idaho desert to the closest hospital. Furthermore, Michaelson expressed his gratitude that he and the community would have access to medications when needed. "It's critical. We've got to have a pharmacy," he said. "When you need medication, you need medication. You can't always drive across the desert for medication."

After the Bengal Telepharmacy success in Arco, the ISU Foundation and ISU College of Pharmacy considered starting similar programs elsewhere in rural Idaho. Huerta knew that the concept of telepharmacy had to overcome a host of barriers, from local buy-in to state approval, but he was confident the groundwork had been laid for future success.

DISCUSSION QUESTIONS

1. Why is it important for Lost Rivers Medical to have a pharmacy in the area? Why is it so difficult to keep a pharmacist on staff at critical access hospitals such as Lost Rivers Medical?

2. What are the advantages and disadvantages of utilizing telepharmacy at Lost Rivers Medical? How does telepharmacy increase access to healthcare in rural areas?

3. Why was there resistance to approving telepharmacy in Idaho? After approval, why was there resistance to providing the service to residents who would benefit from the service?

4. What is the 340B drug program? Why is it important to the Lost Rivers Medical and similar hospitals? Does the program raise questions of fairness because organizations buy medications at wholesale prices but don't pass the savings on to the consumer?

5. What else could Huerta do to increase patronage of Bengal Telepharmacy? Outline several options for him to consider.

6. What differences between the first and second Idaho State Board of Pharmacy presentations might explain why the proposal was approved the second time but not the first time?

ENDNOTES

1. The Joint Commission is the premiere accrediting body that evaluates over 21,000 healthcare organizations and programs in the United States (Joint Commission, 2016).
2. The Medicare Rural Hospital Flexibility Program (or state flex program) was part of the Balanced Budget Act of 1997. It modified Medicare to improve access to healthcare services for rural populations.

REFERENCES

Joint Commission. (2016). About the Joint Commission. https://www.joint-commission.org/about_us/about_the_joint_commission_main.aspx

Pollack, Andrew. (2013). Dispute develops over discount drug program, *New York Times*, February 13, B1. Retrieved from http://www.nytimes.com/2013/02/13/business/dispute-develops-over-340b-discount-drug-program.html

U.S. Government Accountability Office. (2015). Drug discount program: Status of GAO recommendations to improve 340B drug pricing program oversite. GAO-15-455T. Retrieved from http://www.gao.gov/products/GAO-15-455T

U.S. House, Committee on Veterans Affairs. (1992). (H.R. 2890). Medicaid and Department of Veterans Affairs Drug Rebate Amendments of 1992. H. Rept. 102-384, Pt. 2. Retrieved from https://www.congress.gov/bill/102nd-congress/house-bill/2890

20

Structure and Funding of Hospitalist Programs

John E. Paul
University of North Carolina at Chapel Hill

Gillian Gilson Watson
University of North Carolina Hospitals, Chapel Hill, NC

CASE HISTORY/BACKGROUND

The School of Medicine affiliated with Dogwood Academic Medical Center Hospital (Dogwood[1]) has a Section of Hospital Medicine (a "hospitalist program") staffed by physicians from the School of Medicine's Department of General Internal Medicine. Practicing hospitalists are thereby available to Dogwood. According to the School of Medicine's currently proposed budget, the hospitalist program is projected to continue incurring a substantial annual deficit. The School of Medicine has asked Dogwood to continue funding the deficit. Some administrators and clinicians at Dogwood are concerned, however, that a hospitalist program funded this way may have become too expensive and may need to be replaced by another organizational approach, or that the hospitalist program must find ways to become self-funded. Other strategic options for funding the program may need consideration, such as providing new services, expanding patient care provided by nonhospitalists (including perhaps midlevel practitioners), or Dogwood ending the hospitalist relationship with the School of Medicine altogether.

In response, Dogwood and the School of Medicine have asked a consultant to assess the hospitalist program and make recommendations regarding its organization and future, including the level of need and justifiable subsidies.

BACKGROUND TO THE HOSPITALIST SPECIALTY

A hospitalist is defined as a physician who only practices in an inpatient setting (Wachter and Goldman, 1996). Development of this role is one of the most noteworthy innovations in management of hospitalized patients in the United States, paralleling emergence of other inpatient specialties, such as emergency medicine and critical care medicine. Park Nicollet Clinic, a large multispecialty medical group in Minneapolis–St. Paul, established the first hospitalist program in 1994 (Freese, 1999). Hospitals owned by Kaiser-Permanente Northern California began using hospitalists in 1995 (Craig et al., 1999). Teaching hospitals in Boston, San Francisco, and other markets soon implemented similar initiatives in which inpatient care was provided by faculty-led hospitalist teams that included residents and medical students (Brown, Halpert, McKean, Sussman, & Dzau, 1999; Wachter, Katz, Showstach, Bindman, & Goldman, 1998). Since Wachter and colleagues coined the term "hospitalist" in the mid-1990s, the demand for hospitalists has surpassed supply as many hospitals have initiated hospitalist services or expanded their existing programs. The number of hospitalists has now grown to more than 44,000 (Society of Hospital Medicine, 2014). Hospitalists at academic medical centers typically reside administratively in the department of general internal medicine of the affiliated school of medicine.

A number of factors have encouraged use of hospitalists. Diagnosis-related groups and prospective payment incentivize hospitals to save money and resources by reducing lengths of stay and improving efficiency. This effort requires increasing patient throughput and maximizing bed use; hospitalists contribute by applying a combination of clinical skills and organizational knowledge. In addition, hospitalists have more experience with treatment of particular diseases and conditions than other specialists (Meltzer et al., 2002), and thus are presumably more efficient. Unnecessarily long lengths of stay can create a backlog in hospital emergency departments, which results in lower patient satisfaction and even revenue-losing diversions when ambulances are sent elsewhere. Finally, limits on the numbers of hours medical residents are allowed to work have forced some teaching hospitals to add staff, including hospitalists, to cover the physician shortage (Weinstein, 2002).

Hospitalists improve efficiency of inpatient care by: (1) monitoring patients closely; (2) reducing clinically unjustified variation in care; (3) using standardized therapies, testing, and drug regimens; (4) responding quickly to changing clinical needs; and (5) applying their experience in the particular organizational setting. These objectives are accomplished by (1) improved coordination of care between the patient's primary care physician and specialists, with the hospitalist as the "intermediary," (2) more efficient scheduling of tests and procedures, and (3) more informed and better discharge planning due to the nature of the hospitalists' work. Discharge planning is particularly important under the Patient Protection and Affordable Care Act since it includes Medicare reimbursement penalties for readmissions. Moreover, the percentage of Medicare beneficiaries cared for by hospitalists has increased significantly (Kripalani, Jackson, Schnipper, & Coleman, 2007; Kuo, Sharma, Freeman, & Goodwin, 2009).

In terms of outcomes, numerous studies have found that patients managed by hospitalists have (1) shorter lengths of stay with lower total costs than patients in comparison groups (Halasyamani, Valenstein, Friedlander, & Cowen, 2005; Kaboli, Barnett, & Rosenthal, 2004; Myers Bellini, J. Rohrbach, F. S. Shofer, J. E. Hollander, 2006); (2) shorter wait times for surgery or consultation (Batsis et al., 2007; Roy, Heckman, & Roy, 2006); and (3) a greater likelihood of receiving guideline-recommended care (Harrison & Curran, 2009; Lopez, Hicks, Cohen, McKean, & Weissman, 2009; Rifkin, Burger, Holmboe, & Sturdevant, 2007). One study found the greatest reductions in length of stay were for patients requiring close clinical monitoring and for patients requiring complex discharge planning. These results suggest hospitalists could have an effect in reducing mortality or readmission for complex cases (Southern, Berger, Bellin, Hailpern, & Arnsten, 2007), which is important because of the Affordable Care Act. However, despite some supportive evidence, hospital medicine programs generally have had little effect on overall mortality and readmission rates (Dynan et al., 2009; Lindenauer et al., 2007).

HOSPITALIST FUNCTIONS AT DOGWOOD ACADEMIC MEDICAL CENTER HOSPITAL

Establishing a hospitalist program in the School of Medicine's Department of General Internal Medicine was part of a system-wide strategy to improve overall clinical and financial performance. The program is over ten years old. The relationship between Dogwood and the School of Medicine is shown in Figure 20.1. Specifically, hospitalists provided by the School of Medicine contribute to the Dogwood mission through objectives and tactics as shown in Table 20.1. Last fiscal year, the Dogwood hospitalist program was staffed with 12 physicians, who provided the services shown in Figure 20.2 and described next.

Traditional house staff services (patient care and teaching): Hospitalists from the School of Medicine staff one of the ten traditional, resident-based teams at Dogwood. The team includes an attending hospitalist, three residents,

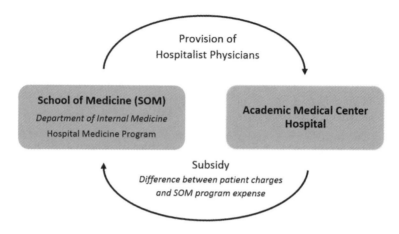

Figure 20.1. Hospitalist relationship between the School of Medicine and the Dogwood Academic Medical Center Hospital.

Table 20.1.   Objectives and tactics of the Dogwood Academic Medical Center Hospital hospitalist program

Objectives	Tactics
Reduce emergency department crowding by increasing bed availability for (1) community patient care providers and (2) hospital-to-hospital referrals, thus enhancing both Dogwood's revenue base and regional referral/tertiary care status	Utilize hospitalists to improve the throughput of inpatient care by reducing length of stay, freeing up space on units, and facilitating earlier discharge
Make up for the limited availability of house staff due to medical residents' work hour limitations, as well as other staffing shortages	Create patient-care-only hospitalist services that focus on inpatient clinical responsibilities
Improve resource utilization; minimize excess costs	Reduce unnecessary and redundant tests and procedures through expertise, communication, and coordination
Optimize revenue and operating margin	Rationalize and standardize coding and documentation
Improve continuity, coordination, and quality of care	Limit unnecessary handoffs in care and improve efficiency; improve access to physician care

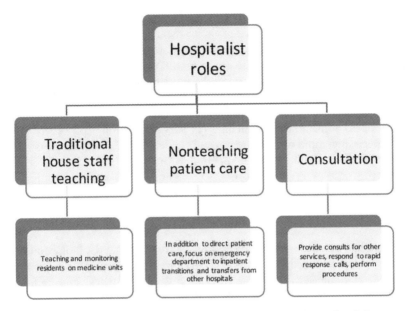

Figure 20.2. Hospitalist roles at Dogwood Academic Medical Center Hospital.

and three medical students. Hospitalists generate patient revenue, participate in medical education, and teach residents efficient and effective hospital medicine as they provide clinical services to inpatients. The number of inpatients treated is determined primarily by availability of residents.

Nonteaching, patient-care-only services: These hospitalist services focus on direct patient care and do not involve supervising residents or medical students. The services are provided 24 hours a day, 7 days a week, and are a response to the resident work hour restrictions described earlier. The hospitalists also improve throughput by serving less-acute and nonteaching cases. In addition to general patient care, night hospitalists (also called nocturnists) (1) oversee the majority of admissions from the emergency department (reducing emergency department crowding, preventing unnecessary admissions, and increasing revenue from patients admitted before midnight as a separate day of care), (2) write orders for night procedures (thus making the procedures billable), (3) provide consultations (not necessarily billable unless the patient is admitted), and (4) answer inquiries from the patient transfer center or referral coordinator (which may lead to admissions, if beds are available). A drawback for the patient-care-only, no research or teaching role is that it may create the perception of a "two-tiered" system with lower status for the hospitalist. If so, lower job satisfaction, retention, and career development may result (Sehgal, Shah, Parekh, Roy, & Williams, 2008).

Consultation services: This team has one hospitalist and one resident and includes a teaching or training role for the hospitalist. The team provides general medicine inpatient consultation at the request of nonmedicine specialists. The consultation team also handles calls from the transfer center or referral coordinator, and admits patients. This 24/7 role is an important feature of the hospitalist program at Dogwood and has generated unanticipated—and generally unreimbursed—demands for their services. Some examples include (1) participating in, and occasionally supervising, rapid response teams and "code blue" teams (increasing quality of care, but adding unpredictably to the workload of the hospitalist at the cost of regular care); (2) providing a backup communication link to commercial laboratories for critical abnormal lab values for non–intensive care unit patients; and (3) handling admissions when the medical residents have reached their mandated maximum hours on duty.

Under the three-pronged approach shown in Figure 20.2, the Dogwood hospitalist program has achieved many of the expected objectives (e.g., improving throughput, covering resident house staff shortages, and reducing emergency department wait times), in addition to unexpected responsibilities (e.g., supervising rapid response teams). However, the degree of program success is not easy to quantify due to the difficulty of attributing time and money for improvements in (1) resource utilization, (2) coding and documentation, (3) quality of care, (4) patient satisfaction, and (5) resident training.

FUTURE STRATEGIC DIRECTIONS

Dogwood and the School of Medicine have discussed two opportunities that are new directions for the hospital medicine program. These opportunities could add revenue for support of the program as well as strengthen intraorganizational relationships. Strategies similar to both opportunities have been successful in other hospital medicine programs.

The first opportunity is to establish a formal bedside procedure service that is staffed by hospitalists. The goals of this service would be to improve medical resident education, provide faster response times for procedures needed prior to patient discharge, and increase revenue for the hospitalist program. Types of procedures hospitalists could perform include paracentesis, thoracentesis, and central line placement. This opportunity would require additional full-time equivalent hospitalists; however, a few procedures per week at current staffing levels could be piloted on the consult service as a "proof of concept" and a preview of revenue potential. In addition to potentially increasing labor costs, a bedside procedure service might require equipment (e.g., a portable ultrasound machine). This need could require capital outlays paid by the School of Medicine or Dogwood,

Table 20.2. Projected reimbursement by procedure type for typical procedures under the procedure service strategy

CPT code	Procedure name	Medicare reimbursement	Estimated commercial reimbursement
32555	Thoracentesis pleura w/ imaging	$113	$338
36556	Insert central venous catheter	$121	$195
49083	Abdominal paracentesis w/ imaging	$109	$385

which would have to be determined. Table 20.2 shows estimated reimbursement by procedure for these typical bedside procedures. Projecting volumes is difficult; among other factors it will take time to familiarize other groups as to available services. Initially, offering one or two procedures per day should be feasible, with potential growth to four or five procedures per day.

The second opportunity involves expanding an existing patient co-management program with the department of surgery. Hospitalists currently consult on postoperative orthopedic patients (primarily hip and knee replacement). As a role expansion, the department of neurosurgery has asked if hospitalists could provide postoperative care for their patients. Co-management for neurosurgery patients is substantially more complicated than for orthopedic patients, however, due to their higher acuity. The School of Medicine and Dogwood are reviewing alternative ways to staff and reimburse for the care of postoperative neurosurgery patients. Having hospitalists co-manage neurosurgery patients would require additional FTE hospitalists. Since the department of neurosurgery is the main service caring for these patients, the primary source of revenue for the hospitalist program in this collaboration would come from inpatient consults. As the source of hospitalists, the School of Medicine Department of General Internal Medicine has considered approaching the Department of Neurosurgery to help pay for the additional full-time equivalent hospitalists since consultation fee revenue alone will not cover salary expense. Details as to the financial and staffing implications for this opportunity are unclear; it is hoped the consultant can provide advice as to options.

FINANCIAL INFORMATION

Income for the hospital medicine program comes from billed patient care services and the Dogwood subsidy ($1.43 million and $2.25 million, respectively, for a total of $3.69 million in the most recent fiscal year). Because income from patient care does not cover the cost of the program, the hospital subsidizes the hospitalist service. In the most recent fiscal year, other program costs included the hospitalist program coordinator salary and midlevel provider salaries, as well as the cost of additional supplies.

Table 20.3. Income and expense of hospitalist program for the School of Medicine, most recent fiscal year

Income	(in $000s)
Reimbursement for patient care services	$1,435
Dogwood Academic Medical Center Hospital subsidy paid to the School of Medicine	2,255
Total	$3,690

Expenses	(in $000s)
Physician salaries and benefits	$3,050
Ancillary and support costs: midlevel provider and program coordinator salaries, supplies, administrative fees	640
Total	$3,690
Surplus (Deficit)	($0)

These costs were added to the salary costs of hospitalists for a total program cost of almost $3.7 million. Income and expenses associated with the program are shown in Table 20.3.

In the most recent fiscal year, growth in billable hospitalists' services was only moderate, and less than anticipated. This shortfall is partly explained by patient volumes that were lower than projected. This may have resulted from a higher percentage of nonreimbursed (thus nonrecorded and nonbilled) "observation" cases seen by hospitalists, compared with other services. Lack of available beds[2] and the fact that hospitalists are often involved in unanticipated (and unbillable) demands may also have contributed to limited growth of inpatient care provided by hospitalists. Additionally, because of their broad perspective, hospitalists are routinely involved in special projects, such as process improvement and quality initiatives. These activities take them away from inpatient, revenue-generating patient care.

To evaluate the success of the hospitalist program, Dogwood compares the variable costs and average length of stay of hospitalists' patients with those of their internal medicine peers. Table 20.4 summarizes comparable cases—where at least one hospitalist and one nonhospitalist had a case in the same diagnosis-related group. This table excludes cost outliers and includes the University Hospital Consortium benchmark.

Table 20.5 is the proposed summary budget for the next fiscal year, without any expansion of the hospitalist program.

OPTIONS FOR HOSPITALIST PROGRAM EXPANSION

Implementing either the procedure service strategy or the neurosurgery co-management strategy would require additional hospitalists. Staffing a Monday through Friday daytime-only service without holiday coverage

Table 20.4. Dogwood Academic Medical Center Hospital average length of stay and direct cost comparisons, most recent fiscal year

Case data	University Hospital Consortium Expected Length of Stay	Dogwood Nonhospitalist Peers	Dogwood Hospitalists
Number of cases, 1,820			
Average length of stay	5.10	4.87	4.54
Direct variable cost per case		$6,267	$6,093
Direct fixed and capital costs per case		$747	$702
Total direct cost per case		$7,013	$6,795
Savings on total direct cost per case			$218
Total savings on direct cost			$397,115

would require approximately 1.4 full-time equivalent hospitalists. Staffing a service 365 days a year would require 2.1 full-time equivalent hospitalists, assuming no additional night coverage. Both the procedure service and the neurosurgery co-management service are needed 7 days a week; offering it only 5 or 7 full days would have to be negotiated. The current average cost of each full-time equivalent hospitalist is $187,500 in salary and $69,637 in benefits. Table 20.2 shows the expected reimbursement by procedure type under the hospitalist procedure service strategy for three typical procedures.

Table 20.5. Dogwood Academic Medical Center Hospital proposed budget for the next fiscal year*

Income		(in $000s)
Reimbursement for patient care services		$1,507
Dogwood subsidy paid to School of Medicine		$2,331
	Total	$3,838

Expense		(in $000s)
Physician salaries and benefits		$3,173
Ancillary and support costs: midlevel provider and program coordinator salaries, supplies, administrative fees		$665
	Total	$3,838
	Surplus (deficit)	($0)

*Without expansion of the hospitalist program and excluding indirect cost savings to hospital.

DISCUSSION QUESTIONS

Dogwood and the School of Medicine want the consultant to provide an unbiased and comprehensive assessment of the hospitalist program, and recommendations for the future.

The following are questions to be considered:

1. Identify key stakeholders. What value or benefits do stakeholders derive? Show the relationships among Dogwood, the School of Medicine, and various stakeholders in tabular or graphical format.

2. Can hospitalist programs at Dogwood be an integral part of cost-effective and efficient inpatient care? Under what circumstances?

3. What information is missing or may be needed for the consultant's initial report?

4. Use the Kaplan and Norton (1996) "Balanced Scorecard" framework and identify specific dimensions and metrics you could use to quantify the impact and performance of the hospitalist program.

5. Identify advantages and disadvantages of expanding the hospital medicine program to include a procedure service. Should co-management services with neurosurgery be considered? What questions must be asked? Explore the School of Medicine and Dogwood perspectives.

6. Identify strategic recommendations for the hospitalist program and suggestions for implementation at Dogwood. Develop recommendations for Dogwood regarding financial arrangements and future development of the program.

ENDNOTES

1. The name of the institution has been changed. This case is based on a consulting assignment by Shoou-Yih (Daniel) Lee, PhD, and student research by Saumya Sehgal, MHA, and Robert Jungerwirth, BSPH.
2. Dogwood's occupancy rate is between 90 and 100+ percent, depending on service.

REFERENCES

Batsis, J. A., Phy, M. P., Melton, L. J., Schleck, C. D., Larson, D. R., Huddleston, P. M., & Huddleston, J. M. (2007). Effects of a hospitalist care model on mortality of elderly patients with hip fractures. *Journal of Hospital Medicine, 2*(4), 219–225.

Brown, M. D., Halpert, A., McKean, S., Sussman, A., & Dzau, V. J. (1999). Assessing the value of hospitalists to academic medical centers: Brigham and Women's Hospital and Harvard Medical School. *American Journal of Medicine, 106*(2), 134–147.

Craig, D. E., Hartka, L., Likosky, W. H., Caplan, W. M., Litsky, P., & Smithey, J. (1999). Implementation of a hospitalist system in a large health maintenance organization: The Kaiser Permanente experience. *Annals of Internal Medicine, 130*(4), 355–359.

Dynan, L., Stein, R., David, G., Kenny, L. C., Eckman, M., & Short, A. D. (2009). Determinants of hospitalist efficiency. *Medical Care Research and Review, 66*(6), 682–702.

Freese, R. B. (1999). The Park Nicollet experience in establishing a hospitalist system. *Annals of Internal Medicine, 130*(4), 350–354.

Halasyamani, L. K., Valenstein, P. N., Friedlander, M. P., & Cowen, M. E. (2005). A comparison of two hospitalist models with traditional care in a community teaching hospital. *American Journal of Medicine, 118*(5), 536–543.

Harrison, J. P., & Curran, L. (2009). The hospitalist model: Does it enhance health care quality? *Journal of Health Care Finance, 35*(3), 22–34.

Kaboli, P. J., Barnett, M. J., & Rosenthal, G. E. (2004). Associations with reduced length of stay and costs on an academic hospitalist service. *American Journal of Managed Care, 10*(8), 561–568.

Kaplan, S. K., & Norton, D. P. (1996). Using the balanced scorecard as a strategic management system. *Harvard Business Review, 74*(1), 75–85.

Kripalani, S. S., Jackson, A. T., Schnipper, J. L., & Coleman, E. A. (2007). Promoting effective transitions of care at hospital discharge: A review of key issues for hospitalists. *Journal of Hospital Medicine, 2*(5), 314–323.

Kuo, Y., Sharma, G., Freeman, J. L., & Goodwin, J. S. (2009). Growth in the care of older patients by hospitalists in the United States. *New England Journal of Medicine, 360*(11), 1102–1112.

Lindenauer, P. K., Rothberg, M. B., Pekow, P. D., Kenwood, C., Benjamin, E. M., & Auerbach, A. D. (2007). Outcomes of care by hospitalists, general internists, and family physicians. *New England Journal of Medicine, 357*(25), 2589–2600.

Lopez, L., Hicks, L. S., Cohen, A. P., McKean, S., & Weissman, J. S. (2009). Hospitalists and the quality of care in hospitals. *Archives of Internal Medicine, 169*(15), 1389–1394.

Meltzer, D., Manning, W. G., Morrison, J., Shah, M. N., Jin, L., Guth, T., & Levinson, W. (2002). Effects of physician experience on costs and outcomes on an academic general medicine service: Results of a trial of hospitalists. *Annals of Internal Medicine, 137*(11), 866–874.

Myers, J. S., Bellini, L. M., Rohrbach, J., Shofer, F. S., & Hollander, J. E. (2006). Improving resource utilization in a teaching hospital: Development of a non-teaching service for chest pain admissions. *Academic Medicine: Journal of the Association of American Medical Colleges, 81*(5), 432–435.

Rifkin, W. D., Burger, A., Holmboe, E. S., & Sturdevant, B. (2007). Comparison of hospitalists and nonhospitalists regarding core measures of pneumonia care. *American Journal of Managed Care, 13*(3), 129–132.

Roy, A. A., Heckman, M. G., & Roy, V. (2006). Associations between the hospital-ist model of care and quality-of-care-related outcomes in patients undergoing hip fracture surgery. *Mayo Clinic Proceedings, 81*(1), 28–31.

Sehgal, N. L., Shah, H. M., Parekh, V. I., Roy, C. L., & Williams, M. V. (2008). Non-housestaff medicine services in academic centers: Models and challenges. *Journal of Hospital Medicine, 3*(3), 247–255.

Society of Hospital Medicine. (2014). Society of Hospital Medicine 2013/2014 Media Information Kit. Philadelphia, PA.

Southern, W. N., Berger, M. A., Bellin, E. Y., Hailpern, S. M., & Arnsten, J. H. (2007). Hospitalist care and length of stay in patients requiring complex discharge planning and close clinical monitoring. *Archives of Internal Medicine (1960)*, *167*(17), 1869–1874.

Weinstein, D. F. (2002). Duty hours for resident physicians—tough choices for teaching hospitals. *New England Journal of Medicine*, *347*(16), 1275–1278.

Wachter, R. M., & Goldman, L. (1996). The emergent role of "hospitalists" in the American health care system. *New England Journal of Medicine*, *335*(7), 514–517.

Wachter, R. M., Katz, P., Showstach, J., Bindman, A.B., & Goldman, L. (1998). Reorganizing an academic medical service: Impact on cost, quality, patient satisfaction, and education. *Journal of the American Medical Association*, *279*(19), 1560–1565.

21

Appian Health Systems

Robert C. Myrtle
University of Southern California, Los Angeles, CA

CASE HISTORY/BACKGROUND

This exercise is a simulation of negotiating a collective bargaining agreement between Appian Health Systems and the Nursing and Health Professionals Union (NHPU). As a member of the health systems' or union's bargaining team, your role is to negotiate a collective bargaining agreement acceptable to the other party. If there is an impasse, the neutral third-party arbitrator will determine the content of the final agreement. Negotiations will begin with the current collective bargaining agreement.

INSTRUCTIONS

Step 1. Those at the negotiations will include the following:

Health system representatives:

- Linn Martin, MBA, Chief Operating Officer, Appian Health
- Terry Howard, DNS, Chief Nursing Officer, Appian Health Systems
- Dale Hardy, Vice President, Finance, Appian Health Systems
- Claire Brown, JD, Vice President, Human Resources, Appian Health Systems

Union representatives:

- Jacque San Miguel, DNS, President NHPU

- Carol Rosenberg, NHPU National Office

- Pat Elliot, Pharm D, Member, NHPU

- Billie Moore, RPT, Member, NHPU

Arbitrator:

- P. J. Appleby, JD, Neutral, Appointed by the American Arbitration Association

Step 2. Read the current collective bargaining agreement (contract; Appendix A), and the descriptions of Appian Health Systems and NHPU (Appendix B). Background information (biographical) and the role member's concerns will be provided by your instructor. That information will ask you NOT TO SHARE YOUR SPECIFIC ROLE INFORMATION with your negotiation team members, but instead use that information as you see relevant when explaining the changes you are making in the contract. These materials, as well as your role, provide the context for your positions and interactions in this simulation.

Step 3. Review the materials and the provisions of the contract with other members of your negotiating team. Decide which provisions should be retained and which should be changed or deleted. Feel free to modify the contract provisions (use Appendix B, a skeletal outline of the current contract, to note your changes to each provision). You may even wish to develop a new contract that is more appropriate to your goals and objectives. Once your team agrees as to which provisions are important, decide your overall approach to the negotiation session(s). Remember, you are trying to reach an agreement the parties can accept. The strategy you use to gain agreement is up to you.

Step 4. Contact those involved in the negotiations to arrange a meeting at which each side can present its proposals and receive feedback.

Step 5. After you meet with the opposing team and understand their position and their reaction to yours, meet privately with your team to develop a response based on what you learned.

Step 6. Arrange further negotiation sessions and private team meetings as appropriate. Try to reach an agreement on a contract acceptable to you and your team.

Step 7. If agreement is reached, each team should prepare a document that details the provisions of the collective bargaining agreement (contract) for signature by the parties.

Step 8. If an agreement is not reached, an impasse is declared. Although several different dispute resolution options are available, this simulation uses binding arbitration.

Step 9. After an impasse is declared, both parties must present their best and final offers to the arbitrator. Be sure your offer is comprehensive and carefully prepared and any provisions you want added or modified are recorded. Once complete, submit your offer to the arbitrator.

Step 10. After reviewing the best and final offer from the parties, the arbitrator will hold a fact-finding hearing to clarify issues, raise questions, or test possible options to resolve the impasse. After the hearing, the arbitrator will provide a final agreement to be signed by the parties.

APPENDIX A

Current Agreement Between Appian Health Systems and The Nurses and Health Professionals Union

January 1, 20XX to December 31, 20XX

Article I
Agreement

This agreement is made and entered into on this 28th day of December 20XX, between Appian Health Systems and the Nursing and Health Professionals Union.

Article II
Recognition

Appian Health Systems recognizes the Nursing and Health Professionals Union (also referred to as the Union or NHPU) as the sole and exclusive bargaining representative certified by the National Labor Relations Board on April 1, 1975, for the following employee classifications: Registered and Licensed Vocational Nurse, Physical, Occupational and Speech Therapists, Medical Social Worker, Clinical Psychologist, Pharmacist, Registered Dietitian, Medical Technologist, and Registered Radiographic Technician.

Excluded from this agreement are all administrative and supervising personnel of Appian Health Systems, including department heads, clinical supervisors, and unit managers.

Article III

During the term of the Agreement, Appian Health Systems agrees to deduct monthly dues and other authorized deductions from the wages and salaries due all members in accordance with provisions of applicable state law. These will be forwarded to the Treasurer of the Union on or before the tenth working day after the conclusion of the month for which the deductions were obtained.

Article IV
Management Rights

Except where specifically provided, the Union recognizes that the operations and administration of Appian Health System, including the right to make rules and regulations, are vested in the Chief Executive Officer or those designated to act as the administrative agents of the organization.

Unless otherwise specified, nothing in this agreement shall be construed as a delegation or waiver of any powers or duties vested in the Chief Executive Officer or those designated to act as an agent for Appian Health Systems.

Article V
Union Representatives
and Privileges

5.1 The Union, its officers and members, shall not engage in union activities, hold meetings on the organization's property, or utilize its facilities in any way which interferes with or interrupts normal operations or the duties and obligations of Union members as employees.

5.2 The Union shall have the right to make reasonable use of the organization's space, facilities, and equipment for proper activities related to its position as the recognized representative of the organization's employees.

5.3 The Union shall have the right to post at appropriate locations in the organization, bulletins and notices relevant to official Union business.

Article VI
Grievance Procedure

6.1 A grievance is defined as any dispute or difference concerning the interpretation, application, or claimed violation of any provision of this Agreement.

6.2 Every attempt will be made to resolve any grievance speedily and informally between the affected parties.

6.3 In the event that informal resolution procedures fail to satisfy the aggrieved party, the following formal procedure is to be followed.

Step 1.

Within ten (10) business days after informal resolution processes have failed, the employee shall file an appeal in writing stating the nature of the grievance and the remedy requested from the immediate supervisor.

Within ten (10) business days the supervisor shall reply in writing to the grievant stating the decision made and the reason for it.

Step 2.

Within ten (10) business days from receipt of the supervisor's written response, the employee may appeal the decision in writing to the supervisor's manager. The manager will have ten (10) business days to discuss the grievance with the supervisor concerned and the employee before reaching a decision. This decision and the reason for the action shall be communicated in writing to the employee.

Step 3.

If the matter is not resolved, the employee may appeal in writing to the Chief Executive Officer within fifteen (15) business days after the manager's decision. The Chief Executive Officer, or a designee that has not been involved in the grievance during the prior appeals, shall make a thorough review of the grievance, meet with the parties involved, and give a written decision, citing the basis for the decision, to the employee within fifteen (15) business days from the receipt of the appeal.

Step 4.

If the matter is not successfully resolved, the Union, acting on behalf of the employee, may file a written appeal within seven (7) business days to the American Arbitration Association (AAA) for binding arbitration under its rules. The arbitration shall be by a neutral arbitrator selected under AAA rules, and the decision of the arbitrator shall be final and binding. The cost of arbitration shall be borne equally by both parties.

Article VII
No Strikes or Lockouts

The Union and Appian Health Systems subscribe to the principle that any and all differences under this Agreement shall be resolved by peaceful and legal means without interruption of services provided to patients or the public. The Union agrees that neither it nor any of its officers, agents, employees, or members will instigate, engage in, support, or condone any strike, work stoppage, or other concerted refusal to perform work by any employees in the bargaining unit during the life of this Agreement.

Appian Health Systems agrees that there shall be no lockout during the life of this Agreement.

Article VIII
Wages and Benefits

8.1 For the period January 1, 20XX, to December 31, 20XX, salaries of members of the bargaining unit shall be adjusted in the following manner:

8.1.1 Each member of the bargaining unit shall have his/her salary increased by an amount equal to 2% of his/her base salary for the period January 1, 20XX, to December 31, 20XX.

8.1.2 In addition, an amount equal to 3% of the base salaries for January 1, 20XX, to December 31, 20XX, of all employees in the bargaining unit shall be allocated to a special merit pool. This pool shall be used to provide additional salary increments to members of the bargaining unit. Decision about the allocation of the merit money rests solely with the Chief Executive Officer of Appian Health Systems based on the recommendations from his/her subordinate managers.

8.2 Employees shall be required to work no more than four (4) of the following nine (9) holidays

New Year's Day	Labor Day
Good Friday	Thanksgiving Day
Easter	Christmas Day
Memorial Day	New Year's Eve
Independence Day	

Decisions as to which holidays an employee shall work are to be understood to be a prerogative of management. When required to work on one of the holidays designated above, employees shall be compensated at one and one-half times their normal hourly rate.

8.3 Employees shall receive paid vacations according to the following schedule:

1st year through 5th year	2 weeks
6th year through 10th year	3 weeks
11th year through 15th year	4 weeks
16th and later years	5 weeks

8.4 Employees are responsible for purchasing and maintaining their own uniforms and personal equipment.

8.5 Employees required to report for duty at all times other than their regularly scheduled shifts shall receive overtime pay of one and one-half their normal hourly rate.

8.6 Appian Health Systems agrees to pay one-half of the tuition and fee expenses, up to a total of $2,500 per employee per year, of any employees enrolled in an approved course of study designed to advance their education or knowledge in their professional field.

8.7 Appian Health Systems shall pay the entire cost of the employee's health insurance premium. The employee shall pay a monthly contribution of $140 to cover members of their immediate family.

8.8 Appian Health Systems shall pay the entire cost of group disability insurance policy for each employee. This policy, selected by Appian Health Systems, shall provide benefits of not less than $2,000 per month to any disabled employee.

8.9 Appian Health Systems shall provide term life insurance at no cost to employees in the amount equal to three (3) times the annual salary of the employee. Choice of a policy and insurance company rests solely with Appian Health Systems.

8.10 Paid sick leave accrues to employees at the rate of five (5) days per year for the first year of employment and ten (10) days per year for each succeeding year. Sick leave may not be carried over from one year to the next.

Article IX
Pension Rights

Appian Health Systems shall contribute an amount equal to 5% of each employee's salary to the Appian Health Systems' Employees' Pension Fund. Each employee shall contribute a minimum of 5% and a maximum of 10% to the Fund. Full pension rights are available at the age of 60 or following 30 years of employment, whichever comes first.

Article X
Maintenance of Practices

The parties agree that there is a body of written policies, and of practices and interpretations of those policies that govern administrative decisions concerning, wages, salaries, hours, workload, sick leave, vacations, grievance procedures, transfers, suspension, and dismissal not explicitly covered in this Agreement. Such policies and practices shall be continued for the life of this Agreement. An administrative action not in accordance with the past application or interpretation of the above policies shall be grievable.

Article XI
Nondiscrimination

Appian Health Systems and the Union, to the extent of their respective authority, agree not to discriminate against a Union member with respect to the application of the provisions of this Agreement because of race, creed, color, gender, religion, national origin, veteran, or handicapped status, or membership or nonmembership in the Union.

Article XII
Contract Period
and Further Negotiations

This agreement shall be binding on both parties for the period January 1, 20XX, to December 31, 20XX. Both parties agree that negotiations to extend or modify this contract for any period beyond December 31, 20XX, shall commence no later than August 31, 20XX.

APPENDIX B

Outline of a Contract between Appian Health Systems and the Nursing and Health Professionals Union

Instructions: The following is a skeletal outline of the current contract between Appian Health Systems and the NHPU. Each number corresponds to a provision in the current contract. Re-type this outline, leaving space in between each provision to indicate in your responses for this exercise. Use this outline to describe the changes you wish to make in each contract section. For each provision, it might be helpful to indicate "retain," "delete," or "modify," depending on how the new contract differs from the current one. Wherever you indicate "modify," provide a brief summary of the changes you want. To help your partners, prepare a written text of the modified provisions, as well as any new provisions you may negotiate or propose, at the end of the outline. Obtain signatures, as required.

I.   Agreement:

II. Recognition:

III. Payroll Deductions and Dues:

IV. Management Rights:

V.   Union Representatives:

VI. Grievance Procedure:

VII. No Strikes or Lockouts:

VIII. Wages and Benefits:

IX. Pension Rights:

X.   Maintenance of Practice:

XI. Nondiscrimination:

XII. Contract Period:

Additional Provisions and/or Text of Altered Provisions:

APPENDIX C

Appian Health Systems

Appian Health Systems is a small healthcare corporation with five wholly-owned subsidiaries. Appian Health Systems operates six hospitals in three states. Appian Health Plan is a federally qualified HMO licensed for operation in five states including the three in which Appian Health Systems hospitals operate. Appian Medical Associates is a multi-specialty medical group affiliated with Appian's acute care facilities. Appian Homecare Services is a home health agency licensed to operate in the five states in which Appian Health Plan has a presence. Appian Hospice is a licensed hospice operating in the southern section of the headquarters' state in which Appian Health Systems is located.

Last year, Appian controlled over $2,682 million in assets. Its total revenue was $264 million with a net total income of $7.1 million. Total operating revenues decreased 4.4% over the previous year, with a 9.4% decrease in total operating expenses during the same period. The decline in total revenue is attributed to increases in the number of uninsured or under-insured patients seeking care. As a not-for-profit provider, Appian Health Systems provided over $364 million in charity and uncompensated care. In some divisions, uncompensated care was 25% of revenue.

Appian Health Systems employs over 7,000 FTEs. Last past year, Appian consolidated life, dental, and health insurance plans system-wide to reduce operating costs. Similar changes in Appian's benefit plans will be explored next year. The continuing shortage of nursing and other healthcare professionals has caused Appian to take several creative actions to address the problem while maintaining standards of care. System-wide, programs and procedures have been revised or streamlined to increase quality. Facilities have revised staffing plans and established differential pay schedules to attract hard-to-recruit staff. Computers are being used more fully and a new medical record system has reduced time physicians and other healthcare workers spend charting and recording clinical information and other activities. The Health Services Division has employed full-time nurse reviewers to analyze patient charts for appropriateness of medications and clinical outcomes and checking the work of colleagues for quality care. Other divisions are using quality improvement to enhance operational performance.

Nursing and Health Professionals Union (NHPU)

The NHPU is one of the largest national unions representing healthcare workers. Although many Appian Health Systems' workers have been unionized for several decades, it was not until mid-1980 that nursing and professional workers voted to be represented by NHPU. The union represents approximately 2,000 workers in Appian Health Systems' facilities. Support for the union among members is high, although there is growing tension among several professional groups in the bargaining unit. They feel that since nurses are the largest professional group in the NHPU their needs and interests override those of other professionals represented by the union. They have been pressing union leadership to be more even-handed in addressing issues affecting all members even if it means taking a hard line in the negotiations and accepting the possibility of work actions, including strikes.

Appian Health System—Union Relations

Until recently, relations between Appian Health Systems and the NHPU were relatively harmonious. In the past, agreements were negotiated smoothly and promptly, with no serious threat of disruption in operations. As competition and managed care organizations have increased, Appian Health Systems, like many organizations, tried to reduce costs of operations. Since most expenses are related to staffing and salaries and benefits, management has been working to reduce these costs to bring them into line with other healthcare providers. As a result, nurses and other direct care providers feel they are required to do much more work than is reasonable to maintain the quality standards so important in the healthcare field. The pressure "to do more with less" has caused some staff members to seek employment elsewhere, or to pursue different career options.

Current Contract Cost

Salary costs can be estimated using the data in Table 1. Additional information to gauge the cost of the 20XX contract, as well as proposals under negotiations, is:

1. Employees required to work overtime must be compensated at one and one-half times their hourly rate. On average, employees work 82 hours of overtime per year.

2. Continuing professional education benefits have been paid for 456 employees. Of these, 322 received the maximum grant of $3,500. The others averaged $2,132.

3. Individual health, disability, and life insurance policies cost $6,635 per employee per year.

   a. The health insurance portion averages $4,390 per year. Family coverage costs $9,530; 1,221 employees chose this benefit.

   b. The base disability insurance policy costs $750 per employee per year. Each $100 per month increase in benefits adds $42.25 to the annual premium.

   c. The term life insurance benefit costs $275 per employee per year with the current benefit structure (see contract provision 8.9). There is a direct relationship between the annual premium per employee and the projected average benefit. If life insurance were to increase to four times an employee's annual salary, the premium would be $490 per employee. An increase to five times an employee's annual salary would raise the premium to $639 per employee per year.

4. The rate of inflation and general economic conditions are the same as prevailing currently.

Table 21.1. Positions, employees, and average salary

Positions	Number of employees	Average annual salary	Total annual wages
Registered nurse	823	$66,220	$54,499,060
Licensed vocational nurse	1,013	$43,448	$44,012,824
Physical Therapist	37	$83,940	$3,105,780
Occupational therapist	27	$75,300	$2,033,100
Speech therapist	6	$66,920	$401,520
Medical social worker	20	$56,820	$1,136,400
Clinical psychologist	8	$83,580	$668,640
Registered dietitian	4	$55,240	$220,960
Pharmacist	33	$116,670	$3,850,110
Medical technologist	45	$63,893	$2,875,185
Registered radiographic technologist	18	$54,620	$983,160
Total wages current fiscal year	2,034		$113,786,739

22

Evolution of the Healthy Communities Initiatives

Barry Ross
St. Jude Medical Center, Fullerton, CA

CASE HISTORY/BACKGROUND

Barry Ross has served as vice president, Healthy Communities, at St. Jude Medical Center (St. Jude) for the last 15 years. His role has been to provide leadership to implement two key parts of St. Jude's vision—promote health improvement and create healthy communities. While many not-for-profit hospitals have a manager to oversee their community benefits efforts, St. Jude is somewhat unique in having this position at the executive team level. Over the last 15 years, Ross has been instrumental in forming or building the capacity of four community collaboratives that partner with St. Jude to create healthy communities. He recognizes that to increase effectiveness of the collaboratives on the health and quality of life in the region served by St. Jude they must have a greater collective impact.

As part of the hospital's strategic review of programs and their effectiveness, St. Jude's community benefits committee asked Ross to respond to the following questions:

1. What are the strengths and weaknesses of our efforts to date?

2. How might the effectiveness of our programs be improved?

3. Within existing resources, what changes might provide a greater impact on improving community health status?

317

ST. JUDE MEDICAL CENTER

To provide a context to the community health initiatives undertaken by St. Jude, it is important to understand how the values of its founders, the Sisters of St. Joseph, have influenced the hospital's approach and emphasis on serving the community. The Order of the Sisters of St. Joseph was founded in 1650 in southern France by a Jesuit priest who asked them to go into the community, find problems of concern, and work with the people to solve those problems. Initially, the Sisters of St. Joseph helped the poor and sick in their homes. Over the years they expanded throughout France and arrived in the United States in 1836 (Sisters of St. Joseph of Orange, 2015).

In 1912, the Bishop of Sacramento invited a group of sisters from LaGrange, Illinois, to establish a school in Eureka, California. In response to the Spanish flu epidemic of 1918 the sisters provided basic healthcare. This led to establishment of their first hospital in California, which further expanded their role in healthcare. In 1922, the sisters determined they could pursue their ministries more effectively by moving the motherhouse to Orange, California. The first ministries of the Sisters of St. Joseph of Orange were in education and healthcare. Today, the congregation engages in ministries beyond healthcare and education: distributing food, providing shelter for the homeless, helping new immigrants, and fostering spiritual development (Sisters of St. Joseph of Orange, 2015).

St. Jude Medical Center, founded in 1957 by the Sisters of St. Joseph of Orange, is one of 14 hospitals in St. Joseph Health (St. Jude Medical Center, 2015). The mission of the St. Jude Medical Center is to bring the healing ministry of Jesus in the tradition of the Sisters of St. Joseph and improve the health and quality of life in the communities it serves. This mission is emphasized by the vision of the organization; vision that brings people together to provide compassionate care, promote health, and create healthy communities. The values of dignity, service, justice, and excellence are achieved through centers of excellence in cardiology, stroke, oncology, orthopedics, rehabilitation, and perinatal services. St. Jude is a 320-bed community hospital with over 13,000 inpatient admissions and over 450,000 outpatient visits. Its annual budget is more than $466,000,000 (St. Jude Medical Center, 2015).

THE COMMUNITIES SERVED BY ST. JUDE MEDICAL CENTER

The focus of St. Jude's community benefits activities is primarily in low-income neighborhoods in four California cities—Fullerton, La Habra, Buena Park, Placentia—as well as the broader communities in Brea and Yorba Linda. These cities have a population over 443,000 and have pockets of wealth and poverty. The cities are home to thousands of undocumented

Table 22.1. Service area demographics—20XX

City	Population	Unemployment rate	Median household income	% Below federal poverty line	% Households renting
Brea	39,638	6.6%	$72,824	5.6%	34.2%
Buena Park	80,795	11.9%	$61,094	5.6%	44.6%
Fullerton	133,771	10.7%	$63,219	11.3%	33.7%
La Habra	68,506	10.8%	$64,700	12.4%	44.8%
Placentia	52,308	8.5%	$79,194	10.4%	33.9%
Yorba Linda	68,795	6.4%	$113,560	2.5%	17.3%
Total	443,813	9.2%	$90,918	8.7%	36.6%

immigrants from Mexico and Latin America who struggle with daily needs. The cities have various community assets: St. Jude, several colleges, strong not-for-profit organizations, service clubs, and chambers of commerce. While considered a part of suburban Orange County, each city has a history and infrastructure that are at least 100 years old. Table 22.1 provides an overview of the demographics of the St. Jude community benefits service area.

Figure 22.1 identifies community needs by zip code using an index developed by Dignity Health and Solucient, a healthcare information

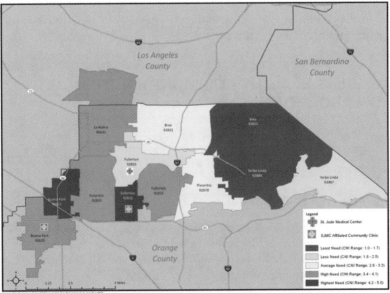

Figure 22.1. Highest-need areas in the service area (1 = lowest need; 5 = highest need).

content company. The index aggregates five socioeconomic indicators: income, primary language, education, insurance status, and housing situation rated on a scale of 1 (low need) to 5 (high need).

ST. JUDE MEDICAL CENTER COMMUNITY BENEFITS EFFORTS

Consistent with the mission, vision, and values of the Sisters of St. Joseph of Orange, St. Jude's community benefits program focuses on meeting needs of the community. Initially, St. Jude's community benefits program was the responsibility of the director of outreach whose primary role was to manage the medical center's mobile health clinic program. After St. Joseph Health revised its vision to incorporate promoting health improvement and creating healthy communities, St. Jude expanded its definition of community outreach.

When Ross became responsible for overseeing the St. Jude Community Benefits Program he embraced the vision developed by the Sisters of St. Joseph of Orange and adopted by the parent organization, St. Joseph Health. The focus on improving health through healthy communities meshed with his educational background in public health and nursing. However, the pragmatist shaped by his MBA recognized that funds available for community benefits were limited, and the current emphasis on cost containment made it uncertain that funding existing programs could be sustained long term. As a result, he wondered if others in the community might be interested in working with St. Jude on its healthy communities initiatives.

BUILDING HEALTHY COMMUNITIES THROUGH COLLABORATION

For 15 years Ross provided leadership and technical assistance to develop several local city collaboratives to partner with St. Jude on its healthy communities' goals (see Table 22.2).

The Fullerton Collaborative

In discussions with the hospital's community outreach program Director Ross learned the Fullerton Public School District had received a healthy start grant that funded a family support center at a local school. As part of the funding requirement, the school district agreed to establish a community collaborative. At the time, the collaborative leader was a part-time

Table 22.2. Summary of work in the collaboratives

Name of collaborative	Year established as community collaborative	Key outcomes
Fullerton Collaborative	2005 (previously an education collaborative)	Move More Eat Healthy Campaign; Faces of Fullerton; Homeless Collaborative; Richman neighborhood revitalization; Summer of Love Fullerton
La Habra Collaborative	2006	Move More Eat Healthy Campaign Teen pregnancy prevention program
Buena Park Collaborative	2007	Move More Eat Healthy Campaign
Placentia Collaborative	2006	Move More Eat Healthy Campaign Community Building Initiative

teacher assigned to this project; representatives from the school district, city government, local colleges, and social service agencies were also included. As Ross began attending meetings he learned Fullerton was a very divided city of 135,000. Low-income residents, primarily Hispanic immigrants, lived in the southern part of the city; upper middle income white and Korean families lived in the north. School performance and health and socioeconomic indicators were strikingly different in these two parts of the city. He concluded that the collaborative should be much more than a grant manager; it could play a role in solving problems facing the city and its residents. He found that others on the board shared his view.

To explore the range of possibilities for the collaborative, Ross invited the collaborative director to join him at a healthy cities conference. The conference broadened their vision as to what was needed to create a healthy city, as well as the role of the collaborative. When the school district grant ended in 2004, members of the collaborative wanted to continue working together, and Ross helped them establish a 501(c)(3) not-for-profit organization. This change in legal status required the collaborative—which had about 20 members at the time—to form a board of directors and raise funds to pay the director's salary. Ross became chair of the collaborative board and St. Jude provided a community benefits grant to fund the group and facilitate its strategic planning.

The original leader Ross worked with entered city politics and, eventually, became the mayor of Fullerton. Later, she became a state assemblywoman. The path to political leadership continued when a subsequent director ran for city council. With this pattern of political engagement, the collaborative began to be viewed as a threat by some in city politics and, by others, as a place for new leadership to emerge.

Today, the collaborative focuses on reducing childhood obesity (also a hospital priority), gang prevention, homelessness, reducing achievement gaps in schools, and bringing together the diverse communities of Fullerton. In its 10th year as a not-for-profit, the collaborative has about 40 organizations that attend regularly, a young and passionate chair who leads a faith-based social services group, and a new executive director who is also a part-time faculty member. While the school district no longer employs the director, it remains active on the board and in the collaborative.

La Habra Collaborative

The effectiveness of the Fullerton Collaborative caught the attention of a community activist from the city of La Habra, another high-need city of 60,000 adjacent to Fullerton. At the time, she was involved with a small networking group formed by the La Habra school district. She asked Ross if he could come to one of their meetings to share what the Fullerton Collaborative was doing. After his presentation he offered to work with the La Habra Collaborative. A strategic planning process Ross led identified their top priorities. With a strategic plan, the head of a small not-for-profit foundation in La Habra agreed to take the lead as chair of the La Habra Collaborative. Ross served as vice chair.

To provide stability during this period, the collaborative contracted with a retired public school principal to be a part-time director of the collaborative. Initially, the school district was displeased with the decision to form a community collaborative from the education collaborative. It felt the actions suggested the education collaborative was taken over. Efforts by the former principal and her previous service as a school board member caused the school district to change its view of the transformation of the educational collaborative.

For the first few years, the collaborative used a local community foundation as its fiscal intermediary. In 2014, the collaborative filed papers to become a 501(c)(3) not-for-profit organization. Today, its priorities are to reduce obesity, prevent gangs, prevent teen pregnancy, and increase reading competence in children. Currently, the collaborative has 50 active members and a board of directors, and it is viewed in La Habra as an asset by all organizations. Annually, St. Jude provides a small grant to support the collaborative's work on obesity.

The City of Buena Park Collaborative

The head of a small Head Start program in Buena Park, which is adjacent to La Habra, came to one of the La Habra Collaborative meetings. She saw the benefit a collaborative involving other organizations could bring to Buena Park. She invited Ross to attend one of her meetings and share his experience and knowledge in developing collaborative relationships with other organizations. Building on his work elsewhere, he assisted this small group of community activists to form the Buena Park Collaborative. To support establishing and developing their collaborative, he secured a community building initiative grant from St. Joseph Health and facilitated development of their strategic plan. To strengthen their role in the city, the Buena Park Collaborative merged recently with a collaborative that works to feed the poor.

The City of Placentia Collaborative

Ten years ago, Ross worked with a small networking group in Placentia, a city of 50,000 with few not-for-profit organizations. He assisted the networking group to obtain a community building initiative grant from St. Joseph Health and facilitated their strategic planning process. As they struggled to become more than a networking group, they became aware of a group in the city that was made up largely of service clubs. A former chair of the Fullerton Collaborative asked Ross to help bring the two small groups together. Ross agreed and asked his healthy communities manager to help the two groups work more closely together. Through the efforts of the healthy communities manager, the groups decided to merge. After merging, the next step was to align their efforts and have the positive impact on their community that both wanted.

THE HEALTHY COMMUNITIES—A JOURNEY GUIDED BY A VISION, VALUES, AND ENLIGHTENED LEADERSHIP

As he reflected on the 15 years he has dedicated to improving the health of communities, Ross is proud of his hospital's and its partners' accomplishments. Yet he wonders about the sustainability of these efforts. For more than 27 years St. Jude has been on a community benefits journey that has resulted in nationally recognized programs and outcomes, including the following:

- Providing more than one million healthcare encounters with low-income persons in 27 years

- Establishing a federally qualified health clinic with five sites in Orange County

- Implementing a model program to serve the homeless

- Acting as a catalyst for four local community collaboratives and a county-wide collaborative to address health disparities

- Developing a long-term care partnership initiative

- Implementing a population-based obesity prevention initiative focused on policy, system, and environmental change

- Reducing rates of asthma, heart disease, osteoporosis, and tobacco use

- Increasing rates of breastfeeding and self-rating of health status

- Revitalizing the Richman neighborhood of Fullerton

At the same time, Ross is concerned about continued success of the community-based collaboratives. Each is at a different stage in its evolution; all are seen as community assets by members and key stakeholders. Each collaborative reflects the unique culture and personality of its city. They have common characteristics, but all depend on their members seeing the value they bring to the organizations they represent and their communities. To be effective, they need more members who will devote time and resources to them. Many collaboratives have memberships that overlap with regional groups, and participation fatigue must be considered. The challenge in years ahead is engaging more community leaders and members and securing funding to sustain the collaboratives' work.

As Ross reflected on his experiences and the need for a strategy to sustain and expand the healthy communities initiatives, he considered the next steps for the collaboratives and the St. Jude Medical Center if they are to achieve the goal of creating healthy communities in the long term.

DISCUSSION QUESTIONS

1. What are the strengths and weaknesses of St. Jude's community benefits strategies?

2. Would the collaboratives have a greater impact on the region if they cooperated? Why? Why not?

3. What strategies do you recommend to Ross to give the collaboratives a greater local and regional impact?

4. Within the limits of existing resources, what changes might Ross consider to have a more notable impact on improving the community's health status?

PART V

Leadership Challenges

23

Hospital Software
Solutions (A)

Elizabeth M. A. Grasby

Jason Stornelli

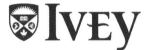

"Sometimes we just have to do things we don't want to do. Now come on, Natalie, stop complaining. I'm busy and you should be too! Get back to work!"

With her manager's words still ringing in her ears after a disastrous meeting, Natalie MacLachlan fell into her chair with a sigh. It was August 2005, and MacLachlan was three months into her tenure at Hospital Software Solutions. Things were not going well—how could MacLachlan's superiors seemingly perceive her as the office "slacker"?

This was certainly not what she had planned for her first job after graduation, and MacLachlan knew she had to fix the situation fast . . . before she was fired.

NATALIE MACLACHLAN

Being labelled as a poor performer was something new for MacLachlan. Before accepting her position at Hospital Software Solutions, she had always been a conscientious student and a high achiever. Originally from Ottawa, Ontario, MacLachlan was attracted to The University of Western Ontario (Western) by the honors business administration (HBA) program at the Richard Ivey School of Business (Ivey), one of Canada's most respected business schools. Because of her strong academic performance and extensive community involvement throughout high school, MacLachlan was pre-accepted into the HBA program before arriving at Western.[1]

During her four years at Western, MacLachlan excelled. She was the recipient of numerous scholarships and awards, including a victory in the Business 020 case competition in her first year. MacLachlan's colleagues at Ivey described her as a good teammate, which was very important in the HBA program, since group work was an important component of the curriculum. Peers considered MacLachlan down-to-earth, articulate, dependable and even-tempered. It was rare to find someone with whom she did not get along. She was ambitious and wanted to do well, but she was not someone who played games to succeed at the expense of others.

MacLachlan extended this sense of thoughtfulness to her activities outside of school. She was active in many charitable, cultural and community organizations in the London area, and she continued to work on behalf of the community when she moved back to Ottawa to begin working for Hospital Software Solutions.

HOSPITAL SOFTWARE SOLUTIONS

History

Hospital Software Solutions (HSS) was founded in 1999 by 10 University of Ottawa software engineering classmates in response to the challenges Ontario hospitals were experiencing when integrating technology into their operations. Deep provincial government budget cuts were forcing hospitals to develop innovative solutions to provide effective and efficient patient care, while keeping costs as low as possible. Many hospitals in Ontario were still using paper systems for tasks such as nursing histories, patient records and medical literature databases.[2] Technology could help streamline these processes and greatly improve service delivery. HSS's customized software solutions promised hospitals an end to the days of lost charts, illegible handwriting and unused capacity with hospital equipment.

Once hospital administrators and physicians were convinced that the computer systems would be as reliable and as easy to use as paper-based methods, HSS's business started to boom. Indeed, the company had uncovered an excellent business opportunity that was easily scalable beyond Ontario. Hospitals around the world were facing similar challenges, and HSS grew very quickly as it expanded into markets in the United States, the United Kingdom and Europe. Much of the company's growth was accomplished through acquisition as the company bought competitors and integrated their operations into the HSS family. By 2005, HSS's financial results were very strong, and the prospects looked good for its future success.

Office Culture

Although HSS had grown significantly, the culture at its Ottawa headquarters had not changed significantly. HSS was still run very much as it had been when the company started—like a small business. Because the original 10 partners knew the business best, all strategic decisions had to be cleared through their offices. They worked very hard, putting in long hours and sacrificing their personal lives to put HSS first. It was not unusual to hear the partners talking about missing an anniversary or a child's birthday, and a few had even come to work on the morning of their wedding day. This devotion to the company was what helped to make HSS a success, and the partners expected everyone on staff to work equally hard to move the company forward. Given the business's success to date, the partners believed they had a winning formula, so they had a strong desire to run the company "as it always had been."

Outside of the partners' offices, the culture at HSS was rather individualistic. Everyone concentrated on their own work, and interaction between employees was infrequent. Most staff communicated through instant messaging programs over the computer, and there were few team meetings. Employees received information on the company's strategic direction through a monthly newsletter, which served as the primary link between the company's partners and its employees.

UNEXPECTED BEGINNINGS

Recruiting season during her final year in the HBA program had been a challenge for MacLachlan. She wanted to work for a company that would give her a position with a significant amount of responsibility and would provide opportunity for advancement within the organization. A few friends of MacLachlan had accepted monotonous jobs, such as data entry, and she knew that she would not be happy unless she was being challenged. MacLachlan had also just married, and a position in Ottawa would allow her and her spouse to be close to both sides of their family.

When MacLachlan saw HSS's posting for a project manager position, she was elated:

> The project manager position had exactly what I wanted. The responsibilities were fantastic, and I could really see myself getting into my work on a daily basis. I've always been interested in computers and technology, and I worked on a large project during HBA that uncovered problems with the installation of a new computer system in a hospital in London, so I was already familiar with the industry. Compensation was more than what I was seeking, which I thought would certainly help with paying back my student loans, and the job was in Ottawa. Not only were our families there, but also, the Ottawa technology community was both tight-knit and growing. I thought the position at HSS would be a great opportunity to make contacts in the industry that would really help me in the future. At the time, I couldn't have asked for anything more.

MacLachlan's interviews with Derek Chow (vice-president, customer care), Marcus Nardi (manager, customer care) and Allan Densmore (vice-president, human resources) went well. All three men expressed numerous times during the interview process how perfect MacLachlan would be for the position. For the most part, the company appeared very laid-back and relaxed, although Chow and Densmore each had to step out of the room a few times to answer phone calls during the interview. MacLachlan left the interview convinced that HSS would be a good fit for her personality.

At the beginning of February 2005, MacLachlan received an offer over the telephone for the project manager position, effective July 1, 2005. Even though the company advised her to take a few weeks to consider, MacLachlan believed the job would be perfect for her, and she insisted on accepting over the telephone. She cancelled her upcoming interviews with other firms the next day.

A few weeks later, Densmore called MacLachlan to tell her that the company was changing its offer: they were now planning to hire her as a Customer Care Team Lead, which was a newly created role. Densmore assured MacLachlan that the team lead position was more prestigious than a project manager job, but he could not to provide her with many details on her expected responsibilities because the job was so new. MacLachlan was reluctant to accept the team lead position:

> It was unclear what I would be doing as a team lead, and I really liked the project manager role. I think Densmore could tell I was upset—he

kept saying on the phone how the team lead job was much better, but he could not give me a firm reason why. I reluctantly accepted, on the condition that they would provide me with a full written job description within two weeks. I don't like to start things when I don't know what I'm getting into.

When MacLachlan received the customer care team lead job description (see Exhibit 1), she had a few concerns, chiefly that she did not have the required three years of support experience with customer service applications; however, she decided not to say anything, fearing Densmore would realize his mistake and rescind the offer.

In early May, MacLachlan and one of her classmates, who had also been hired at HSS, received e-mails from Chow requesting that they start immediately—the office was short-staffed and a client was requesting a complicated software installation. MacLachlan had purposefully booked travel plans before the starting date in her offer, and she really did not want to cancel them. She also wanted to attend her HBA convocation, which was taking place in mid-June. When MacLachlan explained why she would be unable to start work right away, Chow became rather upset. MacLachlan apologized but, at the same time, reminded him that her contract did not begin until July 1. Thankfully, MacLachlan's classmate responded that he was at the end of his vacation and he had a flexible airline ticket, so he could start early. MacLachlan's classmate later told her that Chow had made a point of thanking him for his devotion to the company.

THE FIRST MONTH

No Supervisor

On July 1, MacLachlan arrived at HSS headquarters. Despite the initial issues, MacLachlan was excited to begin the first day of her career; however, her enthusiasm soon waned when she arrived at the reception desk to ask for her manager, Marcus Nardi. She was told he had been fired three weeks earlier. Given her difficulties with Densmore and Chow, Nardi was the only member of the interview team she had not yet disappointed. MacLachlan was told that Chow would be supervising her for the next month until Nardi's replacement, April Worthington, returned from her maternity leave (see Exhibit 2).

MacLachlan proceeded to her desk. Due to a shortage of space, her work area was next to the programming staff area, on the other side of the building from the rest of the customer care team (see Exhibit 3). Chow stopped by soon thereafter; he appeared very rushed and flustered, but he

---

Customer Care—Team Lead

Basic Purpose

This position requires a self-motivated, highly organized and independent individual, responsible for working with Sales and Operations team members to deliver outstanding Customer Service to our Top 150 Public Health Care Accounts. The incumbent will demonstrate productivity, profitability and quality, ensuring excellent customer service is provided to clients at all levels. The incumbent will develop strategies to improve overall Customer Satisfaction Scores. As the "voice of the Customer," the successful person will develop processes to improve internal communication and optimize Help Desk policies and procedures. Key initiatives that derive high value-creating benefit for our customers need to be defined, implemented and measured for their effectiveness. Develop streamlined reporting statistics for Account Management, and work with the Sales Team to articulate the value proposition of maintenance revenues. The successful candidate will have excellent customer service skills and communication skills, coupled with strong technical skills and a positive team player attitude.

Essential Duties and Responsibilities

1. Leadership / Management
   - Streamline processes, increase productivity, gain efficiencies and enhance value.
   - Develop and communicate a clear vision of goals and objectives, philosophies about growth, revenue generation and profitability, in particular the corporate customer care agenda relating to the "Customer is No. 1."
   - Generate, maintain and review with management, annual, quarterly and monthly revenue statistics (leading and lagging indicators) that represent customer satisfaction trends, financial statistics, productivity rates and overall improvement trends.
   - Maintain communications on daily activities, issues and potential challenges.

2. Customer Support / Sales
   - Deliver an effective long-term customer care program for top 150 clients, and implement and maintain client support initiatives.
   - Facilitate in-house training sessions, client training sessions and regional conferences for clients and potential clients.
   - Assist company personnel in the collection and assessment of Customer Care generated client information, and produce documentation relating to program usage, special function, instruction and promotions.
   - Assist in the development and maintenance of competitive intelligence programs and generate industry direction reports to support the development of new features and products.
   - Approve and co-ordinate the administration of customer satisfaction and information gathering surveys and other communication tools.

Exhibit 1. Team lead job description. *Source:* Company files.

(continued)

3. Controlling / Internal
    Review with Management:
    - Annual, quarterly and monthly revenue results/forecasts and costs.
    - Participate in the development of special projects, as well as relationships with various levels of government organizations, other private/public sector organizations (e.g., FTA, State, local government).
    - Participate in the development of internal department policies and programs to support quality and growth.

Education and Work Experience
Bachelor's degree in business or technical field (engineering or IT).
Typically requires minimum three years of customer applications support experience.

Technical and Functional Skills
Excellent customer service skills, including a patient, courteous manner and a clear voice.
Excellent oral and written communication skills.
Managing project-related activities.
Defining and improving processes.
Demonstrated team leadership.
Ownership of issues through to resolution.
Ownership of customer satisfaction and improving scores.
Excellent knowledge of all HSS products, documentation, add-ons and reports.

Equipment and Applications
Knowledge of Hyperion, MS Office, MS Project, Lotus Notes and Maximizer.
Previous experience with incident reporting/bug reporting/call tracking systems an asset.

Work Environment and Physical Demands
General office environment.
Moderate levels of stress may occur at times.
Irregular hours at times.
No special physical demands required.
Travel may be required.

Exhibit 1. (*continued*)

did not mention or appear upset about her refusal to start the job early. Chow told MacLachlan that, unfortunately, he did not have time to train her, since there were too many outstanding projects awaiting completion. In the interim, he was not quite sure what to do with her, so she would have to work on data entry and database cleanup tasks for a few weeks. MacLachlan was disappointed. She believed these menial tasks did not fit with the customer care team lead job description Densmore had given her, and she had been looking forward to developing those required skills right away. Nevertheless, Chow seemed like a reasonable person, and MacLachlan did not want to risk further hindering her relationship with him.

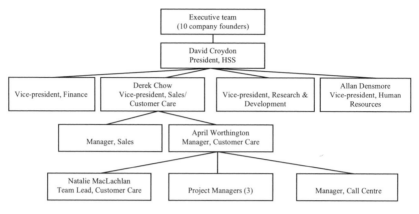

Exhibit 2.   Partial Hospital Software Solutions organizational chart. *Source:* Field.

Data Entry

Like most people beginning a new position, MacLachlan frequently had questions about her tasks, especially surrounding the HSS computer systems, and she often stopped by Chow's office to ask for clarification. He would usually interrupt his typing or phone call to give her a one-word answer and then go right back to work. MacLachlan thought this was odd, but she deduced that Chow was just busy.

After approximately three weeks, MacLachlan was much more comfortable with her tasks. She devised some time-saving measures to make

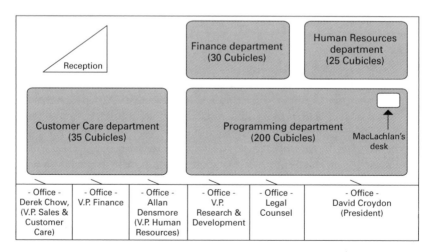

Exhibit 3.   Floor plan of Hospital Software Solutions Ottawa headquarters.

the data entry more efficient, and she was particularly proud of herself when she was able to clean a significant amount of redundant data off the system. Excited about her progress, MacLachlan sent Chow an e-mail highlighting her efforts to date and asking for his feedback on her performance, but Chow replied with a short response reminding her of the importance of following established procedures (see Exhibit 4).

Shortly thereafter, serious problems began to develop with the systems on which MacLachlan was working. She was certain the issues did not relate to her work; nevertheless, she heard from others in the office that Chow was unhappy with her performance. Since she had already asked for feedback in an e-mail and felt that she was bothering Chow, MacLachlan chose not to say anything further.

MacLachlan looked at the pile of data entry sheets sitting on her desk. She believed the established processes Chow had reminded her to follow were redundant, and they were clearly a waste of time. For example, they required a lot of manual checking of figures, when the program had the capability to do that automatically. Chow had asked her to go back and check all her numbers again, which basically meant doing the past three weeks' work over again, even though she knew the numbers were right. "What a waste of my time . . . I don't think I'll bother," she whispered under her breath. This wasn't even what she had signed on for—the customer care team lead position was supposed to help her build skills and give her a significant degree of responsibility, not force her to sit in front of a computer and type in numbers all day.

MacLachlan was very frustrated and, since her work did not require collaboration with others, she decided to start working from home. She assumed this was not a problem, since Chow seemed too busy to spend any time with her and the programming staff (who sat around her) had flexible schedules, often arriving and leaving at odd hours.

THE SECOND MONTH

April Worthington

A few days into MacLachlan's second month at HSS, she met her supervisor, April Worthington, who had returned from her maternity leave.

Worthington had worked at HSS for her entire career (about 10 years), joining the company directly from high school. She held a correspondence diploma in management from a local community college. She had held a number of different positions at the same level within the company over the past three years. As one of the managers of customer care, Worthington was responsible for overseeing many different functions,

TO: Natalie MacLachlan

FROM: Derek Chow

SUBJECT: Re: My performance?

Natalie,

Regarding your request for feedback, unfortunately I have not been able to devote much attention to your work lately, as I have been occupied with other matters.

However, I will remind you to follow HSS's data entry procedures as outlined in your employee manual. These procedures are in place for a reason, and deviating from them may cause data anomalies. Please ensure that the work you have done conforms to these specifications before submitting it.

Regards,

Derek Chow

TO: Derek Chow

FROM: Natalie MacLachlan

SUBJECT: My performance?

Hi Derek,

Just wondering if you could give me some feedback on my performance as of late. I have been working hard on the data entry tasks you gave me, and I think I have come up with a way to tabulate the information without requiring a manual check. This makes the process significantly faster. I have attached the files for your review.

Thanks,

Natalie

Natalie MacLachlan, HBA
Team Lead, Customer Care
Hospital Software Solutions

Exhibit 4. E-mail correspondence between Derek Chow and Natalie MacLachlan. *Source:* Field.

including sales, technical support and complaint resolution. This responsibility required her to develop skills in a number of different areas and, as a result, she often felt overloaded.

Worthington was a very hard worker, and she appeared very dedicated to the company and its processes. It was not unusual to find her at the office late at night after a 12-hour day. Although she had children and a family, she always put her career first. Every task was urgent in Worthington's mind, and she expected the same urgency from her subordinates. She was very ambitious and had mentioned her keen interest in moving up through the organization.

In their first few weeks of working together, the relationship between MacLachlan and Worthington was cordial. Upon Worthington's return to work, MacLachlan was not clear about who she was now working for—Worthington was supposed to be her immediate supervisor, but she still had outstanding projects from Chow. Because she knew both managers were quite busy, MacLachlan decided not to say anything to either Worthington or Chow, and instead decided to complete all her delegated tasks from home, where there were fewer distractions.

The Phone Call

A few days before the end of her second month at HSS, MacLachlan was working through data entry on her home computer when she received a phone call from Worthington. She seemed particularly agitated that MacLachlan was not in the office, and told her that it would be in her best interest to be at her desk immediately. MacLachlan rushed to the office, only to find Worthington standing at her cubicle, waiting for her:

MacLachlan:

> "Hi April. Was there something you needed to talk to me about? The weather wasn't too great this morning, so I felt like working from home today. I have so much on my plate right now."

Worthington:

> "Why don't you know you're not supposed to be working from home? I expect you to be here when I'm here. I really needed your help yesterday and today on the presentation to the executive board, and I haven't been able to find you. You knew this seminar was very important."

MacLachlan:

> "Well, nobody told me I couldn't log in from home. After all, the programmers do it all the time. I think this is going a bit far. I'm kind of

wasting my time at the office doing this data entry stuff anyhow. Do you really want a time sheet from me?"

Worthington:

"No, I don't think I'm that controlling. However, to be honest with you, maybe I should be. I hear your work on the Ontario hospitals database was very disappointing. I've heard you're not following any of the proper procedures."

MacLachlan:

"Well, I wasn't trained. Besides, I was just trying to make things more efficient. I came into this job expecting to take a leadership role, and I was trying to do that by improving the processes. Data entry isn't really what I was expecting, given my job description."

Worthington:

"Your job description is two sentences long. Sometimes we just have to do things we don't want to do. Now come on, Natalie, stop complaining. I'm busy and you should be too. Get back to work!"

As MacLachlan was about to show Worthington the two-page job description from Densmore, Worthington snarled, "If you really want to do something different, do a system format! Have it done by this afternoon." She then stormed off.

Dejected, MacLachlan sat down at her desk. As she turned on her computer, an e-mail from Chow arrived saying that the system problems were getting worse. There appeared to be serious problems with the integrity of the data that needed her immediate attention. In addition to the fact her superiors thought she was a slacker, MacLachlan was now faced with conflicting instructions from two bosses. There was no way she could complete the work for both managers on time.

To add to her troubles, in the course of her data entry, MacLachlan had found problems with the way some of the system processes had been created by the programmers. These processes were unrelated to the data she was entering, but they still affected the computer system as a whole. MacLachlan thought this might be the cause of the problems that had been occurring lately, so she documented her findings. Chow and Worthington probably had no idea there was any problem with the processes, since they had so many other tasks to focus on. Regardless, she was not particularly motivated to share her concerns with either of the two managers, given their recent behavior toward her.

WHAT NEXT?

"Now what?" MacLachlan thought to herself. She knew a town-hall meeting[3] with HSS's president was coming up in a week and that the executive team had specifically asked for feedback on management styles and work processes. This was a meeting for non-management staff only, so Worthington and Chow would not be attending. MacLachlan had met the president a few times in passing, and he seemed like a nice man. She had heard from her colleagues that he was easy to talk to, and he genuinely wanted to do anything that would improve the company. MacLachlan had many ideas about how to improve the workflow at HSS, and she was eager to share them with someone who would listen. She wondered whether she should approach the president at the town hall meeting and raise her concerns. Could this be her chance to make a difference?

"Or maybe I should just talk to Worthington and Chow," thought MacLachlan. After all, a lot of the problems seemed to stem from mis-understandings. After all, Worthington had specifically mentioned that MacLachlan's job description was two sentences long, which was not the case. Had Chow and Worthington thought she was recruited to be doing something different? Maybe a good chat would clear things up. But, what would MacLachlan say? What would be the best way to approach the situation? Should she be threatening? Conciliatory?

MacLachlan knew she could quit, but that would leave her without a job, and she was still paying bills from her wedding and her school debt. It would be very difficult to make ends meet financially. The information technology community in Ottawa was also small, and news of her poor performance and early departure from HSS would surely spread quickly.

MacLachlan knew she had to act quickly. Whatever she decided, she wanted to have a detailed plan of action, with no more mistakes. How could she get herself out of this mess?

ENDNOTES

1. The HBA program was a "2+2" curriculum wherein students undertook two years of university in a field other than business and then entered the HBA program for their third and fourth years of university. Students with exemplary academic and extra-curricular performance could apply at the end of secondary school to have a spot initially reserved for them in the HBA program. Final acceptance into the HBA program was dependent on the maintenance of a high standard of academic and extra-curricular performance in the first two years of university.
2. Canadian Institute for Health Information. *Hospital Report 2002: Acute Care*, pp. 17–18.

3.   "Town-hall" meetings are designed to provide a public link between upper management and front-line personnel. They are usually open to all employees and are often used by management to share corporate strategy or receive feedback from employees in a public forum.

24

The Case of Tim's Last Years

Kurt Darr
The George Washington University, Washington, D.C.

Carla Jackie Sampson
Florida Center of Nursing, Orlando, FL

CASE HISTORY/BACKGROUND

Tim had lived a long and, in many ways, productive and satisfying life. Now, at 86, his situation was diminished by declining physical health. Tim's mental capacity was intact, but his memory was sometimes a bit muddled because of medication. Tim had smoked cigarettes for almost 70 years. One result was chronic obstructive pulmonary disease (COPD). COPD interferes with the lungs' ability to clear phlegm and fluids, and breathing becomes progressively more challenging. Those with COPD have more bouts of pneumonia and respiratory tract problems. Tim's health status was consistent with the usual effects of COPD. Two of his pneumonias required hospitalization. The aftereffects of the pneumonias were, however, a physical decline that resulted in a significantly reduced quality of life. Also, Tim had mild congestive heart failure. In the recent past, he was plagued with urinary incontinence. Other problems that required medical interventions included surgery for a partially blocked carotid artery and setting a broken hip after a fall. Tim's cognition was intact, and he made rational decisions. Behavioral issues became evident after he was admitted to an assisted living facility.

A PROMISING CAREER LARGELY FULFILLED

Tim was born and raised in a small town on the prairie of the U.S. Upper Midwest. His father was an attorney. As was common in those times, his mother was a stay-at-home mom for her two sons. Tim was a typical lad, who led a normal childhood. An early, significant influence was an aunt who taught him the literary classics, some explorations of Greek and Latin, and the importance of attention to detail. As a young man, Tim played sports, had a paper route, and showed a serious interest in birds and the physics of flight. He studied civil engineering as a college undergraduate and proved gifted in mathematics and the sciences. Tim was encouraged to pursue his academic studies and, with the aid of scholarships, completed a master's degree in civil engineering. Another scholarship sponsored his study for the degree of doctor of philosophy in engineering at a prestigious university. The research for his doctoral dissertation produced important new knowledge that earned him a place in his alma mater's pantheon of notable alumni. After completing his doctorate, Tim was employed as a civil engineer with the federal government. There, he undertook design and engineering studies related to managing rivers and streams and oversaw construction of dams, spillways, reservoirs, and canals. After more than two decades of government service, Tim began an academic career when he was recruited by a major East Coast university. There, he taught mathematics and administered academic programs.

Marriage soon after earning his doctorate ended in divorce; the only child from that marriage was raised abroad by her mother. Tim was a loner in the sense that he preferred his own company to spending much time with others. He had numerous acquaintances, but few close friends. Despite being introverted, Tim could be warm, jovial–even courtly–and had a good sense of humor. He read broadly and had a quick wit and an encyclopedic memory. Tim's significant intellect may have been a barrier between him and others. It wasn't clear if he liked people, or only tolerated them. He could not be considered gregarious and was something of a curmudgeon. He was intolerant of those with few intellectual accomplishments and had special disdain for women who, although physically attractive, were superficial and unaccomplished.

At midlife, Tim's early interest in the physics of flight became manifest. He partnered with a faculty colleague to buy a preowned airplane. Tim took pilot instruction and became licensed. In short order, he earned an instrument rating. When his co-owner left the university, Tim purchased the other half interest and became sole owner of the airplane. Weekends with good weather likely found Tim flying a dogleg over rural areas near the airport. He became acquainted with a married couple, both of whom were pilot instructors. After the husband died, Tim continued his friendship with the widow. About two years later, they became more than friends. Tim's long-term intentions regarding the widow were never revealed. Regardless, the romance did not last; the widow ended their relationship after about a year. The break seemed to embitter Tim. Although he spoke fondly of the widow, he seemed to focus much of his anger toward women in general. He was vocal in a negative way about women, who, in passing, seemed vacuous and, in his view, were more objects of pity than affection. The end of his romantic involvement with the widow seemed to put Tim into an even more isolated state of mind; increasingly, he kept to himself.

HOSPITALIZATIONS AND SUBSEQUENT CARE

Tim recovered from the acute phases of his illnesses, but each hospitalization left his physical health something less than it had been. The decline was clear. After being hospitalized with the first bout of pneumonia, Tim was discharged to the rehabilitation unit at Autumn Gold, a life care community. Physical rehabilitation was somewhat successful and Tim ambulated slowly with a walker. He hoped to return to his condominium home after leaving Autumn Gold. He could not, however, perform all the activities of daily living (ADL). His choices were to have 24-hour, 7-day-a-week live-in assistance at home, or remain at Autumn Gold. Consequently, Tim rented an assisted living apartment at Autumn Gold. Additional physical rehabilitation was attempted. Tim had little enthusiasm for rehabilitation and cooperated grudgingly with the therapist.

Insurance coverage for rehabilitation is linked to continued progress in regaining normal function. When his progress plateaued and insurance would no longer pay, Tim ordered it discontinued. When physical rehabilitation ended, Tim could ambulate slowly using a walker.

A few months later, Tim fell in his Autumn Gold apartment and fractured his left femur near the hip. He was hospitalized briefly after the bone was set. Again, he returned to Autumn Gold for rehabilitation, but his recovery was slow and it became clear that he would never return to his condominium. This was a serious blow to Tim's sense of independence. Tim's attorney advised him to rent his condominium to help defray the significant costs at Autumn Gold. That his condominium was rented was a major psychological blow to Tim. It confirmed that he was unlikely to ever return home. This realization saddened him greatly. Tim stopped driving after his first hospitalization. When he became a full-time resident at Autumn Gold, he gave the vehicle to a niece. Psychologically, giving up his car seemed to end hope of ever regaining his independence.

SOCIAL COURSE AT AUTUMN GOLD

Friends hoped living among persons of similar age and circumstance would encourage Tim to engage socially and develop friendships. The dining room and mealtime seemed an ideal setting for these interactions. In his younger years, Tim became an accomplished contract bridge player and playing bridge seemed a promising source of social intercourse at Autumn Gold. This optimism proved a vain hope. He made a few friends at the meal table to which he was assigned. Although he remarked later that he found some at the table stimulating, the potential benefit of spending time in their company was insufficient for him to develop other avenues of social interaction with them. Often, Tim had meals brought to his apartment where he ate alone. Despite efforts to engage him, Tim never played bridge at Autumn Gold. He preferred to stay in his apartment, listen to classical music, and work on a scientific paper, the data for which had lingered in a file drawer for years.

Even before his medical problems and admission to Autumn Gold, Tim had engaged a personal care assistant, Mia, to drive him to medical appointments, shop for personal items and fresh food, and be his companion several hours a week. Mia is married and the mother of three; there was no romantic dimension to their relationship. Tim treasured the time with her and often commented that Mia was scheduled—when she was not—and wondered why she didn't spend more time with him. When reminded that Mia had responsibilities at home and with other clients, Tim acknowledged those commitments, but continued to fret about the limited time he had with her. In a sense, she became a surrogate wife.

CLINICAL COURSE AT AUTUMN GOLD

In assisted living, Tim paid for full-time care. This level of care included regular visits from various members of the Autumn Gold staff who administered medications and nebulizer treatments, took vital signs, provided housekeeping services, and delivered meals on request. Staff members at Autumn Gold have an electronic key that opens all apartments. Most staff members understand they are at a private residence, knock on the door, and ask permission to enter. Others show far less deference and are almost disrespectful in that they consider entry into the apartment a matter of right, not a matter of privilege. This attitude reflects a "I have a job to do, and I'll do it as quickly as possible" attitude. Often, they entered Tim's apartment as would be typical of staff entering a hospital room in which the patient is the object of their attention, not an independent resident who gives them permission to enter a private residence. This attitude of privilege seemed demeaning and rankled Tim. Sometimes, he lashed out at them. There were instances when Tim demanded that they "get out," come back later, or just leave without specifying a time to return. Some staff expressed their dismay at his attitude; others said they were afraid of him because he was sometimes gruff and unfriendly, or even hostile. Staff who had respectful interactions with Tim were treated cordially; others fared less well. His bark was far worse than his bite; he did not become physical except to wave his arm to shoo them from his apartment.

MEDICATIONS

Medications were prescribed and administered to mediate Tim's physical problems, including urinary incontinence, high cholesterol, mild congestive heart failure, and COPD. Nebulizer treatments were used for symptomatic improvement of COPD. Tim had been taking medications for his physical problems for many months. Acquaintances saw no behavioral change with his medication regime at the beginning of Tim's time at Autumn Gold until after the second care conference. This change was noted by friends who visited Tim regularly. A medication commonly prescribed in situations such as Tim's is Ativan (lorazepam).[1] Ativan is prescribed to control behavior attributed to anxiety and the acting out it might cause. His friends speculated that Tim was being given a medication such as Ativan, since his affect definitely changed to one more distant, and less engaged. Most concerning to one of his friends was the fact that Tim was less vibrant. He wasn't himself.

While at Autumn Gold, Tim continued to be seen by his long-time personal physician. Autumn Gold has a medical director, which is a Medicare and Medicaid requirement.[2] That two physicians were treating Tim complicated his care. Those who knew Tim and interacted with him on a regular basis suspected the staff had convinced the medical director to prescribe an antianxiety medication, such as Ativan, to make Tim more controllable and less difficult for staff to handle. Further, although his personal physician could review Tim's chart, he was unwilling to countermand the medical director's medication orders. The change in Tim's affect was especially notable in the significant reduction in what his friends knew was his usual, somewhat feisty, personality. He became more placid and less animated. This change may have helped staff manage Tim, but it furthered neither Tim's independence nor his ability to self-legislate. The patient privacy requirements of the Health Insurance Portability and Accountability Act of 1996 (HIPAA) prevented family and friends from learning about Tim's medications without receiving Tim's express permission.[3] His friends did not want to upset Tim by suggesting they should have access to his medical records to review medications.

CARE CONFERENCES

Several times during his tenure at Autumn Gold, and as required by law, the administration requested a care conference.[4] Care conferences assess the resident and review problems in delivering services. Actions and activities of residents become a topic of discussion. Those present at care conferences include the resident, members of the administration, and family and friends. Tim insisted that his attorney be present by phone or in person, as well. Although desirable to coordinate all aspects of care for the resident—administrative, clinical, service, and comfort care—this was not apparent when the care conferences were requested. The care conferences seemed one-sided and were more a condemnation of Tim's behavior than an effort to integrate observations across the spectrum of care and an effort to consult with family, friends, and the resident, as well as to help the resident achieve the highest practical level of well-being.

Tim's record as related by representatives from the administration included instances in which he had reacted harshly to staff members who entered his apartment. Also mentioned were claims that some staff feared providing care to him because of his gruff, seemingly hostile manner. There were instances when Tim was allegedly rude to staff in the dining room, which may have led to Tim taking some meals in his apartment. The results of Tim's care conferences were that he promised to mend his ways; staff agreed to be more considerate of his privacy and status as a self-legislating resident. The agreement was affirmed by those present, but especially by Tim. One of Tim's friends expressed a more cynical view. He stated that because Tim paid cash for his assisted living and could meet its high costs, it was unlikely he would ever be asked to leave, regardless of issues that arose. Despite the good intentions of the care conferences, the implied threat of eviction was always present. Tim regressed to his usual behavior after them.

CHOOSING TO LET GO

A few weeks after he was discharged from his third hospitalization for pneumonia, Tim seemed to lose hope of ever regaining a quality of life acceptable to him. His difficulty with swallowing that was first evident during the third hospitalization continued after discharge. The swallowing problem was attributed to the likelihood of an undiagnosed minor stroke before or during his hospital stay. His urinary incontinence worsened, and the numerous "accidents" caused staff to insist that Tim wear adult diapers. Wearing diapers embarrassed Tim and reinforced a self-perception that his quality of life had become unacceptably diminished. To help control incontinence, Tim was encouraged to practice exercises that strengthen muscles of the pelvic floor. Known as Kegels, these exercises can reduce urinary incontinence. Tim refused to try.

In the hospital, a speech therapist had worked with Tim to strengthen his swallowing reflex. Speech therapy continued after his discharge to Autumn Gold. Improvement in his swallowing reflex was minimal, and there was continuing fear he would aspirate solids or liquids. Aspiration would likely cause another case of pneumonia. Friends encouraged Tim to practice swallowing on his own. This advice was based on the speech therapist's recommendation that continued practice would likely strengthen the swallowing reflex; Tim complied half-heartedly. Work with the speech therapist ended; guided progress had plateaued.

Tim's caloric intake declined noticeably over the course of his last several weeks. Friends implored him to eat. His private caregiver, Mia, prepared foods she knew Tim relished, including fresh fruit and blueberry muffins. At times, she fed Tim as a parent feeds a child. Tim did not protest this special attention. Despite being pressed and implored to increase his caloric intake, Tim ate very little; his weight loss continued. His physical decline was prolonged because he had gained considerable weight in the first months at Autumn Gold. Friends told him pointedly that failing to eat was a self-imposed death sentence. He ignored them.

HOSPICE CARE AND COORDINATION

It became clear Tim was on a slow, inexorable decline to death. Tim was not dying because of an underlying acute disease process, but because he refused to make efforts to eat. Tim's medical condition was diagnosed as terminal, and he was admitted to hospice at Autumn Gold.

Tim's daughter and family were aware of his situation and came for a final visit. They stayed several days, but Tim's interactions with them were sporadic. Even when awake, Tim had difficulty speaking, and their conversations had little substance. His family's presence pleased Tim but did little to raise his spirits or change his decision about eating; his decline continued. The effort by the family to bid Tim a final goodbye was important, but seemed less than satisfying to them, and, perhaps, to Tim.

As had been their long-time pattern, two of Tim's friends visited weekly. The friends were increasingly distressed to see the general state of Tim's appearance. There were obvious problems with his personal hygiene. Visits during meal times showed meal trays were delivered and placed on the over-bed table. Tim was barely strong enough to feed himself, even if he had been motivated to try. Beyond that, the staff did not encourage him to eat or assist him to do so. Occasionally, he picked at the food. In addition, he was not shaved daily or even every other day and his hair was matted and uncut. He had a disheveled appearance. When staff was asked how often Tim was helped out of bed and seated in a chair, the response was unsatisfactory. It was clear that the comfort care minimally required in hospice was not being provided.

Tim's friends pursued the problems they observed with more senior staff. They learned that hospice at Autumn Gold was neither a specific unit nor a physical place. Instead, hospice is defined as a designated bed in the long-term care unit at Autumn Gold. The unit staff is expected to provide day-to-day care. By definition, the hospice concept offers only comfort care and pain control.[5] In his advance medical directive (AMD)[6] Tim directed there were to be no interventions, such as artificial nutrition or hydration, cardiopulmonary resuscitation, antibiotics for infections, ventilator support, or surgery. Only comfort care and pain control were to be provided.

In addition, Tim's friends learned that Autumn Gold neither owned nor managed the hospice services provided in it. By contract, "hospice beds" at Autumn Gold are managed by Starlite Hospice Services (Starlite). Starlite is an independent, for-profit corporation that manages hospice services at several long-term care facilities in the metro area. Starlite provides a nurse supervisor who reviews the medical record for hospice patients at Autumn Gold and assures they are receiving the care ordered by the Starlite medical director, as limited by the patient's AMD. Day-to-day services and the all-important comfort care are provided by staff at Autumn Gold. One of Tim's friends contacted Starlite directly to voice his concerns about the quality of care and to press for ways to improve his situation.

Following the telephone inquiry by Tim's friend, a visit two days later showed that Tim's hair had been washed and trimmed, and he had been shaved. He was seated in a bedside recliner wearing a bathrobe. This marked change seemed to please Tim and his mood was cheerier than before. The issue with feeding continued. It was unclear if Tim refused food when it was presented by hand feeding, or whether the staff was unwilling to take the time needed to feed him. Regardless, Tim's weight loss and general physical decline continued uninterrupted.

FINAL DAYS

Tim's cognitive abilities decreased as his physical decline continued. He was only occasionally alert. His eyes brightened a bit when someone spoke to him and roused him from the somnolence caused by physical weakness and medications. Tim's ability to eat was nil. His personal caregiver, Mia, visited almost daily and brought fresh fruit which she tried to feed Tim. He accepted her help and ate a small amount of what was offered. He ate too few calories to sustain life.

A few days before he died, Starlite sent a sitter. The sitter provided no care, but, as the name suggests, only sat with Tim. His breathing became agonal and stopped early one morning.

According to his will, Tim's remains were cremated. Family members arranged shipment and interment of his ashes in the family burial plot where he had been raised. As Tim had directed, neither a religious service nor a memorial service was held. This request reflected Tim's dislike of organized religion. Family and friends found Tim's directive consistent with his views but were distressed to be denied the closure that a funeral service or memorial service would bring.

REFLECTIONS AND EPILOGUE

Institutional care has a rhythm. It is a rhythm independent-minded persons may be loath to accept. Rules are needed in congregate living so acceptable care can be provided to all. Rules will likely rankle those whose life and lifestyle choices are diminished when they enter such facilities. Some residents are reluctant to be in a facility in which they are less-than-independent, but are constrained by their physical condition to be elsewhere.

The goal of care that is acceptable care to all residents is a dilemma in managing a long-term care facility. Administration must balance resident idiosyncrasies with equity. All patients receive at least the minimum level of care, but curmudgeons like Tim diminish the resources available to others. Tim was unwilling to submit to the schedule of services offered by the facility. This required additional rounds, which incurred overtime expenses to the facility or extra work for the staff. In addition, his demeanor and the frequency and hostility of his outbursts ensured that some staff feared him, or availed themselves of any opportunity to avoid him altogether. Many staff members at life care communities are paid minimum wage. Some facilities pay fringe benefits. Low wages and few fringe benefits may make staff less than amenable to seeing residents as customers and working to please them. Further, the system and processes may constrain their ability and inherent desire to please the customer-resident. This does not suggest mistreatment of residents; it is to say, however, the incentive of financial recognition for a job well done is absent. It is common that life care communities limit tipping to contributions to an annual holiday fund.

This homogenizes the connection between individual residents and specific staff members. The result is that staff who are kind and patient with residents are treated the same as those who show less compassion and patience.

Persons needing extensive personal care services have few choices; one is to go to a facility such as Autumn Gold that meets those needs. This is a much less expensive alternative than at-home, live-in help. Many persons are reluctant to give up their independence and live in the collective experience of congregate housing. They are less than enthusiastic about being in such a facility. One reaction is a feeling of incarceration. This sense of institutionalization diminishes the psychological benefit of being where they are. Intellectually, residents understand they are in long-term care because they need its services. Emotionally, they don't want to be institutionalized, and this is likely expressed in small, but identifiable ways in their interactions with staff and with one another. Being in a facility is less than desirable; it is not a holiday resort or vacation cruise.

The loss of autonomy and diminished privacy likely make them less than happy with their situation. This unhappiness may cause them to interact negatively with staff who provide services. Some residents have mental changes caused by aging and their lessened physical health. In addition, almost all are taking prescription drugs whose side effects may change personalities and cognitive abilities. The cumulative effects increase the likelihood they will become "difficult" residents. "Difficult" residents tend to be uncooperative and are willing to question the services being provided. Such residents may be further medicated. As an additional side effect, medications may diminish the resident's vigor and vibrancy. The balance for staff is fairly easy: manageable residents are preferred. "Good" patients are easier to work with and will likely receive more attention and remain unmedicated. With the rush of a heavy workload, there is not always time to observe the desired etiquette of giving a friendly greeting, explaining why they want to enter the resident's apartment, and providing services quickly and effectively in a friendly, caring manner. The confluence of residents being less than happy as to their circumstances in assisted living, and hurried, overworked staff members can lead to confrontational and unpleasant interactions, as evidenced by Tim's situation.

The 24/7 care provided to Tim in assisted living was very expensive. In addition to the rent for his apartment, labor costs for round-the-clock care are high. Total charges were over $12,000 per month. Tim was fortunate to have a cash flow sufficient to sustain this outlay. Even with long-term care insurance and significant assets, most residents cannot afford such care for long.

DISCUSSION QUESTIONS

1. Might improved planning and training of staff at Autumn Gold have avoided the problems Tim encountered in assisted living? Why or why not?

2. Consider Tim's decline and discuss the appropriateness of using medications to control the behavior of residents in long-term care. Should family be involved in the decision to use these medications?

3. Suggest how institutional policies can be written to accommodate and define a role for private physicians in seeing their patients in long-term care facilities.

4. Discuss the use of advance medical directives in situations such as Tim's.

5. The case shows a breakdown in care coordination. Suggest at least three steps to prevent similar problems in the future and include a discussion of the responsibilities of Autumn Gold and Starlite Hospice Services, respectively.

6. Nutrition through normal feeding, personal hygiene, and pain control are intrinsic in the concept of comfort care. Hospice services are based on comfort care. What efforts, if any, should be directed to provide nutrition to patients who refuse to eat? Did Tim commit suicide?

7. Tim had no acute, underlying disease process. Although not explicitly known, Tim seems to have decided he did not want to live given his quality of life. In such situations, depression can be an underlying cause of decisions. Was enough done to determine and improve, if necessary, Tim's psychological state to know that he was making a rational choice? Identify the roles of caregivers, and of family and friends, when depression might be an underlying cause of what appear to be irrational decisions.

8. Tim's presence at Autumn Gold raised unique challenges for its management and staff. Draft an argument that Autumn Gold contributed to Tim's death. Further, what more could (or should) have been done to maintain his highest level of functioning?

ENDNOTES

1. Ativan (lorazepam) balances brain chemicals in patients with general anxiety disorders. Ativan causes drowsiness especially in older patients and is not suggested for patients with a history of depression or suicidal thoughts and behaviors. The drug is potentially addictive after only two weeks' use. Possible side effects include dizziness and cognitive impairment.

2. Title 42 of the *Code of Federal Regulations* specifies that long-term care facilities must be capable of maintaining the total well-being of residents. An administrator appointed by the governing board must hold a nursing home administrator state license, if necessary, and is responsible for operation of the facility. A facility not meeting these requirements risks nonpayment by Centers for Medicare & Medicaid Services.

3. The Health Insurance Portability and Accountability Act of 1996 required the Secretary of the Department of Health and Human Services to issue regulations to govern the "privacy of individually identifiable health information," also known as the "Privacy Rule." This rule establishes rights for individuals to protect the use and release of health information. Individuals who cannot exercise this right may designate an authorized person, a personal representative, to access health information and exercise these privacy rights on the individual's behalf. There are situations in which family members, or others involved in the treatment of the incapacitated individual, might get access to private health information directly related to payment or the particular treatment without the designation of personal representative. These circumstances include: to assist in locating a designated personal representative, with the consent of the individual, or if no objection is raised by the individual, or if an inference on no objection can be made (based on professional judgment in the circumstance). 45 *CFR* 164.510(b)

4. "Care conference" is the term used at the life care community in which Tim was a resident. The facility's interdisciplinary team assesses the resident using a resident assessment instrument (RAI). The RAI is required by state and federal regulations and determines the resident's strengths and needs. The result is to assist the resident to achieve or maintain the highest practical level of well-being.

5. Hospice care or palliative care are final-stage comfort care provided for patients with life-limited prognoses. To qualify, the patient must receive two independent physicians' prognoses that fewer than six months of life remain. The interdisciplinary hospice care team manages pain and other discomfort and prepares the patient for the emotional, spiritual, and psychological aspects of death. While under care, which can be inpatient or in-home, the patient may receive speech or physical therapy. All medical supplies, durable medical equipment, and medications are provided by Medicare. Care may include bereavement counseling to survivors.

6. Advance medical directives (AMDs) allow patient participation and control of end-of-life healthcare decisions. When patients are incapable of making decisions, the AMD is used to guide and direct caregivers to provide the care the patient has specified—usually as a limit on care. Patients who have named a personal representative (or healthcare proxy) have someone who acts on their behalf following the directives in the AMD.

BIBLIOGRAPHY

Darr, K., & Sampson, C. J. (2015). Ethical challenges in healthcare (pp. 460–482). In M. Fottler, D. Malvey, D. Slovensky (Eds.), *Handbook of healthcare management*. Cheltenham Glos, UK: Edward Elgar Publishing Ltd.

RxList. (2014) Ativan. Retrieved from http://www.rxlist.com/ativan-drug.htm

U.S. Centers for Medicare & Medicaid Services. (n.d.). Hospice and respite care. Retrieved from https://www.medicare.gov/coverage/hospice-and-respite-care.html

U.S. Centers for Medicare & Medicaid Services. (n.d.). Skilled nursing facility (SNF) care. Retrieved from https://www.medicare.gov/coverage/skilled-nursing-facility-care.html

U.S. Government Printing Office. (2016). Title 42: Public Health Part 483. Requirements for States and Long Term Care Facilities Subpart B. Retrieved from http://www.ecfr.gov/cgi-bin/text-idx?SID=8258bcbb0e4eb2c6faff46861e506d8c&mc=true&node=se42.5.483_175&rgn=div8

U.S. Government Printing Office. (2016). Title 45: Public Welfare Part 164—Security and Privacy Subpart E—Privacy of Individually Identifiable Health Information. Retrieved from http://www.ecfr.gov/cgi-bin/text-idx?SID=d01b258c247bbfc1bad8fba40b905cec&mc=true&node=se45.1.164_1510&rgn=div8

25

Autumn Park

Cara Thomason Embry
University of Southern California, Anaheim, CA

Robert C. Myrtle
University of Southern California, Los Angeles, CA

Brad Douglas, Executive Director of Autumn Park, was tired and frustrated as he once again looked at the resident file of Mildred Puce. Douglas was preparing for the afternoon meeting with Puce and Hannah Meeks, a registered nurse and Director of Assisted Living at Autumn Park. Douglas supported the company's principles, values, and beliefs on how to deal with resident issues and problems, yet everything he is doing with Puce goes against them (see Figure 25.1).

THE HISTORY OF AUTUMN PARK

Autumn Park is one of thirteen properties owned and managed by Abbot Retirement Communities (ARC), which owns and manages high-quality, full-service rental retirement communities nationwide that offer independent living, assisted living, and dementia care. Most are continuing care retirement communities (CCRCs). Regulated by the state, CCRCs offer long-term continuing care services by contract that includes housing and residential services, usually for a resident's life time. ARC is passionate about enhancing the lives of seniors and is committed to delivering exemplary service with integrity, dignity, and compassion.

Statement of Principles, Values, and Beliefs

We are committed to exemplary service delivered with integrity, dignity, and compassion. Our communities for seniors are distinguished by warm, secure, and friendly environments.

We will enhance each resident's lifestyle by:
• Responding immediately to residents' needs and concerns.
• Offering high-quality, creatively designed programs.
• Encouraging independence.
• Promoting a sense of community and friendship.

We the staff are committed to:
• Teamwork
• Being professional
• Open communication
• Fostering a learning environment
• Continuous improvement
• Profitability

We live by a standard of conduct that encompasses honesty, accountability, personal development, and a passion for excellence.

Figure 25.1. These principles, values, and beliefs are referenced whenever important decisions are made at Autumn Park.

ARC is a family-owned company founded in 2001. The President and CEO, Anthony Abbot, was given a retirement property by his family as an investment. The original plan was to manage the property and improve its appearance and services, and then resell it. Abbot became so interested in managing the property he decided to keep it and expand the business.

Abbot had a vision to grow ARC as a unique company dedicated to meeting the changing needs of residents and their families. He wanted to create a working environment in which associates are appreciated and inspired to develop as individuals and in which strengths and abilities are nurtured and rewarded. He wanted to own a company of high-quality retirement communities and services delivered with warmth and friendliness. He was committed to responsible growth, operational excellence, and superior financial results. He did not want the largest company in the industry; just the best.

In 2013, Abbot and his executive team wanted to develop a property from the ground up. Abbot wanted to build a high-end retirement community. The properties he had acquired previously were all middle- to high-end properties, in appearance and price. Abbot was able to meet with the county development planning department for a new, planned city in Southern California. They found a central location for the facility and bought the land. Contemporaneously, ARC moved its corporate office from North Carolina to Southern California.

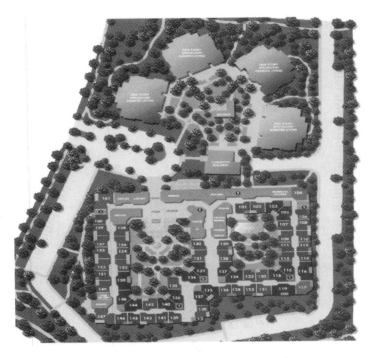

Figure 25.2. Autumn Park Continuum Care Retirement Community.

ARC broke ground for Autumn Park in 2013, with an anticipated opening in March 2014 (Figure 25.2). Autumn Park is a community for independent and assisted living residents, with an additional facility for dementia care. The goal for Autumn Park was to have no more than 40% of residents in assisted living.

BACKGROUND OF MILDRED PUCE

In September 2013, Mildred Puce visited the house trailer that was the marketing office for Autumn Park while it was being built. After several visits with the marketing team about what Autumn Park could provide her, she gave her deposit in November. Puce already lived at another continuing care retirement community (CCRC), yet she was attracted to Autumn Park's centralized location. It would be near shops, restaurants, churches, and grocery stores. Autumn Park offered what she has now, plus access to more services.

Autumn Park's marketing team sought to fill their new property as soon as possible. They took applications and deposits from anyone who was interested and seemed to meet their admission requirements. But, Puce was different. She is younger than 60, lives in another CCRC, and uses a motorized wheelchair because multiple sclerosis limits function to only her head and left arm. Autumn Park accepted her deposit on condition that they would be able to obtain an exception letter from the state because she was under the age requirement to live in a CCRC. In addition, she had special needs and required a Vera body lift, which might limit her ability to live independently (Figure 25.3).

Circumstances delayed Autumn Park's opening to July 2014. In March 2014, Autumn Park received a doctor's order that Puce needed a

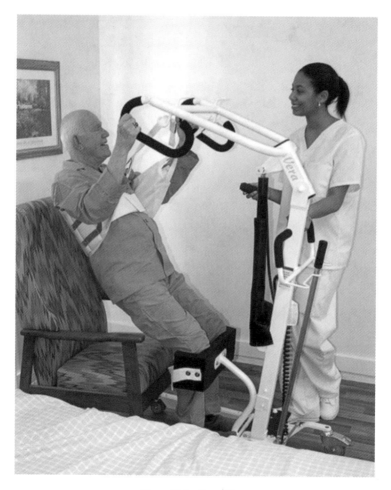

Figure 25.3. Vera Lift.

Vera lift to get into and out of bed, and to the toilet. The orders also stated she could operate the Vera lift with little assistance. She used a motorized chair because of her disability and, therefore, needed a handicapped-access apartment.

The life enrichment assistant coordinator of the CCRC in which she lived also wrote a letter to Autumn Park saying how wonderful a resident Puce was and how sorry they are that she is leaving them.

In May 2014, Autumn Park received another order from Puce's doctor that stated she could self-administer her Interferon Beta injections. The physician disclosed all her disabilities for the clinical staff to examine and consider in their assessment. The marketing department collected the information, but did not share it with the clinical staff to assess at that time.

ARC's policy was to complete an applicant's admission assessment prior to accepting a potential resident's application. The assessment is based on observations of, and conversation with the resident, as well as a physician's assessment of the resident's medications, diagnoses, disabilities, and abilities (see Figure 25.4). If the clinical staff determines that Autumn Park cannot meet the needs identified, the application will not be approved. Consistent with state requirements, ARC's policy states that, following initial assessment, the resident must be reassessed 30 days after move-in.

Puce's assessment prior to admission indicated she required 10 minutes for bathing and showering, 15 minutes for grooming, and 15 minutes for assistance in transfers. This indicated that her care required Level 1, assisted living care. This was in contrast to her personal assessment that she was fully capable of taking care of herself, as well as her two cats.

Autumn Park opened July 1, 2014. During the first month, the executive director resigned and the director of assisted living was dismissed. Corporate brought in regional directors to fill in. By the end of August, Brad Douglas was hired as the new Executive Director of Autumn Park and Hannah Meeks was Autumn Park's new Director of Assisted Living.

At the end of August, 2 months after her admission, Meeks reassessed Puce as a Level III assisted living resident. She was taking 45 minutes of caregivers' time for her showers, which are given three times per week. Also, caregivers spent 20 minutes daily helping Puce with oral care. It was also determined that caregivers were spending an extra 15–30 minutes with Puce each time she used the bathroom. Much of that time was spent helping her in and out of her Vera lift. It also took caregivers 20 minutes to transfer Puce into and out of bed, which they did once each per day.

Each apartment at Autumn Park has two emergency call cords (e-cords): one in the bedroom and one in the bathroom. The e-cords are to be pulled only in emergencies. A pulled e-cord shows on a computer screen at the front desk and the receptionist texts a caregiver to go to that room. A resident who wants nonemergency help calls the front desk, and the

Instructions for Level of Care Assessment

Bathing/Showering:
- 20 minutes—Resident requires daily bathing/showering due to incontinence
- 10 minutes—Requires total assistance, substantial assistance, or standby assistance during bathing/showering including help in and out, supervision/assistance with washing, shampooing, toweling, dressing, and so forth; bath/shower 3×/week; assist with dressing daily
- 5 minutes—Resident requires verbal reminders, clothes laid out, bathing items prepared, some assistance with buttons, zipper, and so forth
- 2 minutes—Resident requires minimal assistance, including reminders and follow-up
  Staff member does not need to be present during bathing and dressing
- 0 minutes—Independent

Oral Care:
- 10 minutes—Total assistance or standby assistance with and/or reminders for oral care including care of dentures, partials, and so forth
- 5 minutes—Reminder and setup only
- 2 minutes—Reminders only and follow-up check daily
- 0 minutes—Independent

Grooming: (includes hair care, shaving, and makeup application)
- 15 minutes—Total assistance or standby assistance daily
- 7 minutes—Reminders, setup, and follow-up only
- 0 minutes—Independent

Toileting/Incontinence:
- 50 minutes—Assistance and/or reminders to resident to use the bathroom every 2–3 hours; assistance with protective undergarments, assistance with removing and/or reapplying clothing; changing bed as needed
- 25 minutes—Reminders and directing only and/or frequent accidents (more than 1×/week)
- 10 minutes—Assist with cleanup of occasional accidents
- 0 minutes—Independent

Medication Management:
- 20 minutes—Total medication administration (4 plus × a day/dosing or more than 6 medications a day)
- 15 minutes—Supervision of medication administration (3× a day/dosing or 3–6 different medications a day)
- 10 minutes—Supervision of medication administration (2× a day/dosing or less than 3 medications per day)
- 5 minutes—Weekly medications setup only, or supervision of medication administration for P.R.N.s only
- 0 minutes—Independent

Mental Status/Behaviors:
- 60 minutes—Disoriented, requires 24-hour supervision and monitoring; occasional redirection

(continued)

Figure 25.4.   Level of care assessment criteria at Autumn Park.

(continued)

- 30 minutes—Disoriented, frequent reminders needed, but some direction or redirection required or depression requiring constant encouragement and frequent individual socialization
- 20 minutes—Mild disorientation, occasional behavior problems, needs reminders daily or depression requiring daily encouragement
- 10 minutes—Mild disorientation, no behavior problems, follows routines or some depression requiring occasional encouragement
- 0 minutes—Independent

Transfers/Ambulation:
- 10 minutes—Always assist with transfers; pushing wheelchair to meals, activities, or standby assistance for ambulation with walker
- 5 minutes—Occasional assistance for wheelchair transport to meals, activities, or standby assistance for ambulation with walker
- 0 minutes—Independent

Other Treatments:
- Other treatments, including follow-up of therapies, dressing changes, customary care, Unna boots, whirlpool treatments, application of ointments, blood sugar, frequent vital signs, or treatment. Record estimated/actual time per day to perform treatment. This includes weights or vital signs, more than once a month, daily bed change due to incontinence, and so forth.

Legend:

0–45	Minutes of care per day is	Level I
46–90	Minutes of care per day is	Level II
91–135	Minutes of care per day is	Level III

Greater than 135 minutes per day might require Alzheimer's care or nursing care. Each additional 40 minutes will be billed as an additional level.

receptionist texts a caregiver to respond. E-calls are considered emergencies and take priority over phone calls. Puce was, however, abusing the process by pulling her e-cord every 30 minutes for caregivers to help with non-emergencies, such as taking out trash, turning on lights, or feeding her cats.

Douglas, Autumn Park's new executive director, and Meeks also noted that Puce was abusing her use of Autumn Park's transportation. Autumn Park owns a wheelchair accessible bus that carries 20 residents and is used for scheduled outings and other residents' activities. Autumn Park also owns a Lincoln Town Car for doctor's visits and unscheduled errands. One hundred and forty residents share these two vehicles. Puce's handicaps limit her to using the bus. Disregarding its use for scheduled activities and groups of residents, she demanded the bus take her to doctor's visits as needed.

Puce complained constantly that caregivers don't understand her Vera lift and don't understand English. She continually pulled the e-cord. When Autumn Park increased her fees due to the time spent on her, she and her attorney claimed discrimination under the federal Americans with Disabilities Act saying that Autumn Park raised only her rate and no other resident's.

When Autumn Park showed her the minutes used for her care, she insisted they were not correct. She dictated to Meeks which caregivers she wanted to care for her. Such a request is considered private duty care in Autumn Park, which necessitates a rate increase. Puce again claimed Autumn Park was discriminating against her and threatened to sue.

In November 2014, which was 5 months after Puce was admitted to Autumn Park, Meeks discovered that the letter describing Puce's health status and disabilities had not been sent to the state. Douglas and Meeks prepared the letter asking the state to decide if Puce would receive an exception to the regulation prohibiting someone younger than 60 from living in a CCRC. If, as Douglas and Meeks hoped, the exception were not granted, the state would no longer allow her to live at Autumn Park. To their dismay, the exception was approved by the state. This meant Puce could remain at Autumn Park.

Also in November, Autumn Park began a 30-day period to record the minutes spent on Puce's care. She was to keep a record and the caregivers were to keep a separate record of the minutes they spent with her. It was discovered that Puce manipulated the caregivers as they documented the minutes used in her care. Puce denied the accusations that she manipulated the caregivers in their documentation of her care. Due to the dispute on how to record and how the minutes reflected care, Puce and Autumn Park redid the evaluation in January 2015. Also, in January, a letter was sent to all residents at Autumn Park stating there was a change in the fee structure for assisted living. Instead of $400 for Level I, and $300 for Levels II and III, it would be $500 for each additional level of care.

In March 2015, a third evaluation of the minutes of care used for Puce was conducted. Puce continued to assert that the minutes documented were not a true reflection of the care she was being given. Once again Puce manipulated the caregivers; many came forward to describe it to Meeks. Also, several caregivers wanted to resign because they no longer wanted to care for Puce. They claimed she was verbally abusive and yelled at them. Puce denied she ever raised her voice to a caregiver or spoke to them in a derogatory way. She said caregivers must have interpreted her requests incorrectly. Also, in only 5 months, three caregivers made workers' compensation claims because they hurt their backs caring for her. Puce continued to demand that only certain caregivers care for her, and now she wanted no male caregivers giving her showers.

By this time, Douglas and Meeks were very frustrated with Puce. They wanted her out of Autumn Park, but didn't know how to evict her without being sued or causing negative publicity. Douglas decided to visit the executive director of the CCRC Puce lived in prior to coming to Autumn Park. The executive director agreed with Douglas about how difficult and manipulative Puce was. She also told Douglas that, "once we got her 30-day move-out notice we were jumping up and down in the halls. We wrote glowing letters about her just to make certain that Autumn Park would take her." Douglas was at a loss as to what to do about Puce. In May 2015, Autumn Park talked to the state ombudsman[2] about the difficulties they were having with Puce. Her demands on Autumn Park and her caregivers were causing a great deal of stress. The ombudsman agreed that Puce is a difficult resident.

In June 2015, Puce complained to the state ombudsman that her privacy rights were being violated because a male staff member was assigned to help her take a shower. The ombudsman called the state licensing authority, which sent an official to Autumn Park to speak to Douglas and Meeks about Puce. The official reviewed Puce's file. It documented the skill level they provided and showed that Puce needed an even higher level.

By this time, Puce had severe edema in her legs because of poor circulation. The edema caused her legs to weigh about 50 pounds each. This increased the risk of caregivers being injured repositioning her legs in her wheelchair or when operating her Vera lift. If the edema persisted, her skin would break down, causing open, weeping wounds. If this happened, she would have to be hospitalized.

California regulations require a residential care facility to give residents 30-day notice to move out if the facility feels it can no longer provide the care a resident needs. Also, state regulations allow a facility to refuse a former resident's request to return to it if, after hospitalization, the facility determines it cannot provide the care the resident requires. The regulations state that a resident in such a facility must have skilled health professionals take care of any open wound, skin tears, or pressure ulcers. Hospitalization may be needed to receive such care, or the facility may have an exception from the state that a home health nurse will care for the resident until the wound heals.

As Douglas reviewed Puce's file, he felt his hands were tied. If Autumn Park gives Puce notice, she will sue Autumn Park under the Americans with Disabilities Act. Puce also threatened to call the local media about Autumn Park's treatment of a handicapped resident. Therefore, Douglas had made certain he told the state licensing official Autumn Park can care for Puce, but not to her unique expectations. Puce needed custodial care not skilled nursing care. Yet, Puce was a victim of her own circumstances since she could not afford the one-to-one care. Community care licensing agents had evaluated Puce. They agreed that Puce was not appropriate for a CCRC and needed a higher level of care.

Douglas also thought about what the ARC corporate staff had told him. They stated that anything is better than negative publicity about Autumn Park or its parent, ARC. "Do what it takes to provide her care; avoid a lawsuit and negative publicity at all costs."

At the meeting with Puce, Douglas plans to offer her three options:

1. Get the level of care she needs from sources such as home health

2. Move to a facility with more skilled care

3. Get 12 hours of one-to-one care daily at a cost of $7,000 a month

DISCUSSION QUESTIONS

1. Are there other options Douglas should suggest to Puce?

2. The state licensing official reviewed the assessment of Puce and agreed the care she needs is beyond that available in a CCRC. Should Autumn Park appeal the state's decision regarding the exception that was made earlier?

3. How does Douglas protect his staff and further the goals of Autumn Park while meeting the directive from corporate to avoid a lawsuit and negative publicity "at all costs"?

4. Identify the process failure(s) that allowed Mildred Puce to be admitted to Autumn Park. Develop an action plan to prevent similar failures in the future.

ENDNOTES

This case used by permission of the authors. Copyright © 2016 by Cara Thomason Embry and Robert C. Myrtle.

1. The California State Long-Term Care Ombudsman Program is authorized by the federal Older Americans Act and its state companion, the Older Californians Act. The program investigates and tries to resolve complaints by, or on behalf of, residents in long-term care facilities (LTCs), including nursing homes, residential care facilities for the elderly, and assisted living facilities. The program investigates elder abuse complaints in LTCs and residential care facilities for the elderly.

26

Appalachian Home Health Services

Kathryn H. Dansky
Pennsylvania State University, University Park, PA

Frances Matthews, the director of clinical services at Appalachian Home Health Services, Inc. (AHHS), was concerned. AHHS needed to hire a nurse quickly. One of the staff nurses had just handed in her resignation because her husband was being transferred out of state. The nurse who was leaving gave AHHS 2 weeks' notice, which complied with the agency policy; however, it still left the agency in a bind. Matthews knew that recruiting and interviewing home health nurses was a time-consuming process, and, even after a nurse was hired, several weeks of orientation were usually required before the nurse could perform independently. She knew that all of the regular staff nurses were working to capacity and that the loss of even one nurse would have major implications. She walked over to Kate Hennessey's office to discuss the situation. Hennessey was the director of administrative services. Matthews and Hennessey had started AHHS 4 years ago. Together, they made all final hiring decisions.

Matthews knocked on the door, saw that Hennessey was sitting at her desk, and walked in. "Sue is leaving. She sure picked a bad time to move!" She laughed halfheartedly, and said, "We need to replace her quickly. Do you have any brilliant ideas?"

Hennessey sighed, and responded, more in the form of a statement than a question, "We don't have any decent applications on file, do we?"

"Nope."

"Great. Well, there's an online RN recruitment site that has been getting good publicity. It's https://www.healthcareers.com/. I'll post something there. Let's also get our ad into the newspaper's online section. Maybe something will turn up."

BACKGROUND

AHHS is a private, not-for-profit home health agency, located in a rural area of a southeastern state. The stated purpose of AHHS is to provide health care services at home to elderly individuals, persons with disabilities, and persons with short-term, specific health care needs that could be handled at home.

AHHS is a "fee-for-service" health care organization; it provides in-home services, then bills for the services, either to a public or private insurance carrier (e.g., Medicare, Medicaid, Blue Cross/Blue Shield), or to the patient directly. AHHS receives all (100%) of its revenue from billed services. As a private organization, it does not receive government subsidies or tax support.

Competition in the home health field is intense, particularly in rural areas, where the need for services fluctuates. Because services are expensive to provide, it is critical for agencies to generate a volume of visits sufficient to cover fixed expenses plus make a small profit. Competition for AHHS comes primarily from Care One, Inc., a multicounty operation that has been established in the area for well over 10 years. AHHS surpassed Care One in total number of visits after its second year of operation and has been steadily growing. Many of the physicians in the area, however, continue to use Care One, and Care One receives more referrals from hospitals outside of its service area than does AHHS.

AHHS currently has 32 employees, including 15 registered nurses (full time and part time), 8 nursing aides, 2 physical therapists, 1 speech-language therapist, and 7 administrative staff. All but two employees at AHHS are female.

REFERRALS FOR SERVICE

Most of the business generated for AHHS is in the form of referrals. Hospitals (social workers, discharge planners) account for more than 70% of patient referrals; of this total, approximately 85% are from the two local hospitals and 15% are from out-of-town hospitals. The second most frequent source of referrals is the general public; former patients, potential patients, family members, clergy, and the like may request services directly. Approximately 20% of referrals come from this source. A small number of referrals come directly from physicians. Although this source is less than 10% of the total, it is important to AHHS, because of the power and status that physicians have in the community.

PATIENTS WHO RECEIVE HOME HEALTH SERVICES

Most of the individuals who receive in-home care are elderly. They usually have a chronic illness that requires monitoring or have a need for rehabilitation therapy following an acute episode, such as a stroke or hip fracture. Some patients have disabilities and require ongoing therapy at home. Some are convalescing from a hospital stay, and need short-term care (e.g., dressing changes). Others have a special type of acute medical need that does not require hospitalization, such as intravenous antibiotics or chemotherapy.

Most of the patients cared for by AHHS are indigenous to the area, live in rural areas, and are religious. Although not all patients fit this description, it is fairly safe to say that the patient population is elderly, traditional, and conservative.

THE ROLE OF THE HOME HEALTH NURSE

The registered nurse is the central caregiver in the home health field. Home health nurses must be able to function independently and comfortably in the patient's home, and must be capable of performing a wide variety of clinical procedures (e.g., giving injections, inserting catheters, obtaining specimens). In rural areas, the nurse may be the only contact that the patient has with the local healthcare system. Therefore, the RN is considered to be both a "case manager" and a "gatekeeper" in coordinating medical, health, and social services (see Table 26.1). This position requires high-level skills in nursing and communications. Due to the incorporation of electronic medical records, as well as remote monitoring (telehealth) services, in the home health industry, computer literacy is also necessary. Nurses with a Bachelor of Science in Nursing (BSN) degree and experience in home health or community nursing are usually sought for these positions.

ANSWERS TO THE AHHS ADVERTISEMENTS

After Matthews left, Hennessey asked the office manager to send a copy of their standard classified ad for a home health nurse (see Figure 26.1) to

Table 26.1. Job description for home health agency registered nurse

DEFINITION
The registered nurse administers skilled nursing services to individuals in their homes, in accordance with a written plan of treatment established by the patient's physician. The incumbent is directly responsible to the Nursing Supervisor and ultimately to the Director of Patient Services.

QUALIFICATIONS
1. Graduate of an approved school of professional nursing
2. Current license to practice as a registered nurse in this state

RESPONSIBILITIES
1. Conduct initial patient assessment and evaluation
2. Evaluate the ongoing needs of patients on a regular basis
3. Initiate the patient's plan of treatment and any necessary revisions
4. Provide those services that require substantial specialized nursing skills
5. Initiate appropriate preventive and rehabilitative nursing procedures
6. Prepare and maintain clinical notes, using the agency's EMR system
7. Coordinate care with allied health professionals
8. Inform the physician and other personnel of changes in the patient's condition
9. Counsel the patient and family in meeting nursing and related health needs
10. Participate in in-service and continuing education programs
11. Supervise and teach other nursing personnel

the local newspaper's office. She also submitted a similar ad to healthcare. com. The next day, the newspaper carried the ad in the classified section, both paper and online. The newspaper and healthcare.com ads ran for 3 consecutive days. Applicants were requested to call the office, or to send a résumé to the director of clinical services.

AHHS received two responses to the ads. (Both responses were from the newspaper online ad). One was a résumé from a student at a nearby technical college. The college had a 2-year (associate degree) registered nurse program, and the applicant was in the last quarter of her second year. She had no experience in the healthcare field but had been caring for her elderly father. After his death, she decided to return to school. Matthews knew, from past experience, that RNs from 2-year programs lacked many of the skills for this type of work. She decided not to interview this applicant.

The other applicant, Margaret Jenkins, called to express interest in this position; the conversation was pleasant and informal because the women knew each other. Jenkins had lived in the area all her life, had family there, and was well known for her community activities.

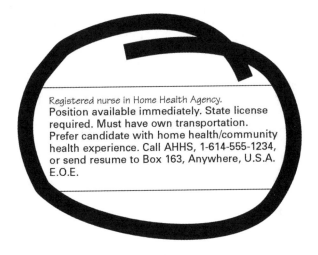

Registered nurse in Home Health Agency.
Position available immediately. State license
required. Must have own transportation.
Prefer candidate with home health/community
health experience. Call AHHS, 1-614-555-1234,
or send resume to Box 163, Anywhere, U.S.A.
E.O.E.

Figure 26.1. Sample classified ad for a home health nursing position.

Jenkins is a registered nurse, with a BSN from the local university. She had most recently worked for 8 years for Dr. Edward Smith, a general practitioner in town. Prior to that time, she had worked at the state mental health center. Written references from both employers indicated that she was hard working, responsible and professional, and got along well with patients, staff, and physicians. Hennessy decided to call Dr. Smith's office to gain additional insight. She spoke to the office manager, who spoke warmly and enthusiastically about Jenkins. The office manager added that Dr. Smith was cutting his hours because he was nearing retirement. Otherwise, they would have rehired Jenkins.

Eighteen months ago, Jenkins was involved in a domestic violence situation in her home. During an argument with her husband, according to the press, Jenkins was physically attacked, and the argument ended in the death of her husband. Jenkins was charged with murder. During the course of the trial, most of the details were made public. Episodes of violence had occurred previously, resulting in a separation of Jenkins and her husband, with a restraining order against the husband. Jenkins testified that on the night of the fatal argument, she was home with her two young children when he appeared and threatened all three of them. While her husband was beating her, she managed to pick up a large kitchen knife and stab him. The court convicted her of involuntary manslaughter and sentenced her to 10 years in prison. While she was in prison, her attorney petitioned for early release, based on her standing in the community and the fact that she was the sole support of two young children. Also during this time, several concerned friends led a successful campaign to have her nursing license reinstated. (The state board of nursing had revoked her license to practice nursing, a standard practice for convicted felons.)

Jenkins' immediate concern was finding employment, since Dr. Smith, her former employer, was not able to rehire her. When she saw the AHHS ad on the newspaper site, she thought it was her answer. Now that she had her license back, she could begin working immediately. But her criminal record weighed heavily on her mind.

THE INTERVIEWS

After initial review of applications by the nursing supervisor, the procedure at AHHS was for all qualified applicants to be interviewed first by the nursing supervisor, then by the two directors, Matthews and Hennessey. Because of Jenkins' good work record and because no other suitable applicants were available, Matthews asked Jenkins to come in for an interview, and set up an appointment for that afternoon.

Jenkins walked into the AHHS offices and greeted everyone warmly. A Caucasian woman of average height and weight, she appeared to be in her mid-thirties. She was on time, was dressed appropriately, and looked nervous. Barbara Jones, the nursing supervisor, introduced herself and led Jenkins into the conference room. A half-hour later, Jones brought Jenkins to Hennessey's office, where the second interview would take place. Jones went in first and briefly summarized her interview. Although she had a positive overall impression, she was concerned about Jenkins' lack of experience with home health procedures, particularly interviewing and assessment skills. Because this part of the job was so important to the overall plan of care, it was essential that RNs have experience in this area. She then left the office and Jenkins went in.

Jenkins sat down with Hennessey and Matthews. The three women discussed AHHS policies and general personnel issues, including benefits. It was clear that Jenkins had the abilities needed, she knew the geographical area well, and could communicate effectively with area physicians. Her only weakness was that she did not have home health experience. Her personal life was not discussed, but she did remark at one point, "You know, I really need this job." At the end of the interview, Matthews thanked her for coming, and said, "You do meet many of the qualifications, but I'm not sure if you're the right person for this job." Jenkins smiled grimly and said, "I wouldn't blame you if you don't want to hire me." With that, she picked up her things and walked quietly from the office.

Matthews and Hennessey looked at each other. "I don't know," Hennessey said. "I don't know either!" responded Matthews. They usually based their hiring decisions on qualifications plus "intuition," and usually agreed on an applicant's suitability. This case was different, however, and neither was sure whether they should hire Margaret Jenkins. Matthews said, "Well, let me know what you decide," and left the office.

Hennessy reviewed the application, references, and notes from the interview. In addition to her lack of home health experience, Jenkins had never had the opportunity to utilize clinical assessment skills, such as auscultation and physical examination. She used a personal computer, but had no experience with electronic medical records.

More importantly, Hennessy wondered about the ramifications of hiring or not hiring a convicted felon. Was discrimination a potential issue? She also felt that some of their elderly patients, who held more traditional views about women's roles, might react negatively to having Ms. Jenkins in their home.

Hennessy searched online to find laws related to discrimination against convicted felons. On https://www.eeoc.gov/laws/practices/ she learned that federal law addresses this question in Title VII (basic employment discrimination law). Specifically, an employer can refuse to hire if the felony conviction directly affects a felon's qualifications. Her search for state laws found http://lac.org/toolkits/standards/Fourteen_State_Laws.pdf.

Kentucky law forbids discrimination by public employers and licensing agencies. However, public employers can consider applicants' convictions if they relate directly to the employment. The statute does not protect persons convicted of "felonies, high misdemeanors, and misdemeanors for which a jail sentence may be imposed," as well as crimes of "moral turpitude." A quick call to their attorney confirmed that AHHS could claim "job relatedness" if they decided not to hire Jenkins.

Hennessy considered her options. She knew she had to make a decision soon.

ENDNOTE

This case used by permission of the author. From Dansky, K. H. (1991). Appalachian Home Health Services. In G. E. Stevens (Ed.), Cases and exercises in human resource management (5th ed., pp. 246–251). Homewood, IL: Richard D. Irwin, Inc.

27

Suburban Health Center

Bruce D. Evans
University of Dallas, Irving, TX

George S. Cooley
Long Green Associates, Inc., Long Green, MD

The situation gave Helen Lawson good reason to pause. She had been supervisor of Metro City Health Department's Suburban Health Center for only 2 months and reflected that things had been going well. Yet, Lawson had one problem that, unfortunately, threatened to overshadow all the positive feedback to her. She was not sure how to solve the problem she had identified.

Dr. Morgan had just left her office, and he had merely added fuel to the fire. He is the staff doctor for a state-funded health project. He had come to plead that Dorothy Wilson be fired. Wilson, it seems, was a problem. As one of Lawson's staff nurses and one of only three in the office with a bachelor's degree in nursing, Wilson had been with the Suburban Center for 3 years. When Lawson was first hired, she had planned to rely heavily on Wilson, but so far she had not been able to do so.

Lawson knew, of course, that she did not have the authority to dismiss Wilson, because they were all municipal employees. She had had trouble convincing Morgan of this. He had been adamant. He had tried previously to have Wilson discharged because his staff was unable to work with her. His staff said her attitude conveyed that they were intruding into her domain and she resented them. Wilson's actions did appear to reflect this attitude.

Morgan had related several incidents indicating Wilson was a weak communicator and that both her resentment and inability to communicate resulted in almost no coordination. Because coordination in community health services is very important, Morgan believed it was essential to replace Wilson with someone more mature who could work effectively with the state agency. Lawson had listened. Although reiterating the limitations of her authority, Lawson promised to look into it further.

Appointments and lunch gave Lawson a brief respite from Morgan's comments. On her return, however, she felt compelled to carry through on her promise quickly. The first step was to review Wilson's personnel file carefully. To do so, Lawson called for her clerk to bring in the file. In passing she said, "Billie, why don't you go to lunch now. Ms. Wilson will be here to cover the phones." Billie replied excitedly, "Oh, no, Ms. Lawson! I'll just wait for the others to get back. Wilson can't handle them. I can never make out messages that she leaves after answering."

With the exchange ended, Lawson turned to the file. She had glanced casually at all the personnel files previously, but she had not looked thoroughly to see what they might reveal. Wilson's job application showed she had held eight assorted jobs in the 8 years preceding her application for her job at the center. Lawson wondered what caused those job changes.

Pertaining to her education, Wilson's file reflected that her degree had been earned only after coursework from five colleges and universities. Also, excessive tardiness had delayed her attaining full employment status at the center. Finally, the most recent performance report by her previous supervisor had been downgraded to "satisfactory" from earlier ratings of "excellent."

Armed with this information, Lawson decided to meet with Lila Murphy, the previous supervisor who had left to take a part-time position closer to her home. At the meeting in her office, Murphy added information. "I confess I wasn't able to handle Wilson," Murphy said. "I was afraid of her and did not want to confront her. After all, she is a big woman and can be intimidating. Certainly, her performance ratings were inflated, but I only did so to avoid trouble. Wilson's work—especially her reports—was often substandard. She often refused to comply with my requests, but others in the office covered for her, so I let it go."

WILSON'S BEHAVIOR

The information developed in the past 2 days' input weighed heavily on Lawson. In subsequent findings, she saw that Wilson's performance continued to be unsatisfactory. As a result, Lawson felt compelled to begin a detailed file on Wilson's performance. Despite the incidents that had been related to her, Lawson found no specific deviations committed to writing. The depth of the problem was highlighted by the fact that it took less than 2 weeks for Lawson to accumulate several memos in Wilson's file. Wilson's less-than-satisfactory performance, it seems, was hardly a rare occurrence.

One thing Lawson noted again and again was that Wilson consistently failed to leave word with anyone when she left the office. Not only did she fail to sign out, but also she failed to even mention where she was going or when she would return. This happened even at peak workload times when the entire staff was needed. Wilson seemed oblivious to these needs and went about tasks that could have been easily scheduled for slower periods.

Lawson also noticed that Wilson always took 2 hours for lunch on Fridays. The staff jokingly seemed to know what she was doing and covered for her. Although Lawson did not object to occasional long lunch hours, the regularity and seeming secrecy bothered her.

In one specific incident, Wilson was gone for more than an hour one afternoon. When she returned, Lawson asked where she had been. "I went to get gas," she said. "I only use this one brand, and there is no station on my way home." Lawson asked her why she could not go out of her way after work. Rather than answering, Wilson appeared hurt and just looked away. Reacting to the awkward situation, Wilson went off to sulk and was moody the rest of the day.

Next, Lawson reviewed Wilson's time sheets and written reports. All employees are required to account for their time and report on the families for whom they are responsible. These reports result from periodic visits to the families' homes. Lawson noted that Wilson's sheet reflected consistently longer transportation and visit times than did those of other staff nurses. Furthermore, Wilson's reports were poorly organized and provided scant information to justify the time spent. The reports did not reflect why she made the visit, what problems, if any, were found, and what actions she took or planned to take to correct them. Rather, she gave a hazy narrative paragraph to show the visit was made.

When Lawson asked her about this, Wilson again seemed hurt, but she also indicated in a rather hostile manner that many of the problems were not her fault. "My district is the most spread out. I also find many families not at home. That's why my transportation time is higher. I can't help that." She also laid much blame on the coordinating agencies. "It's often the agencies' fault. They don't coordinate properly. I can't do it all myself." She said further that she often failed to get proper and adequate information because someone else slipped up.

LAWSON'S PROBLEM

Lawson considered this information for a few days and decided to discuss the situation with Betsy Graham—her immediate superior at the health department—in the hope she could provide useful guidance. Graham began by saying, "Yes, I was aware that Murphy was having a personnel problem at Suburban, but it never officially got to me, so I took no action. My main contact with Wilson came when Murphy decided to leave. Wilson was senior there and could have taken over your supervisory position, but she expressed no interest in it. She apparently had no desire to move up or accept more responsibility. The job remained essentially vacant until you arrived. Everyone pretty much looked after themselves." Graham was neither able to give Lawson more first-hand information, nor did she seem to have concrete advice for Lawson. Lawson puzzled over the facts as she drove back to the office. She realized she had sufficient information to solve the problem, but had been unable to put it together to reach an actionable conclusion. As Lawson reached the office, she tried to sort out the issues, identify the causes of the problem, and decide what to do.

DISCUSSION QUESTIONS

1. Do Wilson's long lunch breaks, failure to sign out from the office, and less efficient home visits suggest she is hiding unacceptable behavior? What other information shows a similar pattern of behavior?

2. When Wilson sulks, is her behavior an extension of always getting her way with her previous supervisor?

3. Why would other staff members cover for Wilson?

4. Is it possible Wilson is a loner who got her way previously and is not willing to change?

5. Outline a course of action for Lawson to address the issues with Wilson's employment. List the steps in order of priority.

ENDNOTE

28

Team Building

From Success to Failure in 24 Hours

Cherie A. Hudson Whittlesey
St. Jude Medical Center, Fullerton, CA

Sara Brown returned to her office and reflected on the team-building activity she had just finished leading with one of the clinical departments. She was pleased with how the session had gone and the active, thoughtful participation of physicians, nurses and other professionals, and support staff. She smiled as she thought about one physician's comment: "This was really helpful; I'd like to do it with my team." To her, this was especially meaningful because she had been worried about his reaction to the workshop; his comments gave her a good feeling.

Brown did not know, however, that after the session one physician sent a highly critical e-mail about the workshop and all the things he felt were wrong with it to his physician colleagues. To make matters worse, he "blind copied" his negative assessment to the clinical staff who had participated. The next morning as Brown was preparing to send a thank-you e-mail to the participants, she received a call from one of them telling her about the physician's e-mail and the negative impact it was having on the department's staff. Since Brown was not copied on the e-mail, this information caught her off guard. As she recovered from the "out of the blue" revelation, she asked the department head if it might be possible to meet with the staff to learn more about the issues and concerns that were emerging. The department head thought the sooner Brown could meet with her team the better. She asked Brown to participate in the scheduled department meeting later that day. When Brown arrived at the department she learned the doctor had called asking for her contact information stating that "he was going to get her." The meaning of the statement was unclear. It is clear, however, this physician is extremely upset and his actions and behaviors were upsetting all who participated in the program. How, she wondered, could something that seemed highly successful the night before become an issue that was unraveling all of the trust and good feelings from the night before. Brown knew she needed to address the issue and the sooner the better. The question was, how?

CASE HISTORY/BACKGROUND

Several weeks before the current controversy the department head had asked Brown to develop a workshop to improve how members of the department worked together. This was something Brown had done with considerable success in other departments. Indeed, it was those successes that led to the request for her assistance. With help from the department head and several physician champions Brown developed an agenda for a two-hour workshop to be held after working hours. This would allow physicians to see their patients and make rounds to ensure postsurgical recovery was proceeding properly.

The workshop was held in a classroom at the education center. Ten round tables were used to facilitate discussion, and participants sat at the table of their own choosing. After the goals of the program were described and the table facilitators introduced, participants were asked to complete a survey about the seven areas the organization had identified as critical for effective departmental functioning. The completed surveys were collected, and participants took a break while facilitators tabulated the results.

After returning from break, participants were asked to join specific tables to ensure a balance of experience and professional backgrounds (physicians, nurses and other professionals, and support staff). The survey results from the previous exercise were shared. After participants asked questions to clarify the process, the next activity was introduced. Using the nominal group technique (Delbecq, Van de Ven, & Gustafson, 1975) participants were asked to list on an index card a barrier or concern that prevented the department from functioning at a high level. After cards were collected, the facilitators sorted them into three categories: people, process, and communication. After they reviewed the results, participants were asked to suggest actions to improve the department's functioning in those areas. Suggestions were recorded. The meeting concluded by outlining the next step: developing plans to implement the actions identified.

REFLECTING ON THE TEAM-BUILDING PROCESS

Brown was puzzled by the negative and unexpected turn of events. This workshop was no different than others she had conducted and which had been very successful. Participants at the others left feeling good about the process and the prospects for developing implementation plans to improve their departments' functioning. As she reflected on the evening's activities Brown recalled that a couple of physicians said the workshop might have been more effective had it used an open forum process rather than following the structured process she had used. Later, when action items were identified, a few physicians wanted to continue the discussion so implementation plans could be developed while participants were still present. Brown felt continuing the process would have been useful, but the agenda developed by the department head and physician champions specified a two-hour, evening session. Thus the meeting ended as scheduled. After all, it was the plan they had developed, the agenda they had created, and the amount of time it seemed reasonable to ask people to spend on this activity—especially after working their shifts that day.

Brown has a problem. What began as a successful workshop to improve organizational functioning is now seen as creating frustration and disillusionment among various staff members.

DISCUSSION QUESTIONS

1. What might Brown have done differently?

2. How should Brown address the disillusionment beginning to permeate the department?

3. What might she do now to get the entire process back on track?

4. Finally, what should her response be to the physician who "wanted to get her"?

REFERENCE

Delbecq, A. L., Van de Ven, A. H., & Gustafson, D. H. (1975). *Group techniques for program planning: A guide to nominal group and Del-phi processes*. Glenview, IL: Foresman.

PART VI

Ethics Incidents

29

Ethics Incidents

Kurt Darr
The George Washington University

ADMINISTRATIVE ETHICS

Incident 1: Borrowed Time

Annabeth Jackson is director for ancillary departments at Healing Hands Rehabilitation, a 120-bed acute rehabilitation center located in the Northwest. Jackson's departments include food and nutrition services (F&NS). Two years ago, she hired Frank Anderson as supervisor for F&NS, a department with 37 full-time equivalent (FTE) employees. Initially, Jackson was very pleased with Anderson's performance. However, problems have arisen over the past 8 months, including being tardy, taking numerous sick days, missing deadlines for employee performance evaluations, socializing (and partying) excessively with members of his staff, and addressing and engaging with staff in ways that are too familiar and casual. Some staff members have told Jackson they are uncomfortable with Anderson's informality and overly friendly behavior. Jackson has verbally cautioned Anderson several times, noted these problems in his performance review, and even written a step one disciplinary memorandum, a copy of which was given to Anderson as well as put into his employment file. These actions to change Anderson's behavior have had no observable effect.

Healing Hands' human resources (HR) policies do not specify the appropriate relationship between supervisors and staff. It is clear, however, that supervisors are expected to treat all staff with respect and maintain a certain distance between themselves and those for whom they are responsible. For example, HR policies specifically prohibit managers from borrowing money from those they supervise. This is to avoid placing staff members in an untenable position if they refuse to lend money, or have to make efforts for repayment if money is lent.

Anderson's use of sick days causes him to use his paid time off (PTO) as quickly as he accumulates it. Employees earn 20 hours per month (240 hours per year) of combined sick leave, vacation, personal days, and bereavement time. Last week Anderson sent an e-mail to Jackson stating that he needed to take an extended medical leave due to the stress of his work. Under the federal Family and Medical Leave Act, Anderson is entitled to take the medical leave (with physician verification of his condition); however, he would have to use PTO hours to continue to be paid while on leave. Knowing that Anderson had only a few hours of PTO left for the year, Jackson wondered how he could maintain his income.

This morning Jackson learned that Anderson had sent an e-mail to three of his staff in F&NS asking them to donate some of their PTO to him. HR policies allow employees to voluntarily donate PTO hours to other staff. Jackson was angry; she saw this as a breach of the appropriate relationship between managers and staff. The situation raised several issues for Jackson. She pondered what course of action to take.

Incident 2: Emergency Department Repeat Admissions— A Question of Resource Use

Matt Losinski finished reading an article that provided grim details of a study of the overuse of emergency services in hospitals in central Texas. He smiled that sardonic half smile that meant there was a strong possibility that County General Hospital (CGH) might have the same problem. As chief executive officer (CEO), Losinski always saw the problems of other hospitals as potential problems at CGH, a 300-bed, acute care hospital in a mixed urban and suburban service area in the south central United States. CGH was established as a county-owned hospital; however, 10 years ago the county wanted to get out of the hospital business and the assets were donated to a not-for-profit hospital system. The new owner has continued a strong public service orientation, even though CGH no longer receives the tax subsidy it did when it was county owned; it must look to itself for fiscal health.

The study data showed that nine residents of a central Texas community had been seen in emergency departments (EDs) a total of 2,678 times over 6 years. One resident had been seen in an ED 100 times each year for the past 4 years. Given that an ED visit can cost $1,000 or more, the nine residents had consumed $2.7 million in resources. These high users of ED services were middle age, spoke English, and were split between male and female. To Losinski, the problem seemed like a manifestation of Wilfredo Pareto's classic 80/20 rule.

Losinski forwarded the article on a priority basis to Mary Scott, his chief financial officer (CFO), and asked her to see him after she read it. Scott stopped by Losinski's office late the next day and began the conversation by asking him why he thought the article was a priority. Scott reminded Losinski that Medicaid paid 75% of costs for eligible ED users and that the cross subsidy from privately insured and self-pay ED admissions covered most of the unpaid additional costs. Losinski had a good working relationship with Scott, but he was a bit annoyed by her rather indifferent response.

Losinski wanted details on use of the ED at CGH. He asked the administrative resident, Aniysha Patel, to gather data to identify use rates for persons repeatedly admitted to the ED. The findings that Patel gave to Losinski two weeks later were not as extreme as those reported from central Texas; however, they did show that a few persons were repeatedly admitted to the ED and accounted for hundreds of visits in the past year. The clinical details were not immediately available, but a superficial review of the admitting diagnoses suggested that most admissions involved persons with minor, nonspecific medical problems—persons commonly known as the "worried well." Although Scott was correct that Medicaid covered the majority of costs, the fact remained that over $200,000 each year was not reimbursed to CGH. Were that money available, it could go directly to the bottom line and could be used for enhancements to health initiatives for the community. In addition, repeated admissions to the ED contributed to crowding, treatment delays, and general dissatisfaction for other patients.

Losinski presented the data to his executive committee, which includes all vice presidents, the director of development, and the elected president of the medical staff. The responses ran the gamut from "So what?" to "Wow, this is worse than I imagined." Losinski was bemused by the disparity of views. He had thought there would have been an almost immediate consensus that this was a problem needing a solution. The financial margins for CGH were already very thin, and the future for higher reimbursement was not bright. A concern echoed by several at the meeting was the requirement of the federal Emergency Medical Treatment and Active Labor Act (EMTALA) that all persons who present at an ED that receives federal reimbursement for services must be treated and stabilized.

Losinski asked his senior management team for recommendations to address the problem of ED overuse.

Incident 3: The Administrative Institutional Ethics Committee[1]

The CEO of Community Health Plan (CHP), a small not-for-profit accountable care organization (ACO), has been approached by a group from "north of the river." This area of the city is economically depressed and has lost many of its health services organizations (HSOs) and physicians to the suburbs in the last decade. North of the river seems to be in a downward vortex with no apparent bottom. An increasing number of uninsured patients means that HSOs are less and less able to continue serving the area. The city-owned hospital has made several ill-fated attempts to serve north of the river with a clinic system, but its efforts have been scandal-ridden. The system is a political football with little credibility in the community.

The representatives from "north of the river" are community leaders, none of whom appear to have political ambitions. They seem genuinely willing to do whatever they can to assist in delivering high-quality health services to the community. They proposed that CHP establish and staff three store-front clinics in the area. The community leaders stated they would get volunteers to remodel the facilities and work in clerical capacities. The CEO described the proposed activity to the administrative institutional ethics committee (IEC), which includes members of governance, managers, and physicians and others from clinical areas. In making the presentation, the CEO stressed the plan's historical role in providing health services to those in need, its not-for-profit status, and its continuing modest surplus. The members listened patiently, but the minute the CEO finished all of them seemed to speak at once. Several were opposed and made the following points about the suggested venture:

1. "North of the river" is the city's responsibility. Providing care to the needy is not something a small, not-for-profit ACO should attempt.

2. They have a primary obligation to enhance benefits for their enrollees, rather than become involved in new schemes. Several of their physicians and many plan members have requested additional services.

3. The modest surplus the plan has accumulated over several years could be consumed easily. The chief financial officer noted CHP is expecting increases in rent and equipment and salary costs in the next quarter.

4. If CHP pulls the city's political chestnuts out of the fire by providing even stop-gap assistance, the city will never get its house in order and develop the system needed "north of the river."

Several spoke in favor of working "north of the river":

1. Helping the "north of the river" community is the right thing to do. The people there deserve health services. It was noted that CHP's own start had come about when several physicians in the community fought the prevailing attitude among their peers about prepaid practice.

2. Those opposed are putting dollars ahead of people's health. They must be willing to assist persons who are less fortunate.

3. Plan members will support such an initiative if it is properly explained to them.

4. The positive publicity will further CHP's interests by increasing the number of patients.

It seems to the CEO that this is a no-win situation. The organizational philosophy is not well developed, and the proposal is a major step. Something should be done to assist the "north of the river" community. The IEC members are raising valid points that merit further discussion.

Incident 4: Bits and Pieces[2]

John Henry Williams really liked his new job in the department of radiology at Affiliated Nursing Homes and Rehabilitation Center. He had recently been appointed acting head when his predecessor, Mary Beth Jacobson, went on maternity leave. As acting head of radiology, John Henry is responsible for two and a half full-time equivalent (FTE) technicians, an appointments clerk, and more than $250,000 worth of equipment. He has authority to purchase radiographic supplies, including certain types of film. The total value of these purchases is approximately $90,000 per year. Most are obtained from three vendors, companies with which the organization has done business for many years.

When Mary Beth oriented John Henry to the demands and responsibilities of the job, she told him that some of the best parts were the meetings with the sales representatives from the three vendors. She said that most of these meetings were held at nice restaurants in the suburban area near the center. Some were held in her office. When that was the case, she said, the sales representatives invariably brought along a "little something." When John Henry asked what that meant, Mary Beth gave examples: perfume, a bottle of French brandy, and a pen set in a leather case. John Henry remembered thinking that his wife might like the perfume.

He asked Mary Beth if there was a policy concerning accepting gifts from vendors. Mary Beth was a little put out by the question, because it seemed to suggest something might be wrong with what she was doing. She responded somewhat curtly that the center's senior management trusted its managers and allowed them discretion in such matters.

Personally, John Henry was more interested in the lunches, because they would allow him to leave the facility occasionally and get away from the dreary cafeteria as well as his sandwiches from home. Mary Beth described the lunches as nothing fancy. She estimated their cost to the sales representative as about the same as the small gifts—$40–50.

John Henry asked if the action might suggest to some members of the staff that her purchasing decisions were being influenced by the gifts and lunches with the sales representatives. Mary Beth's anger flashed. She quickly gave four reasons in justification to John Henry:

1. Taking clients to lunch or providing small gifts is common practice in business relationships.

2. There was no cost to the center because the vendors paid for everything and they could charge it against their expense account, or get reimbursed by the company.

3. At least one of the sales representatives had become a friend over the years and she enjoyed his company on a social level, as well.

4. There was absolutely no possibility her judgment could be influenced by the small gifts and lunches.

Somewhat heatedly, Mary Beth added, "I know you're thinking that somehow this whole thing doesn't look right. But that isn't fair at all. I work long hours as a manager and get paid very little extra. It also takes more effort and time to do the ordering and keep the inventory of supplies at a proper level. If anything goes wrong, it's my neck that's in a noose. These gratuities from vendors are a little something to help compensate me for those activities. My work for the center has been very effective. I'd be happy to talk to anyone who thinks otherwise!"

Incident 5: A Potentially Shocking Revelation

Geraldene Jones had been a nurse before she earned her master of health administration degree and began her trek to the top of the corporate ladder, a trek that sometimes seemed agonizingly slow. Her love of long-term care and improving the way it is provided fuels her goal to become the chief executive officer of a nursing facility. Currently, Jones is the vice president for support services at a large nursing facility. It is part of a for-profit chain that owns more than 100 facilities; most of them are large and have more than 200 residents. The facility has an excellent reputation and there is a waiting list for admission.

Jones's facility is undergoing a major expansion of its physical plant, one that will almost double the number of square feet. The new space will house rehabilitation services and will add a new respite care program and about 50 new private rooms for residents. Jones volunteered to be responsible for the building program, and some of her other duties were reassigned. She volunteered because she believed success in getting the building program completed on time and under budget would bring her to the attention of corporate headquarters and make her more promotable.

One day as Jones walked through the half-completed structure, she overheard a heated conversation between the foreman for the electrical contractor and the county electrical inspector. The inspector was pointing out a long list of discrepancies, which ranged from the number of amperes of overall electrical service at that location to the number and placement of electrical outlets. The contractor stated repeatedly that the inspector was being overly aggressive in applying the county electrical code. After the inspector left, Jones approached the electrical contractor and asked him if there was a problem she should know about. The electrical contractor rubbed two of his fingers and thumb together and said, "Nothing that a little 'grease' won't take care of." It was obvious the contractor was talking about bribing the inspector. Jones expressed shock and was rebuked by the contractor. "Obviously, you're new to the construction game. Payoffs are common; I've dealt with this kind of thing before. I know what to do and it's what we'll have to do if you want this building completed on time. I have an account for just such a contingency, but you may have to add to it if the electrical inspector isn't reasonable."

Jones was stunned. She had no idea what to say or what to do.

Incident 6: Intensive Care Unit Dysfunction

Differing practice methodologies and attitudes of physicians can cause confusion and distress for patients and families—particularly when they receive mixed or even contradictory messages as to prognosis, course of treatment, and use of adjuvant services. Further, the turmoil causes stress for nursing staff and dysfunction in the nursing unit.

Ms. O'Leary, a 65-year-old female with a history of hypertension, depression, and breast cancer was admitted to Community Hospital through the emergency department after she experienced fevers, rectal bleeding, and abdominal pain following a hemicolectomy two weeks prior at another hospital. On admission, Ms. O'Leary was alert and oriented and able to participate in medical decisions regarding her care. Her stay at Community involved treatment for septic shock, numerous blood transfusions, the need for fluid resuscitation because of dehydration, and several surgical procedures for bowel repair. Ms. O'Leary had two cardiac arrests and required several intubations for respiratory failure. She became increasingly unaware of her surroundings in the course of her hospitalization. She was able to follow simple commands, but she did not have the capacity to understand what was happening to her or what was happening around her. Ms. O'Leary did not have an advance medical directive (AMD). Several days after admission, registration documented a request for information on advance care planning, including an AMD. There is no documentation of a follow-up, however.

Three weeks into her hospital stay, and while Ms. O'Leary was intubated in the intensive care unit (ICU), nurses in the ICU and Mr. O'Leary discussed the desirability of a consultation from hospice staff. Mr. O'Leary, who has been married to Ms. O'Leary for 47 years, said he had heard of positive experiences with hospice from acquaintances and wanted to consider the hospice option. The hospitalist, Dr. A, who was attending Ms. O'Leary that day, ordered a consultation with hospice staff; the consultation occurred later the same day. A hospice consultation provides information to patients and families and outlines available services. A hospice consultation is different from a physician's order for hospice, which occurs as part of discharge planning. An order for hospice causes a patient to be discharged to a hospice program with orders for comfort care, only. Community Hospital has no standard operating procedure, policy, or set of criteria to determine when a patient should have a hospice consultation or be referred to a hospice program.

The day following the hospice consultation, another hospitalist, Dr. B., who is Dr. A's partner, made rounds in the ICU. Dr. B told Mr. O'Leary that Ms. O'Leary was not a candidate for a hospice consultation at this time and nursing staff had been wrong to suggest it. Dr. B's comment ignored the fact that his partner, Dr. A, had written the order for a hospice consultation. Dr. B made the nurse involved feel she had overstepped her scope of practice by discussing hospice with Mr. O'Leary. Even afterward, Dr. B was vocal in expressing his criticism of the nurse; this caused a very tense environment in the ICU for a number of days.

Mr. O'Leary and his adult children were angry about the contradictory assessment by Dr. B and felt their decision-making authority had been compromised. Nursing staff bore the brunt of the family's anger and experienced even greater stress from an already stressful situation. All those involved felt the contradictory advice from the physicians had called into question the validity of the care plan for Ms. O'Leary and the quality of care being provided to her.

It is not surprising ICU nursing staff reacted negatively to Dr. B's comments regarding hospice consultation. ICU nurses are at the bedside 24-hours a day and usually develop a personal relationship with patients and families. Nurses believe it is well within their purview and scope of practice to discuss care options such as hospice. Even more frustrating for nursing staff is that the situation with Ms. O'Leary is not an isolated instance in the ICU. On a number of occasions, physicians have written conflicting orders and given contradictory assessments and advice to patients and families.

Given her dire prognosis, Mr. O'Leary asked Dr. A to write an order for Ms. O'Leary to be made "allow natural death" (AND).[3] The status of AND preempted the need for hospice. When the AND order was written Ms. O'Leary was supported by a ventilator. She could not participate in the decision because of her diminished mental capacity.

A week after the hospice consultation issue, and to everyone's surprise, Ms. O'Leary's clinical condition improved enough for her to be discharged from the ICU. Three weeks after discharge from the ICU, Ms. O'Leary remains hospitalized. Despite her complex post-surgical course she began to take food by mouth, which was supplemented by tube feedings. Her mentation improved slowly, but she continued to suffer from encephalopathy. At times, she is agitated and confused. The discharge plan is that Ms. O'Leary will go to a rehabilitation facility when her ability to take food by mouth improves.

CLINICAL ETHICS
Incident 7: Protecting the Community[4]

University Hospital has a unique role. It is not only a tertiary referral hospital for the region, but also a major source of service to the community. In 1977, it experienced an outbreak of *Legionella* (the bacterium that causes Legionnaires' disease). A number of patients were affected; several died.

Legionella affects the respiratory tract and lungs and may cause death if not diagnosed and treated early. It is especially dangerous for the elderly and those with weakened immune systems. A factor requiring even greater caution on the part of hospital management is that, at the time of the outbreak, the laboratory test to identify the organism took several days. Thus, patients were at great risk until a confirmatory diagnosis was obtained. Epidemiological studies showed a relationship between air conditioning cooling towers and the fine mist they give off and spread of *Legionella* through the aerosol. Workers exposed directly to the aerosol have contracted severe cases of *Legionella*. Chlorinating the water in the cooling towers eliminates the organism.

Although a cooling tower was implicated in the 1977 outbreak at University Hospital, the relationship was never confirmed. The infection control committee of the hospital did not develop standing orders or policies after the first outbreak. In May 1982, there was evidence of another outbreak of *Legionella*. The cooling tower was immediately chlorinated and the number of new cases dropped dramatically. An undetected failure in the chlorination system, however, brought a second outbreak of *Legionella* in early June.

When the first cases were detected in May 1982, the administrator was notified. He met with various staff members, including physicians on the attending staff. It was decided that information about the outbreak should be kept from the community, lest there be a panic and a sudden drop in census, as well as loss of public confidence. A confidential letter was sent to staff physicians advising them of the problem and asking that they keep in mind the *potential* for infection when making admissions decisions. Admissions were not limited to emergencies, however, and there was no prospective review of elective admissions to determine whether patients at higher risk for pulmonary infections such as *Legionella* should be sent elsewhere. Nor was there any review of indications for, and necessity of, admission. The medical staff developed a protocol (standing order) stating that unexplained acute-onset pneumonias were to be treated immediately with an antibiotic shown to be effective against *Legionella*. No provision was made, however, for effective review to determine that the protocol was actually followed on a concurrent basis.

Incident 8: Decisions[5]

Mrs. Nickleby is in her mid-forties and has severe multiple sclerosis, a chronic disease that impairs muscular control. She has been a resident of Hightower Nursing Home for almost 3 years. Her two teenage daughters live with her sister in a nearby subdivision and visit her often. She and Mr. Nickleby, a middle-management executive with a local firm, had divorced 5 years earlier.

Mrs. Nickleby has frequent, acute attacks of asthma. To date, they have been caught in time by the nursing staff; on a couple of occasions she had to be rushed to the emergency room at the local community hospital. Her physician, who treats her at Hightower Nursing Home, has ordered "no code" if Nickleby has a cardiac arrest during an acute asthma episode at the nursing home—that is, she will not be resuscitated. (Skilled nursing facilities [and acute care hospitals] use different signals, or codes, that call a resuscitation team over the loud-speaker system to respond to a cardiac arrest without alarming other patients and visitors.)

The nurses understand Nickleby's physician made his decision without discussing it with her or her family. One nurse is very upset because the decision conflicts with her professional values, although she admits privately that, if she were Nickleby, she would find the situation intolerable and she would not want to continue living in those circumstances. None of the nurses has heard Nickleby express the same opinion about her condition, even though she has become increasingly depressed, especially after each asthma attack. The nurses have asked the administrative director of the unit for advice.

Incident 9: The Missing Needle Protector[6]

E. L. Straight is director of clinical services at Hopewell Hospital. As in many hospitals, a few physicians provide care that is acceptable, but not of very high quality; they tend to make more mistakes than the others and have a higher incidence of patients going "sour." Since Straight took the position 2 years ago, new programs have been developed and things seem to be getting better in terms of quality.

Dr. Cutrite has practiced at Hopewell for longer than anyone can remember. Although once a brilliant general surgeon, he has slipped physically and mentally over the years, and Straight is contemplating taking steps to recommend a reduction in his privileges. However, the process is not complete, and Dr. Cutrite continues to perform a full range of procedures.

The operating room supervisor appeared at Straight's office one Monday afternoon. "We've got a problem," she said, somewhat nonchalantly, but with a hint of disgust. "I'm almost sure we left a plastic needle protector from a disposable syringe in a patient's belly, a Mrs. Jameson. You know, the protectors with the red-pink color. They'd be almost impossible to see if they were in a wound."

"Where did it come from?" asked Straight.

"I'm not absolutely sure," answered the supervisor. "All I know is that the syringe was among items in a used surgical pack when we did the count." She went on to describe the safeguards of counts and records. The discrepancy was noted when records were reconciled at the end of the week. A surgical pack was shown as having a syringe that was not supposed to be there. When the scrub nurse working with Dr. Cutrite was questioned, she remembered that he had used a syringe, but, when it was included in the count at the conclusion of surgery, she didn't think about the protective sheath, which must have been on it.

Let's get Mrs. Jameson back into surgery," said Straight. "We'll tell her it's necessary to check her incision and deep sutures. She'll never know we're really looking for the needle cover."

"Too late," responded the supervisor, "she went home day before yesterday."

Oh, oh, thought Straight. Now what to do? "Have you talked to Dr. Cutrite?"

The supervisor nodded affirmatively. "He won't consider telling Mrs. Jameson there might be a problem and calling her back to the hospital," she said. "And he warned us not to do anything, either," she added. "Dr. Cutrite claims it cannot possibly hurt her. Except for a little discomfort, she'll never know it's there."

Straight called the chief of surgery and asked a hypothetical question about the consequences of leaving a small plastic cap in a patient's belly.

The chief knew something was amiss but didn't pursue it. He simply replied there would likely be occasional discomfort, but probably no life-threatening consequences from leaving it in. "Although," he added, "one never knows."

Straight liked working at Hopewell Hospital and didn't relish crossing swords with Dr. Cutrite, who, although declining clinically, was politically very powerful. Straight had refrained from fingernail biting for years, but that old habit was suddenly overwhelming.

Incident 10: To Vaccinate, or Not?

Jenna and Chris Smith are the proud parents of Ana, a 5-day-old baby girl born without complications at Community Hospital. Since delivery, the parents have bonded well with Ana and express their desire to raise her as naturally as possible. For the Smiths, this means breastfeeding exclusively for the first six months, making their own baby food using pureed organic foods, and not allowing Ana to be vaccinated.

The Smiths are college educated and explain they have researched vaccines and decided the potential harms caused by them far outweigh any benefits. They point to the rise in autism rates as proof of the unforeseen risk of vaccines. Their new pediatrician, Dr. Angela Kerr, listens intently to the Smiths' description of their research, including online mommy-blogs that detail how vaccines may have caused autism in many children. The Smiths conclude by resolutely stating they've decided not to vaccinate Ana, despite the recommendations of the medical community.

Dr. Kerr begins by stating that while vaccines have certainly sparked controversy in recent years, she strongly recommends that Ana become fully vaccinated. Dr. Kerr explains that vaccines have saved the lives of millions of children worldwide and have been largely responsible for decreases in child mortality over the past century. For example, the decreased incidence of infection with the potentially fatal *Haemophilus influenzae* type b, has resulted from routine immunization against that bacterium.[7] Similarly, epidemics such as the recent outbreak of measles are usually associated with individuals who have not been vaccinated against that pathogen.

Dr. Kerr goes on to endorse the general safety of vaccines by informing Ana's parents that safety profiles of vaccines are updated regularly through data sources such as the federal government's Vaccine Adverse Event Reporting System (VAERS). The VAERS, a nationwide vaccine safety surveillance program sponsored by the Food and Drug Administration and the Centers for Disease Control and Prevention, is accessible to the public at https://vaers.hhs.gov/index. This system allows transparency for vaccine safety by encouraging the public and healthcare providers to report adverse reactions to vaccines and enables the federal government to monitor their safety. No vaccine has been proven causal for autism spectrum disorder (ASD), or any developmental disorder. On the contrary, many studies have shown that vaccines containing thimerasol, an ingredient once thought to cause autism, do not increase the risk of ASD.[8, 9, 10]

Finally, Dr. Kerr reminds the Smiths that some children in the general population have weakened immune systems because of genetic diseases or cancer treatment, for example. It may not be medically feasible to vaccinate such children. Other children are too young to receive certain immunizations. Instead, these children are protected because almost all other children (and adults) have been vaccinated and this decreases their exposure to vaccine-preventable illnesses (VPIs). This epidemiological concept is known as "herd immunity."[11] As more parents refuse immunization for their healthy children, however, the rate of VPIs will increase. This puts vulnerable children at significant risk of morbidity and mortality. Routine childhood immunization contributes significantly to the health of the general public, both by providing a direct benefit to those who are vaccinated and by protecting others via herd immunity. Dr. Kerr concludes by stating that after considering the risks versus the benefits of immunization, most states require vaccinations before children can attend school.[12] Parents may decide not to vaccinate under specific circumstances, however, which vary by state.[13]

Jenna and Chris Smith confirm their understanding of what Dr. Kerr has explained, but restate that they do not want Ana vaccinated at this time. Dr. Kerr is perplexed as to what to do.

Incident 11: Demarketing to Avoid Bankruptcy[14]

Chris Hines had finally gotten far enough down in the stack of papers on her desk to see last month's emergency department (ED) activity report. She had already digested the grim news about the continued financial hemorrhage affecting Community Hospital. The current deficit was $500,000—and it was only the fourth month of the fiscal year. Because Community served a largely inner-city population, many of whom were uninsured or whose care was paid by a chronically underfunded Medicaid program that reimbursed poorly, there seemed little hope that the financial situation would improve.

Hines knew that more than 40% of Community's inpatient admissions came through the ED, and that about half of those ED admissions arrived by taxi, private automobile, or on foot. The other half was brought in by the city government's ambulance service. Hines had tried to increase the number of elective admissions (and thus improve the payer mix) by encouraging physicians to bring their private patients to Community. This effort failed, however, largely because physicians had difficulty getting their private patients admitted; ED admissions were taking too many beds.

Then, Hines tried to work with city officials to implement a new ambulance routing system to give Community time to improve its financial condition. This effort also failed because city officials were unsympathetic.

Hines knew that Community's endowment would carry the hospital about 3 years, but that it would be forced to close if it were not breaking even financially by then. Because there was nothing that could be done with the city, Hines concluded the key to survival lay in reducing the number of uninsured and Medicaid admissions through the ED.

Hines spoke with several marketing consultants, one of whom offered to work *pro bono* for Community. He seized on the idea of "demarketing" the ED. He reasoned it was the fine reputation Community's ED had in its service area that was largely responsible for the 50% of ED patients who came in other than by city ambulance. Then he identified ways the ED could be made less attractive to potential patients. The plan he developed included reducing ED staffing to a minimum; closing the parking lot near the ED; reducing housekeeping services so the physical plant would be dirty and unkempt; deferring indefinitely all non–safety-related maintenance; changing the triage policies, procedures, and staffing to increase wait times for nonemergency patients; using staff who were most likely to be rude and inconsiderate; and encouraging rumors that closure of the ED was imminent.

The consultant knew there might be repercussions beyond the ED, but Community Hospital was desperate; he believed extreme actions were the only choice.

Incident 12: Something Must Be Done, But What?[15]

Stunned, Carolyn Aubrey, CEO of Metropolitan Hospital, sank into her chair and stared out the window for a very long time. She knew something was wrong when Dr. Midmore's wife had angrily insisted on seeing the CEO. Even in her worst nightmares, however, Aubrey could not have imagined Mrs. Midmore would tell Aubrey she was suing her husband, an orthopedic surgeon, for divorce because she had contracted AIDS from him. As Mrs. Midmore was leaving Aubrey's office, she turned back and said, "I was sure you'd want to know; of course, you'll want to do something."

Fleetingly, Aubrey thought Mrs. Midmore's remarks might be only the ravings of an angry, vindictive wife, but that was not likely. As she considered what she had just learned, she recalled an incident several years ago involving Dr. Midmore and a male transporter. In retrospect, that incident suggested Dr. Midmore might be bisexual. Aubrey thought, too, about the department of surgery meeting late last year when there had been a long discussion about the desirability of knowing the HIV status of surgical patients. The special risks of torn gloves and cuts during orthopedic surgery had been described in detail.

Now it seemed Dr. Midmore's patients were at special risk. Aubrey called operating room scheduling and learned Dr. Midmore was maintaining a full surgical load. Aubrey asked her secretary to call the hospital attorney and the medical director and set up an emergency meeting for 7:00 a.m. the following morning. Mrs. Midmore might have been telling the truth, thought Aubrey. We will have to do something, but what?

ENDNOTES

Incident 6 was written with Jessica Silcox (Children's National Medical Center, Washington, D.C.). Incident 10 was written with Nova Ashanti Monteiro (Sentara Northern Virginia Medical Center, Alexandria, VA).

1. From Darr, K. (2011). *Ethics in health services management* (5th ed., pp. 105–106). Baltimore: Health Professions Press; reprinted by permission.
2. From Darr, K. (2011). *Ethics in health services management* (5th ed., p. 138). Baltimore: Health Professions Press; reprinted by permission.
3. Allow natural death (AND) is the designation currently recommended in lieu of the more commonly used "DNR" or "do-not-resuscitate." AND focuses on patient quality of life and comfort and delineates which aggressive interventions should or should not be used for patients, such as cardiopulmonary resuscitation and intubation for respiratory failure. The American Heart Association recommends ending use of DNR because "resuscitate" gives patients and families a false sense that CPR is likely to be effective in a hospital setting. Similarly, DNR is often confused by patients and families to mean "do not treat." That is not true. Patients who are designated as AND (and DNR) status will receive treatment including antibiotics and alternative forms of feeding http://www.ncbi.nlm.nih.gov/pmc/articles/PMC3241061/
4. From Darr, K. (2011). *Ethics in health services management* (5th ed., p. 206). Baltimore: Health Professions Press; reprinted by permission.
5. Adapted from Aroskar, M. (1977, August). Case No. 461, Case studies in bioethics. *Hastings Center Report*, p. 17; used by permission.
6. From Longest, Jr., B. B., Rakich, J. S., & Darr, K. (2000). *Managing health services organizations and systems* (4th ed., pp. 725–726). Baltimore: Health Professions Press; reprinted by permission.
7. Centers for Disease Control and Prevention. (2016, October 18). *Haemophilus influenzae* type b (Hib) vaccine information statement (VIS). Retrieved from https://www.cdc.gov/vaccines/hcp/vis/vis-statements/hib.html
8. Price, C. S., Thompson. W. W., Goodson, B., Weintraub, E. S., Croen, L. A., Hinrichsen, V. L., Marcy, M., Robertson, A., Eriksen, E., Lewis, E., Bernal, P., Shay, D., Davis, R. L., & DeStefano, F. (2010) Prenatal and infant exposure to thimerosal from vaccines and immunoglobulins and risk of autism. *Pediatrics, 126*(4), 656–664.
9. Hurley, A. M., Tadrous, M., & Miller, E. S. (2010) Thimerosal-containing vaccines and autism: a review of recent epidemiologic studies. *The Journal of Pediatric Pharmacology and Therapeutics: JPPT, 15*(3), 173–181.
10. Ball, L., Ball, R., & Pratt, R. D. (2001) An assessment of thimerosal in childhood vaccines. *Pediatrics, 107*(5), 1147–1154.

11. U.S. Department of Health and Human Services. (2016, June 23). Community immunity "herd immunity." Retrieved from https://www.vaccines.gov /basics/protection/

12. Centers for Disease Control and Prevention. (2016, January 29). State vaccination requirements. Retrieved from http://www.cdc.gov/vaccines/imz-managers/laws/state-reqs.html

13. Centers for Disease Control and Prevention Office for State, Tribal, Local and Territorial Support. (2015, March 27). State school immunization requirements and vaccine exemption laws. Retrieved from http://www.cdc .gov/phlp/docs/school-vaccinations.pdf

14. From Darr, K. (2011). *Ethics in health services management* (5th ed., pp. 293–294). Baltimore: Health Professions Press; reprinted by permission.

15. From Darr, K. (2011). *Ethics in health services management* (5th ed. p. 204). Baltimore: Health Professions Press; reprinted by permission.